**A Practical Approach
to Quantitative Validation
of Patient-Reported Outcomes**

A Practical Approach to Quantitative Validation of Patient-Reported Outcomes

A Simulation-Based Guide Using SAS

Andrew G. Bushmakin and Joseph C. Cappelleri
Statistical Research and Data Science Center
Pfizer Inc.

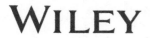

Registered Office
John Wiley & Sons, Inc., 111 River Street, Hoboken, NJ 07030, USA

For details of our global editorial offices, customer services, and more information about Wiley products visit us at www.wiley.com.

Wiley also publishes its books in a variety of electronic formats and by print-on-demand. Some content that appears in standard print versions of this book may not be available in other formats.

Library of Congress Cataloging-in-Publication Data
Names: Bushmakin, Andrew G., author. | Cappelleri, Joseph C., author.
Title: A practical approach to quantitative validation of patient-reported
   outcomes : a simulation-based guide using SAS / Andrew G. Bushmakin and
   Joseph C. Cappelleri.
Description: Hoboken, NJ : Wiley, 2023. | Includes bibliographical
   references and index.
Identifiers: LCCN 2022024236 (print) | LCCN 2022024237 (ebook) | ISBN
   9781119376378 (cloth) | ISBN 9781119376316 (adobe pdf) | ISBN
   9781119376309 (epub)
Subjects: MESH: Patient Reported Outcome Measures | Patient Outcome
   Assessment | Reproducibility of Results | Computer Simulation | Clinical Outcome Assessment
Classification: LCC R853.Q34 (print) | LCC R853.Q34 (ebook) | NLM W 84.41
   | DDC 610.72/1–dc23/eng/20220706
LC record available at https://lccn.loc.gov/2022024236
LC ebook record available at https://lccn.loc.gov/2022024237

Cover Design: Wiley
Cover Image: Courtesy of Andrew Bushmakin

Set in 9.5/12.5pt STIXTwoText by Straive, Pondicherry, India   SKY10037308_102622

Disclosure

Andrew G. Bushmakin and Joseph C. Cappelleri are employees of Pfizer Inc. This book is written for educational and instructional purposes, with emphasis on the methodology of quantitative validation of patient-reported outcomes. Views and opinions expressed in this book are the authors' own and do not necessarily reflect those of Pfizer Inc.

Contents

Preface *xi*
About the Authors *xv*

1 **Introduction** *1*
1.1 What Is a PRO Measure? *1*
1.2 Development of a PRO Measure *4*
1.2.1 Concept Identification *4*
1.2.1.1 Literature and Instrument Review *5*
1.2.1.2 Patient-Centered Input *6*
1.2.2 Item Development *9*
1.2.3 Cognitive Interviews *11*
1.2.4 Additional Considerations *12*
1.2.5 Documentation of Development Process with Conceptual Framework *13*
1.3 Psychometric Validation *15*
1.3.1 Psychometric Evaluation Data *16*
1.3.2 Psychometric Properties *17*
1.3.2.1 Distributional Characteristics *19*
1.3.2.2 Measurement Model Structure *20*
1.3.2.3 Reliability *22*
1.3.2.4 Construct Validity *23*
1.3.2.5 Ability to Detect Change *24*
1.3.2.6 Interpretation *25*
1.4 Learning Through Simulations *26*
1.5 Summary *27*
References *28*

2   Validation Workflow *35*
2.1   Clinical Trials as a Data Source for Validation *35*
2.2   Validation Workflow for Single-Item Scales *39*
2.3   Confirmatory Validation Workflow for Multi-item Multi-domain
       Scales *43*
2.4   Validation Flow for a New Multi-item Multi-domain Scale *45*
2.4.1 New Scale with Known Conceptual Framework *45*
2.4.2 New Scale with Unknown Measurement Structure *47*
2.5   Cross-Sectional Studies and Field Tests *48*
2.6   Summary *49*
       References *49*

3   An Assessment of Classical Test Theory and Item Response Theory *51*
3.1   Overview of Classical Test Theory *52*
3.1.1 Basics *52*
3.1.2 Illustration *52*
3.1.3 Another Look *53*
3.2   Person-Item Maps *55*
3.2.1 CTT Revisited *55*
3.2.2 Note on IRT *56*
3.2.3 Implementation of Person-Item Maps *58*
3.2.4 CTT-Based Scoring vs. IRT-Based Scoring *69*
3.3   Summary *78*
       References *80*

4   Reliability *83*
4.1   Reproducibility/Test–Retest *85*
4.1.1 Measurement Error Model *85*
4.1.2 Two Time Points *87*
4.1.3 Random-Effects Model for ICC Estimation *90*
4.1.4 Test–Retest Reliability Assessment in the Context of Clinical
       Studies *95*
4.1.4.1 Pre-Treatment/Pre-Baseline Data *95*
4.1.4.2 Post-Baseline Data *97*
4.1.4.3 Time Period Between Observations *101*
4.1.5 Spearman-Brown Prophecy Formula *104*
4.1.6 Domain Score Test–Retest vs. Item Test–Retest *109*
4.1.7 Observer-Based and Interviewer-Based Scales *111*
4.1.8 Uncovering True Relationship Between Measurements *113*
4.1.8.1 Accounting for Measurement Error *113*
4.1.8.2 Measurement Error Model with Two Observations *122*

4.2   Cronbach's Alpha   *129*
4.2.1   Likert-Type Scales   *129*
4.2.2   Dichotomous Items   *139*
4.3   Summary   *148*
          References   *148*

5   Construct Validity and Criterion Validity   *151*
5.1   Exploratory Factor Analyses   *153*
5.1.1   Modeling Assumptions   *153*
5.1.2   Exploratory Factor Analysis Implementation   *159*
5.1.3   Evaluating the Number of Factors and Factor Loadings   *165*
5.1.3.1   Scree Plot   *165*
5.1.3.2   Correlated Latent Factors   *168*
5.1.3.3   Parallel Analysis with Reduced Correlation Matrix   *171*
5.1.3.4   Factor Loadings   *175*
5.2   Confirmatory Factor Analyses   *179*
5.2.1   Confirmatory Factor Analysis Model   *179*
5.2.2   Confirmatory Factor Analysis Model Implementation   *183*
5.2.3   Confirmatory Factor Analysis with Domains Represented by a Single
          Item   *192*
5.2.4   Second-Order Confirmatory Factor Analysis   *204*
5.2.4.1   Implementation of the Model with at Least Three First-Order Latent
          Domains   *204*
5.2.4.2   Implementation of the Model with Two First-Order Latent
          Domains   *207*
5.2.5   Formative vs. Reflective Model   *213*
5.2.6   Bifactor Model   *219*
5.2.7   Confirmatory Factor Analysis Using Polychoric Correlations   *227*
5.3   Convergent and Discriminant Validity   *231*
5.3.1   Convergent and Discriminant Validity Assessment   *231*
5.3.2   Convergent and Discriminant Validity Evaluation in a Clinical
          Study   *232*
5.4   Known-Groups Validity   *237*
5.5   Criterion Validity   *242*
5.6   Summary   *247*
          References   *248*

6   Responsiveness and Sensitivity   *251*
6.1   Ability to Detect Change   *252*
6.1.1   Definitions and Concepts   *252*
6.1.2   Ability to Detect Change Analysis Implementation   *255*

6.1.3   Correlation Analysis to Support Ability to Detect Change   *263*
6.1.4   Deconstructing Correlation Between Changes   *268*
6.2   Sensitivity to Treatment   *270*
6.2.1   What Is the Sensitivity to Treatment?   *270*
6.2.2   Concurrent Estimation of the Treatment Effects for a Multi-Domain Scale   *273*
6.2.2.1   Assessment of the Treatment Effect for a Single Domain   *273*
6.2.2.2   Assessment of the Treatment Effects for a Multi-Domain Scale   *279*
6.3   Summary   *292*
         References   *293*

7   Interpretation of Patient-Reported Outcome Findings   *295*
7.1   Meaningful Within-Patient Change   *296*
7.1.1   Definitions and Concepts   *296*
7.1.2   Anchor-Based Method to Assess Meaningful Within-Patient Change   *298*
7.1.3   Cumulative Distribution Functions to Supplement Anchor-Based Methods   *310*
7.2   Clinical Important Difference   *315*
7.2.1   Meaningful Within-Patient Change Versus Between-Group Difference   *315*
7.2.2   Anchor-Based Method to Assess Clinically Important Difference   *316*
7.3   Responder Analyses and Cumulative Distribution Functions   *320*
7.3.1   Treatment Effect Model   *320*
7.3.2   MWPC Application: A Responder Analysis   *323*
7.3.3   Using CDFs for Interpretation of Results   *325*
7.4   Summary   *331*
         References   *332*

Index   *335*

Preface

This book is organized as one volume with interconnected chapters, with each chapter devoted to the methodology of assessments of specific measurement properties of clinical outcome assessments (COAs), which include patient-reported outcomes (PRO), clinician-reported outcomes (ClinRO), observer-reported outcomes (ObsRO), and performance outcome assessments (PerfO). In covering the topics, we made a considerable effort to illustrate the methodology with an extensive number of simulated examples, motivated by and grounded in our experience with practical applications, covering all key topics of the quantitative validation of a COA scale. All simulations are conducted in SAS, the primary software used in the pharmaceutical industry.

Chapter 1 discusses qualitative research including concept identification, item development, cognitive interviews, and other steps in the instrument development process. It is assumed that content validity for the COA instrument of interest has been achieved, and, in doing so, it covers the important concepts of the unobservable or latent attribute under study that the instrument purports to measure. Hence, the content of the PRO (or COA) instrument is taken as an adequate reflection of the construct to be measured. Given this, subsequent chapters focus on the quantitative validation of PRO measures in particular and, when applicable, to COAs in general.

Chapter 2 describes quantitative validation workflows that should be applicable for most realistic scenarios and study designs. The chapter elucidates the distinctive opportunities and challenges when using clinical trials data as the source to psychometrically validate a scale. There is, however, always a possibility that some new scale will need some adjustments to the workflows highlighted and discussed in this chapter.

Chapter 3 provides an overview of classical test theory (CTT) and compares CTT assumptions with the item response theory (IRT) model. A different paradigm on how we think about items in CTT vs. IRT is discussed and illustrated. The relationships between CTT-based scoring and IRT-based scoring are discussed. Based on several examples, this chapter illustrates that both theories are, in general, comparable in terms of the produced scores (which is an ultimate purpose of a measurement scale).

Chapter 4 covers test-retest reliability and internal reliability. Test-retest reliability is introduced based on the basic conventional measurement error model and is discussed in the context of a clinical study. Spearman–Brown prophecy formula is used to contrast the reliability of a single measurement with reliability of an average score. The other major section investigates the methodology behind Cronbach's alpha for Likert-type scales and also includes applications with dichotomous items.

Chapter 5 centers on construct validity. As a method to determine the factor structure of a scale, exploratory factor analysis is analyzed. As a way to test whether a measurement model of a scale fits the data, confirmatory factor analysis is examined. Methodological issues associated with both approaches are discussed at length. The chapter also describes such important properties as convergent and discriminant validity assessment. The longitudinal model for known-groups validity assessment is introduced and detailed. A model using all available data from a clinical study for criterion validity is emphasized.

Chapter 6 centers on the ability to detect change property. An analytic model-based implementation on the ability to detect change is presented, which allows to quantify the relationship between changes in the target PRO (or COA) scale and changes in the anchor (external) scale. Correlational analysis to support an instrument's ability to detect change is investigated. It is shown that correlations between score changes on a pair of variables may provide only adjunct evidence on the ability to detect change on a target scale. The second theme of this chapter relates to an instrument's sensitivity to treatment effects. A framework and an implementation of one unified multi-domain longitudinal model, intended for a scale with multiple domains assessed over time, is discussed in detail.

Chapter 7 discusses the methods and challenges of assessments of meaningful within-patient change (MWPC) and clinical important difference (CID) for a measurement scale. As with the other chapters, this chapter contains methods rooted in the current regulatory documents (especially from the US Food and Drug Administration) and in the existing and more recent literature. Applications of the MWPC and CID for interpretation of the results of treatment effects analyses are highlighted.

As authors, we sought to develop this book to be viewed as a comprehensive guide for all key steps that need to be undertaken in practice during the quantitative validation of a measurement scale. And, for this purpose, it is our aspiration that this monograph can serve as a single, thorough reference that will benefit readers in their research and understanding of the material.

Andrew G. Bushmakin
Joseph C. Cappelleri

About the Authors

Andrew G. Bushmakin earned his MS in applied mathematics and physics from the National Research Nuclear University (former Moscow Engineering Physics Institute, Moscow, Russia). He has more than 20 years of experience in mathematical modeling and data analysis. He is a director of biostatistics in the Statistical Research and Data Science Center at Pfizer Inc. He has co-authored numerous articles and presentations on topics ranging from mathematical modeling of neutron physics processes to patient-reported outcomes, as well as several monographs.

Joseph C. Cappelleri earned his MS in statistics from the City University of New York, PhD in psychometrics from Cornell University, and MPH in epidemiology from Harvard University. He is an executive director of biostatistics in the Statistical Research and Data Science Center at Pfizer Inc. As an adjunct professor, he has served on the faculties of Brown University, University of Connecticut, and Tufts Medical Center. He has delivered numerous conference presentations and has published extensively on clinical and methodological topics. He is a fellow of the American Statistical Association and recipient of the ISPOR Avedis Donabedian Outcomes Research Lifetime Achievement Award.

1

Introduction

1.1   What Is a PRO Measure?

The US Food and Drug Administration defines a **patient-reported outcome (PRO)** as follows: *"Any report of the status of a patient's health condition that comes directly from the patient, without interpretation of the patient's response by a clinician or anyone else. The outcome can be measured in absolute terms (e.g., severity of a symptom, sign, or state of a disease) or as a change from a previous measure. In clinical trials, a PRO instrument can be used to measure the effect of a medical intervention on one or more concepts (i.e., the thing being measured, such as a symptom or group of symptoms, effects on a particular function or group of functions, or a group of symptoms or functions shown to measure the severity of a health condition)"* (FDA 2009).

Similarly, the European Medicines Agency, in its reflection paper on the "Regulatory Guidance for the Use of Health-related Quality of Life Measures in the Evaluation of Medicinal Products," defines a patient-reported outcome as "any outcome directly evaluated by the patient and based on patient's perception of a disease and its treatment(s)" (EMA 2005). A PRO measure that will be used to collect self-reported information from patients may be as simple as a single item or as complex as a multidimensional instrument. (In this book, the terms "instrument," "measure," "questionnaire," and "scale" are used interchangeably; moreover, the terms "item" and "question" are used interchangeably.)

A PRO measure (sometimes referred to as PROM) is an umbrella term that includes a whole host of subjective outcomes such as pain, fatigue, depression, aspects of well-being (e.g., physical, functional, psychological), treatment

A Practical Approach to Quantitative Validation of Patient-Reported Outcomes: A Simulation-Based Guide Using SAS, First Edition. Andrew G. Bushmakin and Joseph C. Cappelleri.

satisfaction, health-related quality of life, and physical symptoms such as nausea and vomiting (Cappelleri et al. 2013). While the term "health-related quality of life" (HRQoL) has been frequently used instead of "patient-reported outcome," HRQoL has a broad and encompassing definition with a number of aspects or dimensions. It consumes a whole array of multidimensional health attributes collectively, including general health, physical functioning, physical symptoms and toxicity, emotional functioning, cognitive functioning, role functioning, social well-being and functioning, and sexual functioning. Health-related quality of life can also involve toxicity and spiritual issues, among other considerations. As such, there is a looseness to the definition of HRQoL.

Health-related quality of life can be viewed as a type or category of PRO measure. Other categories of PRO measures, broadly defined, include functional status (e.g., physical function, cognitive function), which reflects an ability to perform specific activities; symptoms and symptom burden (e.g., pain, fatigue), which are specific to the type of symptom of interest; health behaviors (i.e., smoking, physical activity), which are specific to type of behavior and typically involves its frequency; and patient experience, which concerns satisfaction with healthcare delivery, treatment recommendations, and medication (or other therapies). These broad classifications are neither mutually exclusive nor exhaustive (Cella et al. 2015).

Patient-reported outcomes are, in turn, a type or category of clinical outcome assessments. A clinical outcome assessment (COA) directly or indirectly measures how patients feel or function and can be used to determine whether a treatment has demonstrated efficacy or effectiveness (Cappelleri and Spielberg 2015; FDA 2019a). There are four types of COAs: patient-reported outcomes, clinician-reported outcomes, observer-reported outcomes, and performance outcome assessments. Of the four types of COAs, the first three of these depend on the implementation, interpretation, and reporting from a rater on a patient's assessment – a rater being a patient, clinician, or non-clinician observer.

As depicted and highlighted in Figure 1.1 (FDA 2019b), **patient-reported outcome assessments**, as previously stated, rely on responses to questions on a patient's health condition that come directly from the patient, without any interpretation or judgment on the part of anyone else. An example would be a patient's self-report on a pain scale from 0 (no pain) to 10 (worst possible pain). **Clinician-reported outcome assessments** are reports of a patient's health condition from a trained healthcare professional, a member of the investigator team with appropriate clinical professional training. An example would be a clinician-reported rating scale on severity of a patient's depression (mild, moderate, severe). **Observer-reported outcomes** are reports on a patient's health condition from someone other than a patient or clinician, someone else who is not a specialized healthcare professional training, and based on observable signs, events, or

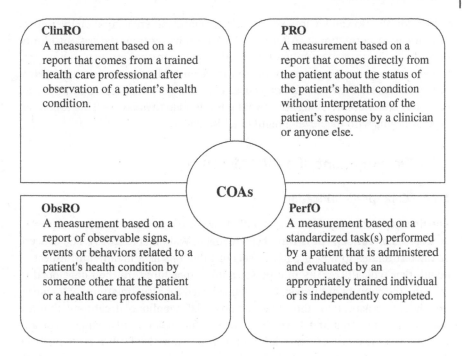

Figure 1.1 COA definitions. *Source:* Adapted from FDA (2019b).

behavior. An example would be a parent's report of infant behavior thought to be caused by pain, such as crying. The fourth type of COA, **performance outcome assessments**, involves measurements of a patient's health condition from a standard task or activity performed actively by the patient and that is administered and evaluated by a suitably trained individual or that is independently completed. An example of a performance-based activity assessment would be an exercise stress test.

Thus, a COA involves volitionally performed tasks or subjective assessments of health status that are patient-focused or centered. Among the categories of COAs, PRO measures distinguish themselves to accommodate health questionnaires whose objective is to measure a patient's self-reported health, be it HRQoL, symptom, satisfaction with treatment, functioning, well-being – whatever the purpose – from his or her perspective rather than from an alternative perspective such as a clinician, observer, or performance activity.

Patient-reported outcomes are often relevant in studying a variety of conditions – including pain, erectile dysfunction, fatigue, migraine, mental functioning, physical functioning, and depression – that cannot be assessed adequately without a patient's evaluation and whose key questions require patient's input on the impact of a disease or a treatment. After all, who knows better than the patient him or herself? To be useful to patients and other decision makers (e.g., clinicians, researchers, regulatory agencies, reimbursement authorities), who are stakeholders in medical care, a PRO measure must undergo a validation process to confirm that it reliably and accurately measures what it is intended to measure. This validation process begins with the development of a PRO measure.

1.2 Development of a PRO Measure

1.2.1 Concept Identification

The first step in the development of a PRO measure is to identify the concept(s) to be assessed or **concept of interest** (FDA 2019b; Walton et al. 2015). The concept of interest relates to how a patient feels or functions as a meaningful aspect of health that typically occurs in a person's life. Procedures are then developed to measure the concept of interest. Concepts selected for assessment in a PRO measure should be aspects of the illness or potential benefits of treatment that are important to patients and have the potential for meaningful change, typically within the context of a clinical trial. Consider the example of self-reported pain as the meaningful health aspect to be measured. The full experience of pain has multiple conceptual faces or characteristics that include intensity, duration, frequency, and sensation (e.g., sharp, burning, stinging). Different disorders may be associated with different pain manifestations. In one disorder, for instance, the concept of interest might be pain intensity, whereas for a different disorder, it might be pain frequency.

Examples of commonly assessed concepts of interest include signs and symptoms of the disease or condition, physical functioning, psychological well-being, activities of daily living, and HRQoL. While all of these concepts may be appropriate for measurement in clinical trials in order to demonstrate treatment benefits that are important to patients, product approvals and labeling claims based on PRO data in the United States are more likely to relate to improvements in symptoms that are proximal to the disease and the drug's mechanism of action (e.g., pain, itch) than those that are more distal and complex (e.g., HRQoL). For the purpose of product labeling, concepts that are considered to be measured more objectively, such as physical function and especially signs and symptoms, also tend to be favored over more subjective concepts, such as satisfaction and self-esteem (Gnanasakthy et al. 2012, 2017). Furthermore, during the time period 2012–2016, the FDA and EMA used different evidentiary standards to assess PRO data for label claims from oncology studies: EMA was more likely than FDA to accept data from open-label studies and broad concepts such as HRQoL (Gnanasakthy et al. 2019).

Researchers recommend that the overall **context of use** for the PRO measure and its resulting endpoint(s) be considered during the concept identification step (Patrick et al. 2011a; Powers et al. 2017). The context of use describes circumstances under which the outcomes of interest adjoined to the PRO measure (or to COAs in general) have been used (i.e., labeled) or are targeted for use (i.e., they have been "qualified" or are part of an ongoing "qualification"). Such "qualification," which also applies to other COAs, is a regulatory conclusion that the PRO is a *well-defined and reliable assessment* of a specified concept of interest for use in adequate and well-controlled studies in a specified context of use (EMA 2009; FDA 2019c). PRO qualification represents a conclusion that within the stated context of use, results of the assessment can be relied upon to measure a specific concept and have a specific interpretation and application in drug development and regulatory decision-making.

Concept identification involves understanding of the disease or condition in the target population; developing an **endpoint model** for the context of use (i.e., developing a diagram of the hierarchy of relationships among the key endpoints, both PRO and non-PRO ones, that corresponds to the clinical trial's objectives, design, and data analysis plan); considering the target population (e.g., language and cultures of patients); considering preliminary issues related to instrument content and structure (e.g., the extent to which respondents will be able to identify and describe symptoms as being specific to their condition); considering the theoretical and qualitative methodologic approach (e.g., using grounded theory methods where ideas for the content of a new measure are developed inductively from the qualitative transcripts); and developing the hypothesized **conceptual framework** (i.e., developing a diagram depicting relationships between the overarching concept, hypothesized domains or sub-concepts, and candidate item content; see Section 1.2.5).

As further elaboration, an endpoint model involves listing the concepts of interest, how they are to be measured, and how the different endpoints are interrelated. For instance, Figure 1.2 illustrates an endpoint model with PRO and non-PRO assessments as key secondary endpoints and a physiologic (non-PRO) measure as the primary endpoint intended to support an indication for the treatment of Disease X (FDA 2009). In this case, the physiologic endpoint would need to show the desired efficacy in a clinical trial before success can be considered to the secondary endpoints in the trial.

1.2.1.1 Literature and Instrument Review

A review of published medical literature and other sources (e.g., practice guidelines, social media) in the relevant therapeutic area can provide a robust background for clinical aspects of the condition, symptoms, and impacts that have been already identified and existing measures that are available (FDA 2019b;

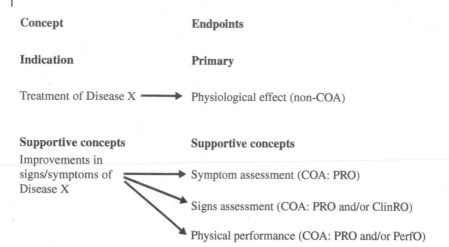

Figure 1.2 Endpoint model: treatment of disease X. *Source:* Adapted from FDA (2019b).

McLeod et al. 2018; Prinsen et al. 2016). In some cases, results of qualitative research or surveys may be available to help begin the process of identifying concepts that are important from the perspective of patients. Furthermore, the literature can provide information related to existing therapies, potential benefits of these therapies, common side effects, and the standard of care, including the role of parents or other caregivers (if relevant).

As potentially important concepts begin to emerge, instruments addressing these concepts should also be reviewed. In addition to instruments identified from previously described sources, the FDA's COA Compendium (FDA 2019d) is an excellent resource for identifying measures with the potential to support labeling claims. There are also instrument databases that can be reviewed to identify potentially relevant measures, along with information regarding the development of these measures and evidence supporting their use, such as the Patient-Reported Outcomes Measurement Information System (PROMIS®, http://www.healthmeasures.net/explore-measurement-systems/promis); the Patient-Reported Outcome and Quality of Life Instruments Database (PROQOLID, https://eprovide.mapi-trust.org/); the Measurement Instrument Database for the Social Sciences (http://www.midss.org/); and Pfizer's Patient-Centered Outcomes Assessment site (https://www.pfizerpcoa.com/).

1.2.1.2 Patient-Centered Input
The most important step in identifying concepts for measurement is the elicitation of input directly from patients (FDA 2019b). Input directly from patients is the cornerstone of content validity, which is the extent to which an instrument covers

the important concepts of the unobservable (latent) attribute or construct – that is, the concept of interest (e.g., depression, anxiety, physical functioning, self-esteem) that the instrument purports to measure. It is "the degree to which the content of a measurement instrument is an adequate reflection of the construct to be measured" (Mokkink et al. 2010a) and thus, how well the PRO instrument captures all of the important aspects of the concept from the patient's perspective. Qualitative work with patients is therefore central to supporting content validity. While quantitative research methods are associated with the gathering, analysis, interpretation, and presentation of numerical information qualitative research methods are associated with the gathering, analysis, interpretation, and presentation of narrative information involving, for example, spoken or written accounts of experiences, observations, and events.

In the qualitative inquiry, participants are asked a series of open-ended questions aimed at furthering the researchers' understanding of the disease, identifying concepts important to patients, and observing patients' word choice when describing these concepts to inform item development (FDA 2019b; Terwee et al. 2018). Qualitative research is a scientific technique that requires a protocol outlining the study details. The protocol should include such elements as inclusion/exclusion criteria, number of subjects, pre-specification if particular sub-groups should be emphasized in recruitment, and information about the questions to be asked by developing a guide for one-on-one interviews or focus groups (or both).

One-on-one interviews or focus groups should be audio recorded to allow transcription and analysis (FDA 2019b). One-on-one interviews involve a discussion on the topic of interest between the research participant and a trained interviewer. They offer opportunities to explore topics in-depth at the individual level using probing questions. One-on-one interviewing can also be used to explore subject areas thought to be too sensitive for a focus group setting. A focus group is a carefully planned discussion conducted among a small group of participants, led by a trained moderator for the task. Group dynamics embedded in a focus group can facilitate additional insights that one-on-one interviews are not equipped for.

Consider the interview guide. It is essential to ensure consistency of questioning, and the questions should be broad and open-ended. For example, if a scale to measure sleep disorders is being proposed, examples of questions can include "How long have you had issues with your sleep?" and "What kinds of sleep difficulties do you experience?". From these broader questions, a researcher can then probe in more detail such as "You said you had problems with staying asleep, can you describe in more detail what specifically these problems are?".

Generally speaking, symptoms that patients mention spontaneously tend to be the most salient compared with those symptoms that are only endorsed in response to follow-up questions; as such, spontaneously reported symptoms may be the most important targets for measurement (McLeod et al. 2018). Additional techniques, such as importance rating and symptom ranking, may also be used to further elucidate the relative importance of concepts elicited from patients. This same line of thinking that applies to symptoms is also relevant more generally to items of a particular concept such as mental functioning or physical functioning.

Input should be elicited from relevant stakeholders, such as caregivers, clinicians and especially patients, to inform PRO development in order to identify the core concepts to target for potential inclusion. In the development of a PRO instrument, the relevant stakeholders should be queried about important aspects of the disease or condition through one-on-one interviews, focus groups, or both – this process is referred as **concept elicitation**.

The number of patients needed for the concept identification (elicitation) stage varies depending on the amount known about the condition, the variability of disease characteristics and symptoms, the number of subgroups of interest, and the potential complexity of the PRO measure (McLeod et al. 2018). For example, the elicitation of concepts for a measure being developed to address the severity of a single symptom experienced by all (or nearly all) patients with a given disease will require a smaller sample size than a measure being developed to assess HRQoL within a diverse patient population. As a general rule, the concept elicitation process should continue until **concept saturation,** the point at which no new information is being elicited, is reached. The achievement of concept saturation should also be documented by developing a detailed table that shows the concepts elicited in each interview (or focus group) and the number of new concepts elicited in later interviews compared with earlier ones.

Once the data have been collected, analysis of the verbatim transcripts is then conducted, involving sorting quotes by concept and could be aided by using software (e.g., Atlas.ti). Such software also allows easier analysis by a specific patient characteristic (e.g., gender or disease severity) to determine if there are differences in the conceptualization of the issue under discussion.

This sorting process will lead to the development of a coding scheme whereby similar concepts are given a code name, forming a cluster. For example, if the discussion is about fatigue and how patients described this symptom, then codes might be tiredness and unrested. Direct quotes from subjects related to these specific terms would then be added under these code names, which allow the researcher to see how such terms were used and how many times the term was used. The codes are usually developed iteratively, changing as the data are analyzed, always through discussion among researchers who are generating the codes to cover the content of the transcripts from the interviews or focus groups.

This aforementioned approach is based on Grounded Theory methods (Glasser and Strauss 1999), whereby ideas for the content of a new measure are developed inductively from the qualitative transcripts. This method involves developing codes to allow the key points of the data to be gathered, which will then be grouped into concepts, and from these concepts, a theory about the data is developed. From this process, a conceptual framework will emerge, a visual depiction of the concepts, sub-concepts, and items and how they interrelate. Other qualitative research approaches are phenomenology, ethnography, case study, discourse analysis, and traditional content analysis; a comparison of these approaches has been discussed (Lasch et al. 2010). Choice of approach will be dependent on the type of research question(s) but, for PRO development, Grounded Theory is generally preferred (Kerr et al. 2010; Lasch et al. 2010).

While patient input reigns supreme in the development of a PRO measure, input from experts in the therapeutic area or condition under study can be extremely useful throughout the development process. For example, clinical experts can facilitate concept identification by providing additional background about the condition, offering insight regarding key symptoms and impacts based on interactions with patients, and identifying unmet needs and desirable treatment attributes based on their experience.

It should be noted that qualitative data can combine and therefore complement quantitative data in collecting and analyzing the patient experience. Mixed methods research addresses a set of research questions via a hybrid approach using both qualitative (narrative) and quantitative (numerical) evidence and methods, which could be analyzed and interpreted together before a conclusion is reached. As an example of mixed methods research, a group of patients is given a survey or questionnaire with both open-ended questions (perhaps accompanied by an interview) and close-ended questions with distinct response options to quantify information for numerical analysis. Information on mixed methods research is found elsewhere (Creswell and Clark 2007; FDA 2019b; Johnson and Christen 2017; Teddlie and Tashakkori 2009).

1.2.2 Item Development

Once the concept or set of concepts to be assessed by the PRO measure has been identified, the focus of the question writing process should be on facilitating patient understanding, yielding proper response, and minimizing measurement error (FDA 2019b). Questions should be succinct and based on the language used by patients, maintain an accessible reading level, and naturally relate to the response options. Items should be comprehensible and generalizable to the total target population, independent of education level, with difficult words and complex sentences avoided, such that anyone over 12 years of age can understand them (Streiner et al. 2015). Item developers should be careful to avoid asking two or more questions masquerading as a single question that addresses more than one concept, which might have different or conflicting answers. For example, an item may ask if a person has trouble walking or jogging. When answering this item, an individual who can walk but not jog must determine which component to answer and which to ignore (McLeod et al. 2018).

Response options should be both comprehensive and mutually exclusive; it is also important that patients be able to clearly differentiate among each option. Responses with multiple meanings should be avoided. For instance, the word "fair" can mean "pretty good," "honest," "plain," and "according to the rules" (de Vet et al. 2011). Careful attention must also be given to the recall period to ensure that patients are able to accurately remember relevant information and formulate an accurate response without complex computations. Thus, it should be clear to which period of time the question refers. Should the patient respond to current pain, pain during the past 24 hours, or pain during the previous 7 days? While very short recall periods (e.g., past 24 hours) and frequent administration have been recommended by the FDA for assessing symptoms with the potential to vary from day to day, as well as within a day, there may be situations in which a longer recall period and less frequent administration are more appropriate. Lengthier recall periods may be appropriate for the assessment of symptoms, behaviors, and functions that are slow to change or require an extended period to assess accurately, such as, for example, using four weeks to assess erectile functioning.

In the context of clinical trials, measures need to be designed to evaluate treatment benefits. As such, patients' experiences (and, consequently, their responses to the PRO items) must have the potential to change over the time course of a clinical trial. Patients typically make multiple measurements over time across multiple PRO instruments. Therefore, the PRO measure should be brief in order to minimize patient burden and allow for flexibility in the mode of administration. For example, a PRO measure being developed for electronic administration on a daily basis should not include more items than patients are willing to answer consistently; the individual items should be brief enough to display clearly on a small screen (e.g., hand-held device or smartphone).

Multiple items may be drafted for each concept of interest so that variable question wording and response scales can be tested in cognitive debriefing interviews and psychometric evaluation to identify what version of the item or its response scale (or both) is most easily understood and answered by patients. In the measurement of pain, for instance, it is not expected that patients can reliably discriminate between 65 and 67 mm of pain or even between 65 and 67 mm on a continuous (interval) 100-mm line visual analog scale (0 = no pain to 100 = worst imaginable pain). Instead, a numeric rating scale with 11 discrete (ordinal) categories would be preferred (0 = no pain, 10 = worst imaginable pain). Of related concern is to set the number of categories on an ordinal scale based on how many categories are relevant.

In addition, it is helpful to consider potential scoring rules during item development. Consider the item "Rate your current level of pain." Including a category for "no pain" can be justified as the lowest (most favorable) score for patients who do not have pain; however, if a "not applicable" response option is offered instead, this response may be chosen by patients who do not experience pain or by patients who restricted their activity to avoid pain, creating measurement error in the item score.

This subsection provided a few examples of requirements in formulating adequate items and responses. A more detailed exposition on the essentials for adequate formulation of questions and answers can be found elsewhere based on principles used in survey research methodology (Bradburn et al. 2004; Fowler 1995; Presser et al. 2004; Schwarz and Sudman 1996; Stone et al. 2000; Sudman et al. 1996).

1.2.3 Cognitive Interviews

Cognitive interviews involve incorporating follow-up questions in a field test interview to gain a better understanding of how patients interpret questions asked of them. Cognitive interviews are a qualitative research tool used to determine whether concepts and items are understood by patients in the same way that instrument developers intend. In this method, respondents are often asked to *think aloud* and describe their thought processes as they answer the instrument questions (FDA 2019b). In general, cognitive interviews are debriefing sessions that focus on the cognitive processing involved when participants read, interpret, and determine their responses to the draft questions.

Insights gained through evaluating this processing step are then used to refine instructions, question-wording, response categories, formatting, and other aspects of the PRO measure to remove aspects that are unclear or influence participants to interpret the items in a way that was not intended; the process is iterative and should continue until evidence is established that no further revisions are warranted. Cognitive interviews typically involve the collection of supplemental data to further support content validity and inform future use of the final measure. As with the concept elicitation interviews or focus groups, cognitive interviews should be accompanied by a semi-structured interview guide; doing so will ensure consistency among cognitive interviews. Additional information on the conduct and analysis of data collected during cognitive interviews can be found in multiple sources and the references cited therein (FDA 2019b; Willis 2005, 2015).

The goals of cognitive interviews are essentially a twofold process: (i) to ensure that the most important concepts are included in the final PRO measure; and (ii) to ensure that respondents understand how to answer each item based on clear instructions, the appropriate recall period, item meaning, response scale, and any other features, such as paper versus electronic mode of administration (Patrick et al. 2011b; Powers et al. 2017). In addition, if subscales are desired for specific concepts of interest, gaining an understanding of how patients perceive relationships among the items will help inform the structure of the PRO scale and the development of initial scoring algorithms. It is also useful to pose specific questions to ascertain what amount of change on the individual items and sets of items is meaningful to patients in order to facilitate the development of Meaningful Within-Patient Change definitions for applications in future clinical trials.

As with the concept elicitation step, cognitive interviews will vary in the number of patients needed as a function of the complexity of the concepts to be measured and variability across the patient population. In general, however, three or four iterative sets of interviews, each comprised of 6–10 patients (for a total of 18–40 additional patients), are typically sufficient to help refine and finalize the items. As a general rule, the cognitive interviews are complete when no additional item changes are identified by subsequent interviews (McLeod et al. 2018).

An **item tracking matrix** is a record of the development (e.g., additions, deletions, modifications, and reasons for the changes) of items or tasks used in an instrument. The item tracking matrix is commonly requested by FDA reviewers and describes the item wording for each version of each item (question) tested, reasons for revisions to retained items, and reasons for the omission of items during the process (FDA 2019b). Moreover, the item tracking matrix provides evidence that further refinements are not needed by documenting subsequent interviews that attest to sufficient understanding, with no feedback identifying weaknesses or suggesting revisions to clarify the wording of the questions or response choices.

1.2.4 Additional Considerations

It should be noted that the steps outlined in the preceding sections are intended to be a general guideline and not prescriptive. As such, suppleness is required when developing a PRO measurement. While not intended to provide an exhaustive or a complete list of special circumstances, this subsection highlights some additional considerations.

For example, if a PRO measure is meant to address a single concept (such as the severity of a particular symptom), or if a great deal is already known about the concepts that need to be measured based on prior research, it may be reasonable to combine the concept identification and cognitive interviewing steps. Interviews would begin with a comprehensive concept elicitation phase in addition to refining the existing item set in supporting the content validity of the final measurement. Such an approach may also be appropriate if interest centers on modifying an existing PRO measure rather than developing a new measure.

The development process often needs to be tailored when working with special populations, such as children and individuals with cognitive or sensory impairments. Recommendations for the conduct of qualitative research in such patient populations have been provided (DeMuro et al. 2012).

If a PRO measure is meant to be administered in international trials, the development process should ideally be completed in multiple countries. It is very common, however, for the initial development of a PRO measure to be limited to a single country. In such cases, translation and cultural adaptation are then performed later in preparation for administration in international studies.

When instrument development takes place in a single country, but the measure is expected to be used in international trials, it is often useful to conduct a translatability assessment. This assessment includes an evaluation of the draft items by translation experts to identify any potential issues with the item wording (language or concepts) and response options/scales. Translatability assessments should be conducted during the item refinement process so that modifications suggested by translators can be tested with participants in additional debriefings from cognitive interviews. For these activities, methodology has been recommended (Wild et al. 2005).

Considerations related to the development of a PRO measure for electronic administration (ePRO) are analogous to those pertaining to its development in multiple languages (McLeod et al. 2018). Ideally, the development process involves cognitive interviewing of ePRO versions of the items with patients using the device slated for use in clinical trials. This process negates the need to demonstrate measurement equivalence between different modes of administration (e.g., ePRO with paper), as the ePRO version is the original and only version of the measure. Nonetheless, the development of a paper-based PRO measure that is later migrated to an electronic platform or migrated from one type of electronic platform to another (e.g., web-based to hand-held) is not uncommon. Much like translation and cultural adaptation processes, ePRO migration must follow a rigorous process to ensure that the content validity and psychometric properties of the final version are maintained. The evidence required to support measurement equivalence between paper-based and ePRO versions has been described elsewhere (Coons et al. 2009).

1.2.5 Documentation of Development Process with Conceptual Framework

It is important to document all steps involved in the PRO development process from the literature review, expert feedback, qualitative research and cognitive interviews for concept elicitation and modification, item development and refinement, endpoint model diagram, and, eventually, current concept and instrument selection up until that point in the process. In addition, from this multi-staged process, a **conceptual framework** for the new measure should be depicted and described. The conceptual framework of a PRO instrument is an explicit description or a diagram for an instrument showing the relationship among items (i.e., questions or tasks) included therein, domains (domain-level concepts), and concepts measured, along with the scores produced by the instrument (FDA 2009, 2019b).

As instrument development evolves, the conceptual framework evolves in tandem and its concepts measured by domain or total scores should be derived using patient input to ensure that the conclusions drawn using instrument scores are valid. Of interest is how individual items are thought to be related, how items may be related within a domain, how multiple domains may be related to each other, and the general concept of interest as reflected in the conceptual framework of the PRO instrument. Figure 1.3 depicts a generic example of a conceptual framework where Domain 1, Domain 2, and Overall Concept each represent related but separate concepts of interest. Conceptual frameworks apply generally to the four types of COAs, not just PRO instruments.

Related to but distinct from a conceptual framework is a **measurement model**, which examines the relationship between the latent variables (domains) and their observed items or variables or questions **(indicators)**. In a **reflective model,** a latent variable drives the indicators (known as **effect or reflective indicators**), which involves a majority of measurement work in the social and health sciences.

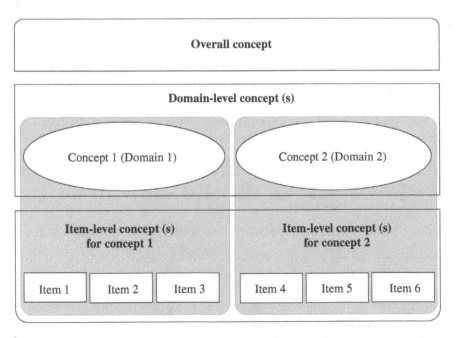

Figure 1.3 Diagram of the conceptual framework of a PRO instrument. *Source:* Adapted from FDA (2019b).

Here, the latent variable drives its effect indicators; in other words, all items should change in the expected way when the concept or construct changes (i.e., items should **reflect** the changes in the concept – hence the name of the model). For instance, as the construct of anxiety changes, so do the items that measure it such as tension, fears, and insomnia.

In a **formative model,** on the other hand, the indicators (also called **causal or formative indicators**) influence its concept; therefore, a change in an indicator affects a change in the concept or construct (rather than the reverse). At the same time, not all causal indicators may change to affect the construct – a change in one of the items may suffice to change the concept, and not all items need to be related. Side effects are an example of variables that are causal indicators in relation to a construct of overall health-related quality of life. More detail on reflective models and formative models are found elsewhere (de Vet et al. 2011; Fayers and Machin 2016) and will also be discussed in detail in Chapter 5 (specifically in Section 5.2.5).

The conceptual framework could be as simple as a single item addressing the severity of a single symptom such as pain intensity or as complex as groupings of items underlying various domains of HRQoL. If the concept of interest is a general one like physical function or clusters of specific symptoms and signs, which includes multiple items and domains, a single-item PRO endpoint will be inadequate to support labeling claims about each of the different aspects of the general concept.

The conceptual framework provides an initial glimpse into possible scoring for the PRO measure based on the development phase (e.g., which items belong to which domain in forming a domain-specific score, and which domains are combined in forming a total score) and may be refined based on the results of the quantitative (psychometric) phase in which the relationships among item scores are evaluated empirically. Documentation of the development process, including the conceptual framework, should be part of the regulatory dossier to facilitate review and agreement that the PRO measure under consideration is fit for purpose – that it is a suitable measure in the proposed context of use for supporting medical product labeling.

1.3 Psychometric Validation

Several guidance on psychometric validation of PRO measures are available from regulatory documents (EMA 2005; FDA 2009, 2019b), books (Bartolucci et al. 2016; Cappelleri et al. 2013; de Vet et al. 2011; DeVellis 2017; Fayers and Machin 2016; Mair 2018; Streiner et al. 2015; Walters 2009), and articles (Calvert et al. 2013, 2018, 2021; Chassany et al. 2002; Mokkink et al. 2010a, 2010b;

Reeve et al. 2013; Revicki et al. 2007a). They center around essentially the evaluation of reliability, validity, and ability to detect change (often referred to as responsiveness) as the psychometric groundwork for the PRO measure as part of good measurement science, especially to support product and labeling claims or, simply, to conduct good measurement science. **Reliability** is the extent to which the measure yields reproducible and consistent results (when it should), **validity** is the extent to which an instrument measures what it is intended to measure and can be useful for its intended purpose, and **ability to detect change** is the ability of the measure to identify differences in scores over time in groups or individuals who have changed with respect to the measurement concept. In general, the quantitative assessment of assessing these measurement properties should be made within the same context of use as planned for the pivotal clinical trials to support labeling claims (if the intention is a label claim).

Generally, the same set of measurement properties should be evaluated regardless of the intent of the PRO measure or whether the PRO measure is newly developed or an existing measure being used in a different condition or for a different purpose. For a PRO instrument that is intended to support product approval or labeling, the amount of evidence required is substantial in order to ensure that the measurements of concepts important to patients are reliable, valid, and have the ability to detect change, as well as be capable of detecting a known treatment benefit.

1.3.1 Psychometric Evaluation Data

Preliminary psychometric evaluations are suggested using a non-interventional study, which is typically based on cross-sectional data, outside of the clinical trial program. In addition, a comprehensive psychometric evaluation of a PRO instrument, including using longitudinal data, should be conducted during a Phase 2 randomized controlled trial. It is important for the Phase 2 study, as well as a non-interventional study, to include additional measures that can support the psychometric evaluation: measures of similar constructs, global assessment of disease status, and global change in disease status relative to baseline. Whenever possible, given the subjectivity of PRO measures, a trial with complete blinding is the first choice.

The PRO measure evaluated before Phase 3 should be administered at key time points aligned to the intended time points for future pivotal randomized controlled trials in Phase 3, which can provide supplemental and confirmatory psychometric information based on previous studies. In general, it is too much of a risk to rely on pivotal Phase 3 studies to establish the major psychometric characteristics of a PRO measure (unless the intention is to seek a label claim on a PRO measure from a Phase 4 study as may occur, for instance, through a supplemental new drug application). In Phase 2, these time points should provide

opportunities to evaluate change in the proposed scores where change is anticipated (assuming a known relative treatment effect from the experimental intervention compared with the control intervention) and to evaluate the stability of
scores where change is not expected (during the pre-treatment stage, before
randomization).

Sensitivity, the ability of a measure to detect differences between groups of
patients, is important in clinical trials as a PRO instrument that cannot differences
in patient outcomes between randomized groups would have little value. Selection
of the number of additional measures should be prudent and not increase patient
burden unnecessarily. Furthermore, it is important that the selected study has
adequate sample size for the methods planned (Chen et al. 2014).

1.3.2 Psychometric Properties

The psychometric evaluation should be guided by a formal and prespecified
psychometric analysis plan. If the psychometric evaluation is performed using
clinical trial data (e.g., Phase 2 data), the psychometric analysis plan on the PRO
instrument should be a separate document from the main statistical analysis plan
designed to guide the evaluation of efficacy and safety for the clinical trial. If the
PRO measure or measures are part of the multiple testing procedures of the efficacy outcomes (both PRO and non-PRO) implemented to preserve type I error
(i.e., the chance of incorrectly or falsely declaring a statistically significant result),
such detail should be part of the main statistical analysis plan.

The psychometric statistical analysis plan should describe the psychometric
and statistical methods to be conducted, including prespecified analytic samples
and subgroups of interest. The psychometric (statistical) analysis plan should
provide a detailed description of analyses to assess reliability, validity, and ability
to detect change and, in interventional studies, thresholds for the clinically meaningful between-patient difference and especially clinically meaningful within-
patient change. It should be noted that problems with content validity (Section 1.2)
cannot be rectified by testing other measurement properties; content validity is an
indispensable prerequisite for a proper quantitative evaluation.

While content validity is of particular interest during the qualitative phase,
construct validity is of particular interest during the quantitative stage.
Construct validity consists of evidence that relationships among items, domains,
and concepts conform to a priori hypotheses concerning logical relationships that
should exist with other measures or characteristics of patients and patient groups
(FDA 2009). Generally, the statistical analyses at baseline and post-baseline
(follow-up) would combine all treatment groups as one unit rather than having
analysis for each treatment group. Table 1.1 provides an overview of typical analysis methods for each of the key psychometric properties.

Table 1.1 Key psychometric properties assessed.

Psychometric property	What is assessed?	Evaluation method
Distributional characteristics	Descriptive assessment of the target PRO measure on item-level and scale-level scores at key time points	Mean, median, standard deviation, minimum, maximum, percentage missing, frequency distribution
Measurement model structure	To assess if the measurement model of a multi-item scale fits the data	Confirmatory factor analysis
Reliability		
Internal Consistency	Consistency of responses to items on the same multi-item scale, where the items are intended to tap into different aspects of the same underlying concept	Cronbach's coefficient alpha
Test-retest	Stability of scores over time when no change is expected in the concept of interest	Intraclass correlation coefficient
Validity		
Content	Evidence that the instrument measures the concept of interest including evidence from qualitative studies that the items and domains of an instrument are appropriate and comprehensive relative to its intended measurement concept, population, and use	Qualitative evaluation of stakeholders (especially patients) involving interviews or focus groups and cognitive interviewing to evaluate patient understanding
Construct	Evidence that relationships among items, domains, and concepts conform to a priori hypotheses concerning logical relationships expected to exist with similar or dissimilar measures Includes at least two major elements: 1) strength of correlation testing a priori hypotheses (convergent validity with similar measures and divergent or discriminant validity with dissimilar measures) and 2) degree to which the PRO instrument can distinguish between or among groups hypothesized a priori to be different (known-groups validity)	Correlational analyses, anchor-based analyses, effect size statistics

Table 1.1 (Continued)

Psychometric property	What is assessed?	Evaluation method
Ability to detect change	Evidence that a PRO instrument can identify changes in scores over time in individuals or groups who have changed with respect to the measurement of concept	Anchor-based analyses complemented with correlational analyses, effect size statistics
Meaningful change and difference	Thresholds for meaningful within-patient change and, separately, between-group difference on the target PRO measure	Anchor-based analyses, cumulative distribution function plots, probability density functions, effect size statistics

Note: PRO, Patient-reported outcome.

1.3.2.1 Distributional Characteristics

Key demographic and sample characteristics at baseline should be tabulated to describe the sample used in the psychometric evaluation. Standard descriptive statistics (including mean, median, standard deviation, minimum, maximum, and percentage missing) should be reported at baseline and, for an interventional study, key post-baseline time points for scores on the targeted PRO measure.

A floor effect is defined by a high proportion of subjects selecting the minimum category or score (e.g., more than 15% select the minimum possible score for scales with a wide range of scores like the SF-36 [McHorney and Tarlov 1995; Terwee et al. 2007]). Alternatively, a ceiling effect is defined by a high proportion of subjects selecting the maximum possible score (e.g., more than 15% select the maximum possible score for scales with a wide range of scores like the SF-36 [McHorney and Tarlov 1995; Terwee et al. 2007]). For reflective indicators (items), both floor effects and ceiling effects can indicate that the PRO measure may not have the measurement range necessary to differentiate and show change. For instance, because patients tend to be homogeneous in their responses at baseline, before treatment intervention, such responses across patients typically have less covariation with a restricted range of scores stemming from a circumscribed inclusion and exclusion criteria. For formative indicators, such as symptoms, a floor or ceiling effect on an item may still be extremely important for descriptive or evaluative purposes (Fayers and Machin 2016).

Given that the magnitude of correlations between variables is a function of their variability (all other factors equal, a restricted range or less variability yields a smaller or attenuated correlation in absolute value), baseline is usually not the ideal time for psychometric evaluation. Under the assumption of a beneficial treatment effect, the range of data expands at post-baseline and the larger estimate of the correlation coefficient (in absolute value) is more accurate reflection of the true correlation coefficient (Bland and Altman 2011; Crocker and Algina 1986; Nunnally and Bernstein 1994).

Thus, if a majority of subjects tend to select an extreme category (or categories) for pain severity at baseline, as a result of the inclusion and exclusion criteria, the estimated correlation coefficient between a targeted PRO pain measure and a related supportive measure would be expected to be lower and attenuated relative to what it would be during the treatment phase when the responses are expected to be more diversified and varied owing to treatment benefit. A careful review of the concept addressed by the item and the characteristics of subjects who endorse extreme categories should be examined to more accurately determine whether an item is only applicable to a certain segment of patients in the target population or simply an artifact of the sample owing to the circumscribed inclusion and exclusion criteria. Therefore, exploration of potential reasons for the observed floor effect or ceiling effect will help to inform decisions on removing, revising, or retaining an item under consideration.

Review of the distributional characteristics provides a general evaluation of compliance and suitability of the PRO measure. Evidence of good compliance (i.e., minimal missing data across items and time points) provides support that patients are capable of completing the measure and that the patient burden of completion is acceptable. The appropriateness of scale-level and item-level scores are judged by the distribution of response categories across time points. Supportive evidence is defined by distributions where all categories are selected by at least a small proportion of subjects without evidence of floor and ceiling effects.

Evidence that the distributions for the PRO instrument and its supporting measures behave as expected provide an initial quantitative understanding for the target PRO measure. For example, if there is little variability in both the target PRO measure and in a related supportive measure, then the concern may shift to the relevance of the sample or overall context of use. On the other hand, if the supporting measures have the expected distributions but the target PRO measure does not – especially during post-baseline assessments with a beneficial intervention – the initial descriptive statistics for the target PRO measure may foreshadow problems with other measurement properties (McLeod et al. 2018).

1.3.2.2 Measurement Model Structure
For multiple items with the potential for subscales, the conceptual framework provides a description of the item-level relationship based on the qualitative phase of the development process and how the items form potential domains.

To inform scoring, this framework is further refined by evaluating the quantitative relationships among the items through inter-item correlation coefficients and dimensionality analysis (e.g., factor analysis).

Methods such as **exploratory factor analysis** have been recommended when these frameworks are preliminary and alternative item groupings have been considered (Finch 2020). In exploratory factor analysis, there is initial uncertainty as to the number of factors (latent variables or domains) being measured, as well as which items are representing those factors. Exploratory factor analysis is suitable for generating hypotheses about the structure of distinct concepts and which items represent a particular concept. Moreover, exploratory factor analysis can further refine an instrument by revealing what items may be dropped from the questionnaire, because they contribute little to the presumed underlying factors.

That said, however, we recommend that, for modern development of PRO instruments, we should already know from the qualitative research and conceptual framework which items belong to which domain. Thus, based on the qualitative research and conceptual framework, we should perform confirmatory factor analysis rather than exploratory factor analysis. Confirmatory factor analysis facilitates the evaluation of a proposed structure (Brown 2015). In this type of analysis, the number of factors and the items that should load on each factor are prespecified. Items are grouped based on the conceptual framework to form hypothesized domains. In confirmatory factor analysis, factor loadings are coefficients that indicate the strength of the relationship between an item and the latent factor (or how well an item reflects changes in the latent factor). These coefficients are important because they signify the nature of the variables that most strongly relate to a factor; the nature of the variables helps to capture the nature and meaning of a factor.

Confirmatory factor analysis is a hypothesis-confirming technique relying on a researcher's hypothesis that requires pre-specification of all aspects of the measurement model: the number of factors, the pattern of item-factor relationships, and so forth. Confirmatory factor analysis tests whether the pre-specification measurement model fits the data.

It is important to stress that baseline data from a clinical trial is not the best or only choice to validate a PRO measure due to the restricted range expected in the data at baseline, as noted previously. Having a wider net of responses (owing to a presumed treatment benefit), post-treatment visits should be especially considered and, relative to baseline, are expected to be more representative of the underlying covariation and, as such, better suited to assess psychometric properties of the scale.

In addition, Rasch modeling and other types of item response theory modeling are useful tools to evaluate the performance of individual items (Andrich 1988; Cappelleri et al. 2014; Edelen and Reeve 2007). These methods can be used to assess the relationships among items, how the items relate to an underlying construct, and redundancy in item content, making the methods informative for item reduction and subscale (domain-level) refinement.

1.3.2.3 Reliability

Reliability is defined as the extent to which an instrument is free of measurement error and can consistently measure a subject's true score, which is the average score that would be expected if the subject completed parallel forms of the instrument many times (Hays and Revicki 2005). A perfectly reliable scale would be a reflection of the true score and nothing else. It is important to evaluate the reliability of a PRO measure in order to provide evidence for the reproducibility of its reported scores under stable conditions. For PRO measures, internal consistency reliability and test-retest reliability are the most relevant forms of reliability.

Internal consistency reliability applies to the consistency of responses to items on the same multi-item scale, where the items are intended to tap into the same construct (or complementary interrelated aspects of it). This form of reliability uses the correlation and covariance among items on a multi-item PRO scale to assess the homogeneity (similarity) of its items at a particular time and refers to the extent to which the items are interrelated and covary. Internal consistency reliability is typically estimated for a group of items whose responses sum to form a single score (a domain score) using Cronbach's coefficient alpha (Cronbach 1951; DeVellis 2017).

Cronbach's alpha presumes that all items adjoined to a multi-item PRO scale reflect a single (latent) concept or construct of interest and is therefore unidimensional, such as scales on anxiety, cognitive ability, and physical function. Thus, Cronbach's alpha coefficient is intended for a PRO measure whose items are intended to summarize distinct aspects of a condition or disease that are related (e.g., different items for measuring anxiety) and not for a PRO measure whose items may not be related (e.g., differing symptoms that are indicative of a disease or condition but may not typically present together).

Test-retest reliability provides an evaluation of reliability by comparing scores for subjects who are classified as stable on the measured construct across at least two time periods where no change is anticipated. The PRO scale is measured at one time (test) and then at least at one other time (retest). Selecting the right period between test and retest, or between times or occasions, is crucial. Typically, a stable group predefined naturally as exhibiting no change during the pretreatment period in clinical trials or may be based on a criterion measure that is judged to be able to adequately assess patients' status in clinical studies.

An intraclass correlation coefficient (ICC), is then computed using the scores for the stable subgroup at specified time points in order to quantify test-retest reliability (McGraw and Wong 1996; Qin et al. 2019; Schuck 2004). An ICC is the ratio of the between-subject variability to total variability. If this ratio is high, there is little measurement error (within-subject variability) to be accounted for by the measurements on the different occasions and the reproducibility (i.e., test-retest reliability) of the measure is high. Values of ICC of at least 0.70 for multi-item scales are recommended to support adequate test-retest (Nunnally and Bernstein 1994; Reeve et al. 2013).

1.3.2.4 Construct Validity

Construct validity is defined as the degree to which the scores of a measurement instrument are consistent with hypotheses, for example, with regard to internal relationships, relationships with scores of other instruments, or differences between relevant groups (de Vet et al. 2011; Mokkink 2010a). Without adequate evidence to support content validity (Section 1.2), most regulatory reviewers will dismiss a measure for further review of the other aspects of validity. These additional aspects of validity use quantitative data and methods grounded in construct validity to build upon the qualitative evidence and prior or preliminary quantitative evidence to further support the content validity of the PRO instrument. Two major types of construct validity are (i) convergent and divergent validity and (ii) known-groups validity.

Convergent/divergent validity describes the prespecified relationships among multiple indicators (items or questions) of constructs (concepts of interest) and the degree to which the scores from these indicators follow predictable patterns. The goal of these analyses is to demonstrate stronger relationships among measures addressing similar constructs (defined as "convergent" validity) compared with measures addressing more disparate or dissimilar constructs (defined as "divergent" or "discriminant" validity). Typically, correlational analyses are conducted to examine these relationships using data at baseline and other key time points. Specifically, the psychometric analysis plan should outline a priori hypotheses that specify the anticipated direction and magnitude or strength of correlations between scores on the target PRO measure and scores on other supporting measures included in the trial (i.e., other PRO measures of both similar and different constructs, other types of clinical outcome assessments, or both). Correlation analyses are then conducted, and their magnitudes and patterns are compared against a priori hypotheses. In most circumstances, a correlation larger than 0.4 is reasonable to support evidence for convergent validity, less than 0.3 to support divergent validity, and between 0.3 and 0.4 as inconclusive evidence to support convergent or divergent validity.

Known-groups validity, another form of construct validity, is based on the principle that the PRO measurement scale of interest should be sensitive to differences between specific groups of patients known to be different in a relevant way. For instance, if a PRO instrument is intended to measure visual functioning, its mean PRO scores should be able to differentiate sufficiently between subjects with different levels of visual acuity (mild, moderate, and severe). Again, these assessments begin with a priori hypotheses that are then evaluated empirically in terms of their predicted direction and magnitude. The magnitude of the separation between known distinct groups is more important than whether the separation is statistically significant, especially in studies with small or modest sample sizes where statistical significance may not be achieved.

While known-group validity and convergent/divergent validity are among the most common forms of construct validity (Table 1.1), other forms of construct validity also have their relevance (Cappelleri et al. 2013; de Vet et al. 2011; Mokkink et al. 2010a). One of them is **structural validity** (i.e., **measurement model structure**): the degree to which the items of a measurement instrument are an adequate reflection of the dimensionality of the construct to be measured, which is assessed by confirmatory factor analysis.

Cross-cultural validity, another type of construct validity, involves the extent that the performance of items on a translated or culturally adapted PRO instrument is an adequate reflection of items in the original version, which is often assessed after the translation of the questionnaire.

Another form of validity, which is sometimes grouped with construct validity but more often is left distinct, is criterion validity, with its two types being **concurrent validity** and **predictive validity**. **Criterion validity** involves assessing a PRO measurement instrument against the true value or against another standard indicative of the true value of measurement, which provides an adequate reflection of a gold standard: **concurrent validity** involves an assessment of scores from the targeted PRO measure with the scores from the gold standard (or quasi-gold standard) at the same time, while **predictive validity** involves an assessment of how the targeted PRO measures predict the gold standard (or purported gold standard) in the future.

1.3.2.5 Ability to Detect Change

The **ability to detect change** – or **responsiveness** – refers to evidence that a PRO instrument, as with other COA instruments, can identify differences in scores over time in individuals or groups who have changed with respect to the measurement concept (FDA 2009, 2019b). In its draft guidance (as of this writing), the FDA reviews the ability to detect change on an instrument as follows: "*FDA reviews a COA's ability to detect change using data that compares change in COA scores to change in other similar measures that indicate that the patient's state has changed with respect to the concept of interest. A review of the ability to detect change includes evidence that the instrument is sensitive to gains and losses in the measurement concept and to change across the entire range expected for the target patient population. When patient experience of a concept changes, the value(s) for the COA measuring that concept also should change*" (FDA 2019b).

Therefore, one way to assess the ability to detect change is to map change from baseline in the target PRO measure with change from baseline on another measure known as an **anchor measure**, an external measure (which can be another PRO measure or other COA measure) that should be clearly interpretable and appreciably correlated with the target PRO measure (FDA 2019b; King 2011). An example of an anchor measure includes the patient global impression of severity – for instance, "Please choose the response that best describes the severity of your overall status over the past week: none, mild, moderate, severe, very severe." Another example of an anchor measure is patient global impression of change – for instance, "Please choose the response that best describes the overall change in your overall status since you started taking the study medication: much better, a little better, no change, a little worse, much worse." Of these two types of measures, the former one which is based on a static and current global impression of severity is recommended at minimum. It is less likely to be subject to recall error than the latter one, which is based on retrospective global measure of change, which can be used as secondary anchor in sensitivity analysis.

1.3.2.6 Interpretation

Unlike well-established clinical measurements such as survival and blood pressure, which are generally understood and can be measured directly, the latent or unobserved concepts captured by PRO measures may be unfamiliar to many healthcare professionals and patients. Patient-reported measures may lack sufficient data or experience or clinical understanding to draw from to properly interpret what, for example, is a 10-point change means on a 0–100 PRO scale.

While PRO endpoints in clinical trials are commonly assessed through the statistical comparison of group means, the results of these comparisons are not always easy to interpret. In addition, statistical significance alone is not sufficient to demonstrate clinically important benefits. As such, characterizing meaningful change for individual patients and meaningful difference at a group level provides the ability to further evaluate, interpret, and communicate PRO results to regulators, patients, and prescribers.

Individual within-patient change is different from between-group mean difference or treatment effect. From a regulatory standpoint, FDA is more interested in what constitutes a meaningful within-patient change in scores from the patient perspective (i.e., at the individual patient level). The between-group mean difference is the difference between the average change score (or average score) between two study arms that is commonly used to evaluate treatment difference, but it does not address the individual within-patient change that is used to evaluate whether a meaningful score change is observed; therefore, a between-group treatment effect is different from a meaningful within-patient change (FDA 2019b).

The literature related to interpretation of change and difference on PRO measures is vast and many terms have been used to characterize them, often interchangeably. For individuals, the terms "responder definition," "responder threshold," and "clinically important change" are among those used; for groups, the terms "minimal important difference," "minimal clinically important difference," and "clinically important difference" are among those used (Cappelleri and Bushmakin 2014; Cook et al. 2015; Coon and Cook 2018; Coon and Cappelleri 2016; Crosby et al. 2003, 2004; FDA 2009, 2019b; Giesinger et al. 2020; King 2011; Marquis et al. 2004; Revicki et al. 2007b, 2008). Given the variety of methods and labels, it is essential to define, understand, and formulate the level of change or difference unambiguously.

1.4 Learning Through Simulations

This book is intended for researchers in the biopharmaceutical and healthcare industry, government, and academe involved in health measurement scales, especially PRO measurement and analysis. Intended readers of the book include statisticians, statistical programmers, psychometricians, and other researchers such as epidemiologists and those involved in outcomes research.

The ensuing chapters provide a detailed description of key steps needed for quantitative validation of PRO measures. Exposition covers major aspects of psychometric validation methodology on PRO measures, including exploratory and confirmatory factor analysis, reliability assessments, longitudinal analysis, and meaningful changes and differences on PRO measures.

This simulation-based guide is intended to give the reader an in-depth understanding on how initial simulated values, various data patterns, and different assumptions affect the results. Much comprehension can be gained by applying computer simulation methods to teach statistics (Good 2005; Mair 2018; Morris et al. 2019; Wicklin 2013) including psychometrics (Beaujean 2018; Feinberg and Rubright 2016). In the chapters that follow, common themes are covered such as how to structure the data before PRO analysis, how to implement an analysis in a step-by-step fashion using simulation examples, and how to delve deeply into concepts by modifying assumptions and parameters.

In order to accomplish these topics of instruction, the book centers on providing a deep understanding and enriched learning environment of quantitative validation methods for PRO measures via simulated data and analytic implementations using the SAS® software. Given that the biopharmaceutical industry is the major sponsor of PRO measures – and that the SAS software is the standard software used in this industry (including by regulatory agencies) – the use of the SAS®

software is a natural choice. In academic settings, faculty members and students generally have free access to SAS software. And, in August 2021, the SAS Institute created a cloud-based version that is available for everyone who would like to learn, even though it is still titled as "SAS OnDemand for Academics": https://www.sas.com/en_us/software/on-demand-for-academics.html. An independent learner simply will need to create a free account with the huge advantage that nothing is needed to be installed on your computer, as everything will be done in the cloud. All that is needed is a compatible web browser. The website https://www.sas.com/en_us/software/on-demand-for-academics.html also provides a lot of additional resources to learn SAS and SAS programming, such as, for example, 10-minute video "Getting Started With SAS Studio" or the free e-learning course "SAS Programming 1: Essentials."

1.5 Summary

This chapter is intended to be general in highlighting the definition and context of PRO measures. The development of a PRO measure is discussed and grounded in concept identification, item development, cognitive interviews, and other considerations. The chapters provide a general view of the instrument development process through the conceptual framework.

After the crucial and indispensable role of qualitative research is described as the basis content validity, the chapter covers psychometric validation of a PRO measure by describing the type of studies and data needed; the measurement properties investigated in terms of reliability, construct validity, and ability to detect change; and methods for interpretation of meaningful scores. Broadstroke elements in an SAP are noted. The role of simulation-based learning using the SAS software for understanding psychometrics is emphasized. Subsequent chapters cover psychometric themes that are conceptualized and explained and then illustrated and augmented through simulation-based learning activities.

In what follows, this book assumes that the PRO instrument of interest has achieved (or is in the process of achieving) content validity, chiefly through qualitative research, in that it covers the important concepts of the unobservable or latent attribute under study (e.g., depression, anxiety, physical functioning, self-esteem) that the instrument purports to measure. Hence the content of the PRO instrument is taken as an adequate reflection of the construct to be measured. Given this backdrop, subsequent chapters focus on the quantitative validation of PRO measures in particular and, when applicable, to COAs in general.

References

Andrich, D. (1988). *Rasch Models for Measurement*. Newbury Park, CA: SAGE Publications, Inc.

Bartolucci, F., Bacci, S., and Gnaldi, M. (2016). *Statistical Analysis of Questionnaire: A Unified Approach Based on R and Stata*. Boca Raton, FL: Chapman & Hall/CRC Press.

Beaujean, A.A. (2018). Simulating data for clinical research: a tutorial. *Journal of Psychoeducational Assessment* 36: 7–20.

Bland, J.M. and Altman, D.G. (2011). Correlation in restricted ranges of data. *British Medical Journal* 342: d556.

Bradburn, N., Sudman, S., and Wansink, B. (2004). *Asking Questions: The Definitive Guide to Questionnaire Design – For Market Research, Political Polls, and Social and Health Questionnaires*, 2e. San Francisco, CA: Jossey-Bass Inc.

Brown, T.A. (2015). *Confirmatory Factor Analysis*, 2e. New York: Guilford Press.

Calvert, M., Blazeby, J., Altman, D.G. et al. (2013). Reporting of patient-reported outcomes in randomized trials: the CONSORT PRO extension. *JAMA* 309: 814–822.

Calvert, M., Kyte, D., Mercieca-Bebber, R. et al. (2018). Guidelines for inclusion of patient-reported outcomes in clinical trial protocols: the SPIRIT-PRO extension. *JAMA* 319: 483–494.

Calvert, M., King, M.T., Mercieca-Bebber, R. et al. (2021). SPIRIT-PRO Extension explanation and elaboration: guidelines for inclusion of patient-reported outcomes in protocols of clinical trials. *BMJ Open* 11: e045105. https://doi.org/10.1136/bmjopen-2020-045105.

Cappelleri, J.C. and Bushmakin, A.G. (2014). Interpretation of patient-reported outcomes. *Statistical Methods in Medical Research* 23: 460–483.

Cappelleri, J.C. and Spielberg, S.P. (2015). Advances in clinical outcome assessments. *Therapeutic Innovation & Regulatory Science* 49: 780–782.

Cappelleri, J.C., Zou, K.H., Bushmakin, A.G. et al. (2013). *Patient-Reported Outcomes: Measurement, Implementation and Interpretation*. Boca Raton, FL: Chapman & Hall/CRC Press.

Cappelleri, J.C., Lundy, J.J., and Hays, R.D. (2014). Overview of classical test theory and item response theory for quantitative assessment of items in developing patient-reported outcomes measures. *Clinical Therapeutics* 36: 648–662.

Cella, D., Hahn, E.A., Jensen, S.E. et al. (2015). *Patient-Reproted Outcomes in Performance Measurement*. Research Triangle Park, NC: RTI Press.

Chassany, O., Sagnier, P., Marquis, P. et al. (2002). Patient-reported outcomes: The example of health-related quality of life – a European guidance document for the improved integration of health-related quality of life assessment in the drug regulatory process. *Drug Information Journal* 36: 209–238.

Chen, W.C., McLeod, L.D., Nelson, L.M. et al. (2014). Quantitative challenges facing patient-centered outcomes research. *Expert Review of Pharmacoeconomics & Outcomes Research* 14: 379–386.

Cook, K.F., Victorson, D.E., Cella, D. et al. (2015). Creating meaningful cut-scores for Neuro-QOL measures of fatigue, physical functioning, and sleep disturbance using standard setting with patients and providers. *Quality of Life Research* 24: 575–589.

Coon, C.D. and Cappelleri, J.C. (2016). Interpreting change in scores on patient-reported outcome instruments. *Therapeutic Innovation & Regulatory Science* 50: 22–29.

Coon, C.D. and Cook, K.F. (2018). Moving from significance to real-world meaning: methods for interpreting change in clinical outcome assessment scores. *Quality of Life Research* 27: 33–40.

Coons, S.J., Gwaltney, C.J., Hays, R.D. et al. (2009). Recommendations on evidence needed to support measurement equivalence between electronic and paper-based patient-reported outcome (PRO) measures: ISPOR ePRO Good Research Practices Task Force Report. *Value in Health* 12: 419–429.

Creswell, J.W. and Clark, V.L.J. (2007). *Design and Conducting Mixed Methods Research*. Thousand Oaks, CA: SAGE Publications, Inc.

Crocker, L. and Algina, J. (1986). *Introduction to Classical and Modern Test Theory*. Belmont, CA: Wadworth.

Cronbach, L.J. (1951). Coefficient alpha and the internal structure of tests. *Psychometrika* 16: 297–334.

Crosby, R.D., Kolotkin, R.L., and Williams, G.R. (2003). Defining clinically meaningful change in health-related quality of life. *Journal of Clinical Epidemiology* 56: 295–407.

Crosby, R.D., Kolotkin, R.L., and Williams, G.R. (2004). An integrated methods to determine meaningful changes in health-related quality of life. *Journal of Clinical Epidemiology* 57: 153–1160.

de Vet, H.C.W., Terwee, C.B., Mokkink, L.B., and Knol, D.L. (2011). *Measurement in Medicine: A Practical Guide*. New York: Cambridge University Press.

DeMuro, C.D., Lewis, S.A., DiBenedetti, D.B. et al. (2012). Successful implementation of cognitive interviews in special populations. *Expert Review of Pharmacoeconomics & Outcomes Research* 12: 181–187.

DeVellis, R.F. (2017). *Scale Development: Theory and Applications*, 4e. Thousand Oaks, CA: SAGE Publications, Inc.

Edelen, M.O. and Reeve, B.B. (2007). Applying item response theory (IRT) modeling to questionnaire development, evaluation, and refinement. *Quality of Life Research* 16: 5–18.

EMA (European Medicines Agency), Committee for Medicinal Products for Human Use (2005). Reflection paper on the regulatory guidance for us of health-related quality of life (HRQOL) measures in the evaluation of medicinal products. European Medicines Agency. www.emea.europa.eu/pdfs/human/ewp/13939104en.pdf (accessed 15 April 2020).

EMA (European Medicines Agency), Committee for Medicinal Products for Human Use (2009). Qualification of novel methodologies for drug development: guidance to applicants. European Medicines Agency. www.ema.europa.eu/pdfs/human/biomarkers/7289408en.pdf (accessed 15 April 2020).

Fayers, P.M. and Machin, D. (2016). *Quality of Life: The Assessment, Analysis and Reporting of Patient-Reported Outcomes*, 3e. Chichester, UK: John Wiley & Sons Ltd.

FDA (Food and Drug Administration) (2009). Guidance for industry on patient-reported outcome measures: use in medical product development to support labeling claims. *Federal Register* 74 (235): 65132–65133. https://www.fda.gov/media/77832/download (accessed 15 April 2020).

FDA (Food and Drug Administration) (2019a). Clinical outcome assessments (COA): frequently asked questions. https://www.fda.gov/about-fda/clinical-outcome-assessments-coa-frequently-asked-questions (accessed 15 April 2020).

FDA (Food and Drug Administration) (2019b). Patient-focused drug development guidance series for enhancing the incorporation of the patient's voice in medical product development and regulatory decision making. Draft guidance documents. https://www.fda.gov/drugs/development-approval-process-drugs/fda-patient-focused-drug-development-guidance-series-enhancing-incorporation-patients-voice-medical (accessed 15 April 2020).

FDA (Food and Drug Administration) (2019c). Clinical outcome assessment (COA) qualification program. https://www.fda.gov/drugs/drug-development-tool-ddt-qualification-programs/clinical-outcome-assessment-coa-qualification-program (accessed 15 April 2020).

FDA (Food and Drug Administration) (2019d). Clinical outcome assessment (COA) compendium. https://www.fda.gov/media/130138/download (accessed 15 April 2020).

Feinberg, R.A. and Rubright, J.D. (2016). Conducting simulation studies in psychometrics. *Educational Measurement: Issues and Practice* 35: 36–49.

Finch, H.W. (2020). *Exploratory Factor Analysis*. Thousand Oaks, CA: SAGE Publications, Inc.

Fowler, F.J. Jr. (1995). *Improving Survey Questions: Design and Evaluation*. Thousand Oaks, CA: SAGE Publications, Inc.

Giesinger, J.M., Loth, F.L.C., Aaronson, N.K. et al. (2020). Thresholds for clinical importance were established to improve interpretation of the EORTC QLQ-C30 in clinical practice and research. *Journal of Clinical Epidemiology* 118: 1–8.

Glasser, B.G. and Strauss, A.L. (1999). *The Discovery of Grounded Theory: Strategies for Qualitative Research*. Chicago, IL: Aldine Publishing Company.

Gnanasakthy, A., Mordin, M., Clark, M. et al. (2012). A review of patient-reported outcome labels in the United States: 2006–2010. *Value in Health* 15: 437–442.

Gnanasakthy, A., Mordin, M., Evans, E. et al. (2017). A review of patient-reported outcome labeling in the United States (2011–2015). *Value in Health* 20: 420–429.

Gnanasakthy, A., Barrett, A., Evans, E. et al. (2019). A review of patient-reported outcomes labeling for oncology drugs approved by the FDA and the EMA (2012–2016). *Value in Health* 22: 203–209.

Good, P.I. (2005). *Resampling Method: A Practical Guide to Data Analysis*, 3e. Boston, MA: Birkhäuser.

Hays, R.D. and Revicki, D. (2005). Reliability and validity (including responsiveness). In: *Assessing Quality of Life in Clinical Trials: Methods and Practice* (ed. P.M. Fayers and R.D. Hays), 25–39. Oxford, UK: Oxford University Press.

Johnson, R.B. and Christensen, L. (2017). *Educational Research: Quantitative, Qualitative, and Mixed Approaches*. Thousand Oaks, CA: SAGE Publications, Inc.

Kerr, C., Nixon, A., and Wild, D. (2010). Assessing and demonstrating data saturation in qualitative inquiry supporting patient-reported outcomes research. *Expert Review of Pharmacoeconomics & Outcomes Research* 10: 269–281.

King, M.T. (2011). A point of minimal important difference (MID): a critique of terminology and methods. *Expert Review of Pharmacoeconomics & Outcomes Research* 11: 171–184.

Lasch, K.E., Marquis, P., Vigneux, M. et al. (2010). PRO development: rigorous qualitative research as the crucial foundation. *Quality of Life Research* 19: 1087–1096.

Mair, P. (2018). *Modern Psychometrics with R*. Switzerland: Springer International Publishing AG.

Marquis, P., Chassany, O., and Abetz, L. (2004). A comprehensive strategy for the interpretation of quality-of-life data based on existing methods. *Value in Health* 7: 93–104.

McGraw, K.O. and Wong, S.P. (1996). Forming inferences about some intraclass correlation coefficients. *Psychological Methods* 1: 30–46.

McHorney, C.A. and Tarlov, A.R. (1995). Individual-patient monitoring in clinical practice: are available health status surveys adequate? *Quality of Life Research* 4: 293–307.

McLeod, L.D., Fehnel, S.E., and Cappelleri, J.C. (2018). Patient-reported outcome measures: development and psychometric validation. In: *Biopharmaceutical Applied Statistics Symposium: Design of Clinical Trials*, vol. 1 (ed. K.E. Peace, D.-G. Chen and S. Menon), 317–346. Springer Nature Singapore Pvt Ltd: Singapore.

Mokkink, L.B., Terwee, C.B., Patrick, D.L. et al. (2010a). The COSMIN study reached international consensus on taxonomy, terminology, and definitions of measurement properties for health-related patient-related outcomes. *Journal of Clinical Epidemiology* 63: 737–745.

Mokkink, L.B., Terwee, C.B., Knol, D.L. et al. (2010b). The COSMIN checklist for evaluating the methodological quality of studies on measurement properties: a clarification of its content. *BMC Medical Research Methodology* 10: 22.

Morris, T.P., White, I.R., and Crowther, M.J. (2019). Using simulation studies to evaluate statistical methods. *Statistics in Medicine* 38: 2074–2102.

Nunnally, J.C. and Bernstein, I.H. (1994). *Psychometric Theory*, 3e. New York: McGraw-Hill.

Patrick, D.L., Burke, L.B., Gwaltney, C.J. et al. (2011a). Content validity – establishing and reporting the evidence in newly developed patient-reported outcomes (PRO) instruments for medical product evaluation: ISPOR PRO good research practices task force report: part 1 – eliciting concepts for a new PRO instrument. *Value in Health* 14: 967–977.

Patrick, D.L., Burke, L.B., Gwaltney, C.J. et al. (2011b). Content validity – establishing and reporting the evidence in newly developed patient-reported outcomes (PRO) instruments for medical product evaluation: ISPOR PRO good research practices task force report: part 2 – assessing respondent understanding. *Value in Health* 14: 978–988.

Powers, J.H. III, Patrick, D.L., Walton, M.K. et al. (2017). Clinician-reported outcome assessment of treatment benefit: report of the ISPOR clinical outcome assessment emerging good practices task force. *Value in Health* 20: 2–14.

Presser, S., Rothgeb, J.M., Couper, M.P. et al. (2004). *Methods for Testing and Evaluating Survey Questions*. Hoboken, NJ: Wiley.

Prinsen, C.A.C., Vohra, S., Rose, M.R. et al. (2016). How to select outcome measurement instruments for outcomes included in "Core Outcome Set" – a practical guideline. *Trials* 17: 449.

Qin, S., Nelson, L., McLeod, L. et al. (2019). Assessing test-retest reliability of patient-reported outcome measures using intraclass correlation coefficients: recommendations for selecting and documenting the analytical formula. *Quality of Life Research* 28: 1029–1033.

Reeve, B.B., Wyrwich, K.W., Wu, A.W. et al. (2013). ISOQOL recommends minimum standards for patient-reported outcome measures used in patient-centered outcomes and comparative effectiveness research. *Quality of Life Research* 22: 1889–1905.

Revicki, D.A., Gnanasakthy, A., and Weinfurt, K. (2007a). Documenting the rationale and psychometric characteristics of patient reported outcomes for labeling and promotional claims: the PRO evidence dossier. *Quality of Life Research* 16: 717–723.

Revicki, D.A., Erickson, P.A., Sloan, J.A. et al. (2007b). Interpreting and reporting results based on patient-reported outcomes. *Value in Health* 10: S116–S124.

Revicki, D., Hays, R.D., Cella, D., and Sloan, J. (2008). Recommended methods for determining responsiveness and minimally important differences for patient-reported outcomes. *Journal of Clinical Epidemiology* 61: 102–109.

Schuck, P. (2004). Assessing reproducibility for interval data in health-related quality of life questionnaires: which coefficients should be used? *Quality of Life Research* 13: 571–586.

Schwarz, N. and Sudman, S. (ed.) (1996). *Answering Questions: Methodology for Determining Cognitive and Communicative Processes in Survey Research*. San Francisco, CA: Jossey-Bass Inc.

Stone, A.A., Turkkan, J.S., Bachrach, C.A. et al. (ed.) (2000). *The Science of Self-Report: Implications for Research and Practice*. Mahwah, NJ: Lawrence Erlbaum Associations.

Streiner, D.L., Norman, G.R., and Cairney, J. (2015). *Health Measurement Scales: A Practical Guide to Their Development and Use*, 5e. New York: Oxford Univeristy Press.

Sudman, S., Bradburn, N.M., and Schwarz, N. (1996). *Thinking About Answers: The Application of Cognitive Processes to Survey Methodology*. San Francisco, CA: Jossey-Bass Publishers.

Teddlie, C. and Tashakkori, A. (2009). *Foundations of Mixed Methods Research: Integrating Quantitative and Qualitative Approaches in the Social and Behavioral Sciences*. Thousand Oaks, CA: SAGE Publications, Inc.

Terwee, C.B., Bot, S.D.M., de Boer, M.R. et al. (2007). Quality criteria were proposed for measurement properties of health status questionnaires. *Journal of Clinical Epidemiology* 60: 34–42.

Terwee, C.B., Prinsen, C.A.C., Chiarotto, A. et al. (2018). COSMIN methodology for evaluating the content validity of patient-reported outcome measures: a Delphi study. *Quality of Life Research* 27: 1147–1157.

Walters, S.J. (2009). *Quality of Life Outcomes in Clinical Trialsand Health-Care Evaluation: A Practical Guide to Analysis and Interpretation*. Chichester, UK: Wiley.

Walton, M.K., Powers, J.H. III, Hobart, J. et al. (2015). Clinical outcome assessments: conceptual foundation – report of the ISPOR clinical outcomes assessment – emerging good practices for outcomes research task force. *Value in Health* 18: 741–752.

Wicklin, R. (2013). *Simulating Data with SAS®*. Cary, NC: SAS Institute Inc.

Wild, D., Grove, A., Martin, M. et al. (2005). Principles of good practice for the translation and cultural adaptation process for patient-reported outcomes (PRO) measures: report of the ISPOR task force for translation and cultural adaptation. *Value in Health* 8: 94–104.

Willis, G.B. (2005). *Cognitive Interviewing: A Tool for Improving Questionnaire Design*. Thousand Oaks, CA: SAGE Publishing, Inc.

Willis, G.B. (2015). *Analysis of the Cognitive Interview in Questionnaire Design: Understanding Qualitative Research*. New York: Oxford University Press.

2

Validation Workflow

The previous chapter covered some key elements useful in the developmental phase of validating a patient-reported outcome (PRO) measure, which includes pilot testing and field testing. Pilot testing of the measurement instrument entails an intensive qualitative analysis of the items in a relatively small number of patients representative of the target population. Field testing of a multi-item measure involves a quantitative analysis in a sufficiently large number of patients (e.g., a few hundred) and concerns item reduction and data structure and, therefore, examines dimensionality and ultimately the definitive selection of items per dimension (domain). As noted in Chapter 1, after the development phase completes, the final measurement instrument is evaluated for its reliability and validity in non-interventional observational studies and in clinical trials.

In this chapter, it is assumed that a well-conducted qualitative work has been satisfactorily performed and that content validity has been established on the PRO (or clinical outcome assessment) measure. Specifically, we describe and characterize the validation workflow for clinical trials, cross-sectional studies, and field tests. We compare and contrast the validation workflow for single-item scales, the confirmatory validation of multi-item multi-domain instruments and validation of new instruments. In this last situation, a further distinction is made between a new measure with multi-item domains having a known conceptual framework and not having one. The psychometric themes highlighted in the set of validation workflows are described in-depth as topics in subsequent chapters.

2.1 Clinical Trials as a Data Source for Validation

The use of clinical trial data presents unique opportunities and, at the same time, distinctive challenges when used as a source to quantitatively validate a scale. A clinical trial will have data for the population of interest not only for

A Practical Approach to Quantitative Validation of Patient-Reported Outcomes: A Simulation-Based Guide Using SAS, First Edition. Andrew G. Bushmakin and Joseph C. Cappelleri.
© 2023 John Wiley & Sons, Inc. Published 2023 by John Wiley & Sons, Inc.

one snapshot in time but also will provide longitudinal profiles. Having a beneficial treatment alongside a placebo or control treatment will likely create substantial differences in responses between subjects, which will likely lead to a considerable spread of scale scores desired for robust and accurate analyses (ideally, a full range of scale scores is vital for meaningful analyses). Among the challenges of clinical trial data is the logistical difficulty to include a comprehensive set of additional scales needed for validation of the target scale of interest, as the frequency of data collection could be driven by patient burden and operational requirements. Another challenge is that due to the entry criteria such as age or gender, validation results may not be easily generalizable beyond the population studied.

To be able to comprehensively execute a psychometric validation of a new scale or perform a validation of an existing scale to confirm its properties, for example, in a different population, it is not enough just to collect data for the scale under investigation. There are several properties of a measurement scale (which will be discussed at length in upcoming chapters) for which it is essential that a set of additional measures also be included in a study. For example, to assess convergent validity (Chapter 5), we seek a collection of additional existing measures that are expected to be related to the target scale.

Another important decision to make during the planning of a clinical trial is when data should be collected – for not only the target scale but also other scales, which are needed to assess different properties of the target scale. Of particular note is that the distance in time between time points when data for the target scale are collected should be larger than the recall period for this scale. If a recall period is four weeks, for instance, data for this scale should not be collected weekly; otherwise, such data cannot be taken as independent. In this case, every measurement that covers a given period will also overlap and hence be at least partially covered by the previous measurement.

But what about the timing of those additional scales? Let's continue with our example of the scale under investigation with a four-week recall or reference period and collected in a study every four weeks. Let's say that to examine convergent validity, we also collect an existing scale with only a one-week recall period. A naïve approach would be to collect this other scale at the same time points as the target scale, that is, with the same frequency. But in this case, the additional scale will only partially cover the recall period of the target scale. While perhaps somewhat counterintuitive, this additional scale should be collected weekly, that is, four times as often as the target scale. Then, as a part of the convergent validity assessment, the four consecutive weekly observations of the other scale should be averaged to create a score that will cover the same recall period as the score on the target scale. There are countless scenarios depending on the reference periods, but in every situation following two important points should be recognized: (i) the recall period should not overlap and (ii) when analyses are based on data from two or more scales, their scores should reflect the same period of time. And this period is likely to be the period corresponding to the largest recall period of scales involved in this analysis.

Among all-time points in a study, baseline data is distinct from all other post-baseline time points for purposes of psychometric validation. Generally, in clinical studies, baseline data are skewed due to the entry criteria and, because of this, often have limited variability. Consequently, many psychometric evaluations based on cross-sectional data – such as convergent and discriminant validity, internal consistency reliability, and confirmatory factor analyses, can produce erroneous results (which will be examined at length and with examples throughout this book). But, on the other hand, we recommend using baseline data jointly with screening data as the most suitable data for the assessment of the test-retest reliability (Chapter 4). Care should be taken in the collection of the baseline data, as in many pertinent analyses, the change from baseline is used (e.g., for the ability to detect change) and, if a subject does not have baseline data, then his or her data cannot be used for this type of analysis.

The main advantage of a clinical study is its ability to include longitudinal data for not only the target scale of interest but also additional scales needed to help validate the target scale. For example, to assess the ability to detect change (Chapter 6), we need to have "data that compares change in COA (clinical outcome assessment) scores to change in other similar measures that indicate that the patient's state has changed with respect to the concept of interest" (FDA 2019). A longitudinal clinical study with a beneficial treatment will likely generate sufficient change from baseline to the end of the study for the target scale ("change in COA scores") and also for the anchor scale ("change in other similar measures"), which is an external measure, related to the target scale, that is fundamental for the assessment of the ability to detect change on the target scale. The same condition also applies to assess sensitivity to treatment (Chapter 6).

Among the additional scales required for validation, the FDA also recommends including two global scales: (i) a static, current-state global impression of severity scale (e.g., PGIS) and (ii) a global impression of change scale (e.g., patient global impression of change or PGIC). Figure 2.1 gives a generic example of a PGIS scale. In a real study, <disease> should be replaced by description of the target disease, such as "atopic dermatitis." Figure 2.2 presents a generic example of a PGIC scale. It is also noted that "a static, current state global impression of severity scale is recommended at minimum … since these scales are less likely to be subject to recall error than global impression of change scales; they also can be used to assess change from baseline" (FDA 2019).

It should be stressed that Figures 2.1 and 2.2 represent generic global assessments and that "global scales can be used for other types of COAs; however, the

Please choose the response below that best describes the severity of your <disease> now.

☐ None

☐ Mild

☐ Moderate

☐ Severe

Figure 2.1 Example of the generic patient global impression of severity (PGIS) scale.

Please choose the response below that best describes the overall change in your < disease >

since you started taking the study medication.

☐ Much better

☐ A little better

☐ No change

☐ A little worse

☐ Much worse

Figure 2.2 Example of a patient global impression of change (PGIC) scale.

instructions and question stems would need to be modified appropriately. The appropriateness of the PGIS scale used depends on the context of use (e.g., patient population)" (FDA 2019). Those two types of scales are discussed and used throughout this book, and they are especially relevant for the assessment of meaningful within-patient change (MWPC) (discussed in detail in Chapter 7).

Thus far we discussed the advantages of the clinical trial data for validation. At the same time, however, data from clinical studies for some diseases can be challenging. Many analyses for the assessment on the psychometric properties of a target scale are implicitly based on the assumption that data are representative of the population at large for the particular disease and, as such, that the data from a variety of subjects with different severity of disease are present. Psychometric analyses, such as exploratory and confirmatory factor analyses (Chapter 5) and Cronbach's alpha estimations (Chapter 4), require meaningful variability in data at a particular time point. In certain studies (e.g., specific cancers, Alzheimer's disease, Duchenne muscular dystrophy, etc.), it is anticipated that the initial state of subjects will not change meaningfully. Yet, for analyses such as the estimation of MWPC and the assessment of the ability to detect change, it is required that a sufficient number of subjects change appreciably over time (either substantial improvement or substantial deterioration, depending on the disease). In this type of situation, the strategy should be to anticipate this and have a prospective plan to include data from other studies, if available, with subjects representing dissimilar severities of the same illness.

In some studies, it is unethical or not feasible to have a placebo arm. As a result, if a drug is beneficial, most subjects will be improving, but their scale scores would still likely have a restricted range, which can impair a psychometric evaluation. For this type of study to increase variability of scale scores for the purpose of (say) a confirmatory factor analysis, a data set can be constructed by dividing subjects randomly in two equal groups, then for subjects from the first group baseline data will be used and for subjects from the second group data at the end of the study will be used. A research team from such a study should be aware that assessments of all psychometric properties for a scale are not possible. In this case, a separate study should be planned to assess the remaining psychometric properties.

Validation of a scale consists of a set of psychometric analyses which assesses a set of measurement properties. It is noteworthy to state that validation should be viewed as a collection of analyses, not as a series of statistical tests. For example, test-retest assessment (Chapter 4) plays an indispensable role on how data will be used in other validation analyses. If an intraclass correlation coefficient (ICC) of a single measurement is less than a desirable value (say, 0.7), then we can average several observations on it to have reliable measurement. The point here is that we should not test whether an ICC value for a single measurement is less than a specific value. We estimate an ICC value and use it as a guidance on how a single measurement should be addressed and viewed. The same can be said about estimating a value for Cronbach's alpha – we simply calculate Cronbach's alpha coefficients and interpret them.

Another example is the estimation of a value for MWPC. We do not (statistically) test an estimated MWPC on whether it is different from some predefined value. And, when MWPC is used to interpret the results of a study, then FDA (draft) documents (2019) specifically state that it is not a test (Chapter 7). While it is traditional to provide confidence intervals or p-values for certain properties, these inference statistics should serve only as a guidance to judge the soundness of results.

2.2 Validation Workflow for Single-Item Scales

A single-item scale can serve as the introductory example of the simplest validation pathway. The first step in the validation of a single-item scale will be assessment of test-retest reliability (Figure 2.3). The circle with digit 1 inside

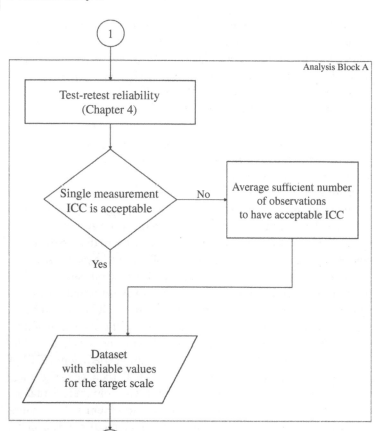

Figure 2.3 Workflow for test-retest reliability assessment.

represents the flow chart *connector*, and in Figure 2.3, it is simply the starting point of the validation. The rectangle "Test-Retest Reliability" in Figure 2.3 represents the flow chart *process* and, in this case, the process is the assessment of an ICC value for a single measurement. After an ICC value is estimated, the important decision should be made on how many single measurements will be used later for validation (the flow chart *decision is* represented by rhombus in Figure 2.3). Generally, for single-item scales, it is expected that test-retest reliability will be low, meaning that a single measurement cannot be considered as a reliable measure of an outcome. Note that it does not necessarily mean that this scale is flawed; it could be that a scale is measuring a symptom that, given a disease, naturally varies over time and is not expected to be stable. In this case, averaging of several observations over time can help to overcome this issue (Chapter 4). For example, based on a single measurement for ICC it may be concluded that at least three observations should be averaged to have acceptable test-retest reliability. If we assume that data are collected daily, then data from every three consecutive days can be averaged.

But, from the logistical standpoint, a week of data can be more convenient to use and practical to interpret. By doing so, we only increase the reliability of the measurements, and it is worthwhile to note that these data should be interpreted as weekly results (akin to a scale with a recall period of a week). If this weekly averaging approach is selected, then an ICC value for a single measurement can also serve as the basis for the number of observations that should be present or completed in the past seven days (or, stated differently, up to how many missing observations are allowed during the past seven days). In the aforementioned example, then, at least three observations (not necessarily consecutive) from a maximum of seven observations should be present in order to have a reliable scale score. In two practical real-life examples, evidence indicates that, for patients with fibromyalgia, at least two daily measurements on a single-item numeric rating scale on pain and, separately, on sleep quality are needed to be averaged to obtain acceptable scale reliability of at least 0.70 (Cappelleri and Bushmakin 2020, 2021).

If, based on a single measurement of ICC, five measurements should instead be averaged to have a reliable measurement, then a maximum of only two observations from seven observations can be missing. Thus, the result of the test-retest analysis is not just about estimating an ICC value: It is also about creating a dataset (the flow chart *data* are represented by parallelogram in Figure 2.3) with scale scores that are considered reliable measurements with these scale scores being used in subsequent validation analyses.

After establishing what is considered a reliable measure for a target scale (be it a single measurement or an average of several observations), a series of analyses represented by Figure 2.4 should be performed. Simply performing all those analyses is not the end of the psychometric validation, however. The results of those analyses need to be interpreted. Do they all support the conclusion that the target scale provides valid measurement? And, if not, then it should be examined and explained why not. For example, suppose the results of convergent and discriminant (divergent) validity are supportive for all post-baseline observations but results at baseline are inconclusive or opposite to the hypothesized relationships. Do those results support convergent and discriminant validity for the target scale? In the case of a clinical study, the explanation can often be the limited range of data at baseline due to entry criteria, which attenuates and impairs correlation coefficients. Given this explanation, then, the overall conclusion here is that convergent and discriminant validity is supported. But in other types of studies, this assumption about the restricted range of data at baseline may not be true.

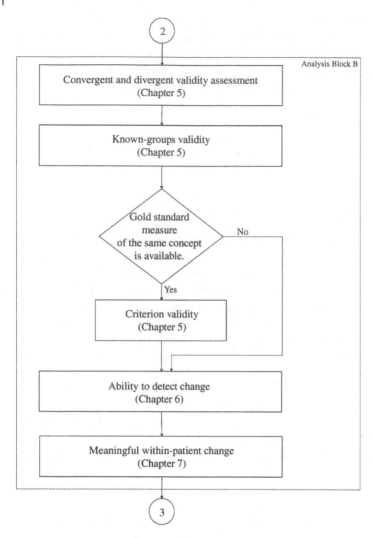

Figure 2.4 Workflow for required analyses.

Therefore, the correct interpretation or at least plausible explanation should be addressed on a case-by-case basis.

Figure 2.5 represents three additional analyses that need consideration. For example, the clinical important difference, which is discussed in detail in Chapter 7, can be important for the research team, patients, some regulators, and other stakeholders. Sensitivity to a treatment is another such assessment (Figure 2.5). It provides information on which domains of a target scale improve, which domains worsen, and which domains did not change for a particular drug

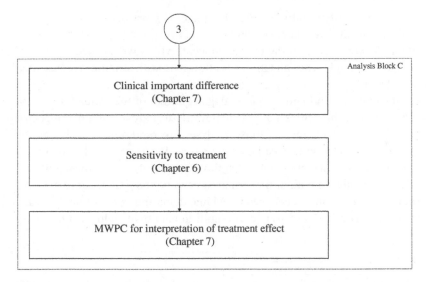

Figure 2.5 Workflow of optional analyses.

or intervention. The last element in Figure 2.5 is on MWPC to aid the interpretation of treatment effects, which is suggested by FDA to be part of submission documents (FDA 2019) (discussed in detail in Chapter 7).

2.3 Confirmatory Validation Workflow for Multi-item Multi-domain Scales

In the previous section, the validation flow for a single-item scale was described. For a measure or questionnaire having multiple domains each with multiple items (i.e., multi-item, multi-domain scales), the validation flow will include the steps discussed in the previous section, but also some additional analyses need to be performed. There is also a difference between a newly developed scale, which is not yet quantitatively validated, and an existing scale, which is planned to be used for a different purpose, for example, in a different population (vs. originally performed validation). In this section, we consider the latter situation, with the former being considered in the next section. The distinguishing feature of this type of validation is that the measurement structure of a scale is established, meaning that we know a priori which items belong to which domains. We simply need to confirm that psychometric properties, including the measurement structure of the scale, are still adequate in the population of interest.

Consider a multi-item multi-domain PRO (or COA) instrument, as was represented by Figure 1.3. There are two domains, and every domain is represented by three items. There exists also the overall concept, which we consider as a third domain in this example. The validation workflow in this illustration is represented by Figure 2.6.

The validation flow in Figure 2.6 is analogous to that of the validation flow of the single-item scale in Figures 2.3–2.5, but now those analyses should be repeated for every domain. In Figure 2.6, those analyses are represented, as before, by "Analysis Block A" (B and C) (see Figures 2.3–2.5). But Figure 2.6 has two additional analyses: internal consistency reliability (Chapter 4) and confirmatory factor analysis (Chapter 5). Both of those analyses can be thought about as analyses that examine the relationship between individual items and domains on this scale. Cronbach's alpha evaluates items in every multi-item domain, while confirmatory

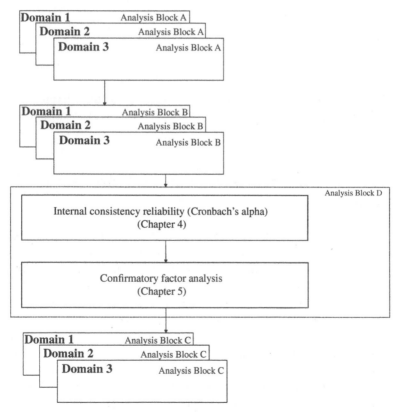

Figure 2.6 Workflow for a confirmatory validation of a multi-item multi-domain PRO instrument.

factor analysis evaluates whether the data (at item and domain level) fit the measurement structure of the PRO instrument.

2.4 Validation Flow for a New Multi-item Multi-domain Scale

2.4.1 New Scale with Known Conceptual Framework

In the previous section, we used an example from Chapter 1, but with assumption that the scale was already established, and we only perform confirmatory validation, for example, for a new context of use such as a new population of interest. As a result, it is assumed that the structure (i.e., which items represent which domains) of the scale is known and immutable. Analysis Block D, in this case (in Figure 2.6), can be done at any point during the validation, for example between Analysis Block A and Analysis Block B.

But if it is the first time for a scale to be quantitatively validated, then the relative position or order in the validation workflow of certain analyses is critical. Figure 2.7 depicts the general workflow for the validation of a new scale. Here the validation of a new scale starts with a question about its structure. Do we have a sound conceptual underpinning on how many domains are on this measure and which items represent those domains? As discussed in Chapter 1, as a part of scale development for the use in clinical trials, a conceptual framework should be constructed in order to depict relationships between items and domains in a multi-item multi-domain scale. This conceptual framework will serve as a starting point in the validation.

Thus, for the top decision rhombus, *"Measurement model is specified"* for a scale with determined conceptual framework, the answer is *Yes*, which next leads to the analyses represented by the Analysis Block A for every domain. Recall that Analysis Block A is related to the test-retest analyses. The outcome of those analyses is not just an estimation of an ICC but also the evaluation of how many observations are needed to obtain a reliable measure. For a multi-item domain, it is unlikely that more than one measurement would be required. However, if more than one measurement turns out to be needed at the domain level, then average domain scores should be used for other psychometric analyses. This averaging (to create a reliable measure for a domain score) of measurements across time has a major effect on the data at the item level. Because we are averaging domain scores in the analyses represented by Analysis Block B and C, then, for consistency, averaged item scores should be used in analyses represented by the Analysis Block D.

The next step in the validation process is the Analysis Block D (internal consistency reliability and confirmatory factor analysis), as displayed in Figure 2.7.

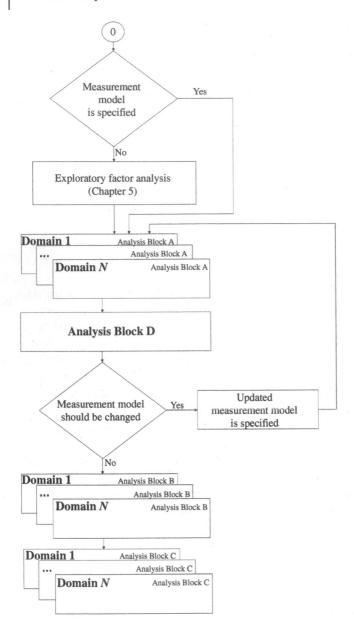

Figure 2.7 General workflow for a newly developed scale.

Because it is supposedly the first time a quantitative validation of a scale is underway, the results of the Cronbach's alpha assessments and confirmatory factor analysis of a postulated measurement model based on a conceptual framework may indicate that some items can be considered for exclusion, or it can be realized that certain items should belong to a different domain. The decision rhombus *"Measurement model should be changed"* symbolizes this point in the workflow. If no changes to the measurement structure is needed, then the analyses represented by Analysis Blocks B (and optionally C) are performed, which will conclude the validation. But if a measurement structure needs to be changed, then based on the results of the Analysis Block D a new, updated structure should be developed (represented by rectangle *"Updated measurement model is specified"*). Analyses represented by Analysis Block A should be repeated using the new, updated measurement structure of the scale.

2.4.2 New Scale with Unknown Measurement Structure

As previously noted, a modern newly developed scale for use in clinical trials should have a conceptual framework depicting the relationships between items and domains. Nonetheless, it is possible that a new measure is developed without a conceptual framework, despite it being recommended by the FDA guidances as good clinical practice for a regulatory label (2009, 2019). It is likely, in this situation that there is no initial information on the measurement structure of the scale (perhaps only a set of items is currently available). Thus, for the top decision rhombus, *"Measurement model is specified"* for a scale with an undetermined measurement model, the answer is *No*, which leads to the analyses represented by the rectangle "Exploratory Factor Analysis" (see Figure 2.7).

There are two important properties of a scale that needs to be known to successfully execute quantitative validation: (i) the number of latent concepts/factors/domains and (ii) which items represent these latent concepts. Exploratory factor analysis can be used in this case to try to find out those two properties. However, the results of those analyses should be carefully evaluated. Researchers need to be critical when using exploratory factor analysis, because it *always* produces *a solution*. Typical outcomes of this analysis are (i) the estimated number of factors and (ii) the allocation of items to factors, alongside (iii) with the possible recommendation to exclude some items from a scale.

It should be first evaluated whether the revealed factors and items representing them make methodological sense. Can items representing a factor be viewed as representing a domain-level concept of the overall concept (as discussed in Chapter 1; see Figure 1.3)? Then, do *all* those newly developed factors correspond to clear and coherent domain-level concepts? The point is that the results of the exploratory factor analysis should not be treated as the final "truth" but rather as an initial step in the understanding of the measurement model.

Exploratory factor analysis and confirmatory factor analysis are methodologically very different. But here, we would like to highlight one major difference with important implications. The factor structure produced by exploratory factor analysis is based on so-called common variance, that is, the amount of variance that is shared among a set of items (which is always smaller than the total variance). This "loosely" means that a factor structure is based on only a part of data for every subject – the part that is apportioned to represent a common variance. The most profound consequence of this realization is that if a just extracted measurement structure from an exploratory factor analysis will be tested with confirmatory factor analysis using the same dataset, then there is a chance that this measurement model will not fit the data because confirmatory factor analysis uses *all* item information and data. As noted in Chapter 5, results of the exploratory factor analysis should be treated as hypothesis-generated results about the underlying structure of the data; this suggested structure should be tested with confirmatory factor analysis.

Another typical outcome of exploratory factor analysis is the identification of items that do not load on any of the generated factors. In Chapter 5, it is discussed in detail that those items should not be simply removed from a scale without due consideration. If items are grounded in well-conducted qualitative work, all those items may be important enough for subjects and cannot be simply dismissed outright.

2.5 Cross-Sectional Studies and Field Tests

Outside of the clinical trial environment, cross-sectional studies are much more commonly employed for the initial validation of newly developed scales. In this case, the workflow represented by Figure 2.7 will not work as the test-retest analyses cannot be performed. If later analyses support the use of a single measurement as a reliable measure of the outcome, the results of analyses based on cross-sectional data can be useful. Earlier discussed issues linked to the possible differences in the recall periods of existing scales used, for example, for convergent validity also can lessen the usefulness of results from cross-sectional analyses.

Longitudinal validation studies in a natural environment (field test) are sometimes also used. These studies from the validation standpoint are close to clinical studies, and, as such, the same workflow (Figure 2.7) can be applied, although with some reservations. If there is no treatment intervention, in many cases, there will be no changes in the disease severity state of subjects in the study; therefore, such analyses as the ability to detect change or MWPC estimations will be difficult to perform. The same will happen if all subjects are already taken medicine for their illness that keeps their severity state stable throughout the course of the study. The most productive approach is (i) to have subjects with all levels of illness severity (which will provide variability in data for severity) and (ii) to have a meaningful number of subjects who are willing to start to use a study medication (which may provide meaningful change in the disease severity on a subject level).

2.6 Summary

This chapter gives general recommendations on the quantitative validation workflow under different scenarios, which should be applicable for most cases. There is, however, always a possibility that some new scale will need some adjustments to the workflows highlighted and discussed in this chapter.

In this chapter, the section on clinical trials as a data source covered some of the distinctive opportunities and challenges when using this source to psychometrically validate a scale. The section on the validation workflow for single-item scales presented the core validation pathway involving test-retest reliability, construct validity (convergent and divergent, known-groups), criterion validity, ability to detect change, and meaningful within-patient change, clinical important difference, sensitivity to treatment, and meaningful within-patient change for interpretation of treatment effects. Extending on this sequence of validation steps, the section on confirmatory validation workflow for existing multi-item multi-domain instrument (for its quantitative validation in a new setting), emphasized additional steps that include assessments using internal consistency reliability and confirmatory factor analysis. The next section advanced the validation workflow for a new multi-item multi-domain instrument, distinguishing between such a measure with a known conceptual framework, where all of the aforementioned analyses are considered, and a measure without it where exploratory factor analysis should be initially used. The last section briefly highlighted some advantages and disadvantages of cross-sectional and field tests for validation purposes.

Each of the psychometric themes captured in the workflows found in this chapter is discussed and analyzed at length in subsequent chapters.

References

Cappelleri, J.C. and Bushmakin, A.G. (2020). Test-rest reliability of a 11-point pain intensity numeric rating scale for patients with fibromyalgia. *Biopharmaceutical Report* 27 (2): 15–19. https://community.amstat.org/biop/biopharmreport (accessed 25 August 2022).

Cappelleri, J.C. and Bushmakin, A.G. (2021). Test-retest reliability on the sleep quality numeric rating scale for patients with fibromyalgia – how many measurements are enough? *Biopharmaceutical Report* 28 (1): 6–10. https://community.amstat.org/biop/biopharmreport (accessed 25 August 2022).

FDA (Food and Drug Administration) (2009). Guidance for industry on patient-reported outcome measures: use in medical product development to support labeling claims. *Federal Register* 74 (235): 65132–65133. https://www.fda.gov/media/77832/download (accessed 15 April 2020).

FDA (Food and Drug Administration) (2019). Patient-focused drug development guidance series for enhancing the incorporation of the patient's voice in medical product development and regulatory decision making. Draft guidance documents. https://www.fda.gov/drugs/development-approval-process-drugs/fda-patient-focused-drug-development-guidance-series-enhancing-incorporation-patients-voice-medical (accessed 15 April 2020).

3

An Assessment of Classical Test Theory and Item Response Theory

Classical test theory (CTT) and item response theory (IRT) are two useful methods to provide a quantitative assessment of items in multi-item scales during the content validity phase of a clinical outcome assessment (COA) (or PRO) measure and a subsequent phase of estimating scale scores in clinical studies (Cappelleri et al. 2014).

In general, scale items are necessary because many constructs cannot be assessed directly. In a sense, items that constitute a scale or measure are proxies for phenomena that cannot be directly observed. A measurement theory is a theory about how the scores generated by items represent the construct to be measured (de Vet et al. 2011; Edwards and Bagozzi 2000). Moreover, only unobservable (latent) constructs require a measurement theory. For observable characteristics, which may be the case with certain one-item scale (e.g., frequency of episodes of itching), it is usually obvious how the observed items contribute to the construct of interest, and thus no measurement theory is needed. Consider, for instance, the assessment of physical activity. Knowing the frequency, type of activity, and its intensity can provide the total energy expenditure that defines physical activity.

On the other hand, unobservable constructs are more challenging to measure. In this case, the underlying phenomenon or construct that a scale is intended to quantify is generally referenced as the latent variable. A latent variable is unobservable by definition. For a given patient, its magnitude can change in time, with an active treatment intervention, and other factors. Patient-reported outcome measures of complex concepts, like physical or emotional functioning, are typically latent and measured via multiple items.

There are two well-known approaches to measurement theory: CTT and IRT (Cappelleri et al. 2014). In the following two sections, we provide a brief overview of CTT and a specific application of IRT for person-item (or patient-item) maps based on the Rasch model as an illustration of IRT.

A Practical Approach to Quantitative Validation of Patient-Reported Outcomes: A Simulation-Based Guide Using SAS, First Edition. Andrew G. Bushmakin and Joseph C. Cappelleri.
© 2023 John Wiley & Sons, Inc. Published 2023 by John Wiley & Sons, Inc.

3.1 Overview of Classical Test Theory

3.1.1 Basics

Classical test theory is a foundation to measure constructs that are not directly observable. Information about an unobserved construct is obtained by assessing items that are manifestations of the construct and, in the case of patient-reported outcomes, these items can be captured through answers from patients to statements or questions. Thus, CTT is suitable for the measurement of constructs that follows a reflective model such that, as the construct changes, the items change in unison.

Classical test theory distinguishes *true score* from *observed score*. A true score is a theoretical value that each subject has on the construct or conceptual variable of interest. A person's unobservable true score at a given time is defined as his or her expected score over (hypothetically) an infinite number of independent administrations of the scale at that time. An observed score, in contrast, is the score actually derived from the measurement process. It is assumed that each subject has a true score on the construct of interest that is not directly observed. Rather, the unknown true score is inferred from the observe score, which is a function of the observed item scores. If we assume that the set of items completely covers the concept of interest and the scores for observed items are perfectly reliable and valid, which is typically not the case, the observed score will equal the true score.

The basic formula of CTT can be written as

$$v_{ij} = F_j + e_{ij} \qquad (3.1)$$

where

v_{ij} is the observed score on item i for patient j,
F_j is the "true" score of the construct for patient j, and
e_{ij} is the error term on item i for patient j (Crocker and Algina 1986; DeVellis 2006, 2017; Furr 2018; Lord and Novick 1968; Nunnally and Bernstein 1994; Spector 1992).

This formula is foundational for many simulated examples throughout the book and will be discussed in depth and used frequently in the following chapters (especially pertinent for Chapters 4 and 5). The formula states that a patient's item score is the sum of the unobservable construct (a fixed entity constant across items for a particular individual at a given time) plus the associated unobservable error term (a random quantity that varies across items for a particular individual).

3.1.2 Illustration

Suppose interest centers on monitoring the severity of atopic eczema (dermatitis) using the Patient Oriented Eczema Measure (POEM) (Charman et al. 2004).

This patient-reported questionnaire consists of seven symptoms (represented by variables $v_1, v_2, \ldots, v_7$), each of which is rated on a five-point ordinal scale for the frequency of occurrence over the last week ($0 = $ no days, $1 = 1\text{--}2$ days, $2 = 3\text{--}4$ days, $3 = 4\text{--}5$ days, $4 = $ every day). The item responses on POEM are summed to give a maximum total score of 28; the larger the score, the more severe the disease state. If a patient scores the first item, "How many days has your skin been itchy because of your eczema" (v_1), it will give an indication on the severity of atopic eczema for this patient. But it would not be a perfect indication on the true level of atopic eczema severity (a latent construct representing the true F for this patient), suggesting that this measurement will be accompanied by a distinct value for this patient's random error term (e_1).

The observed score for this patient on the second item, "How many nights has your sleep been disturbed because of your eczema" (v_2), like all remaining items on POEM, can again be subdivided into the same true score F plus another distinct value for the error term (e_2). All seven items on POEM can be seen as repeated measurements of the latent attribute called severity of atopic eczema. It is also important to stress that every item in a measurement scale is not just another measurement of the true score, which differs only by error term. Otherwise, we could have had just a one item and ask a patient to respond to this item many times. Because latent constructs that we attempt to measure are complex in nature, the items should "cover" different aspects of the same measured construct.

3.1.3 Another Look

It is important to note that Eq. (3.1), by itself, is not unique to CTT of educational or psychological phenomena. Eq. (3.1) is behind almost any kind of measurement. For instance, if we want to measure a weight of a subject, there is no true directly observable weight available (in a sense, then, weight is a latent entity). An instrument such as a beam balance scale is needed to measure weight, and this scale will have random error associated with every use. It should be clear that this measurement process can be described by the same Eq. (3.1) with F representing true weight, v representing the observed weight produced by the scale, and e representing the error in measurement. Note that this phenomenon is not exclusive to measurements related to humans; the same can be said about measurements of any physical object. One can even say that the ultimate unobservable (latent) variable is time. Physicists often debate on what time really is, but humanity over millennia has created instruments to measure time and used those measurements to improve lives.

In some instances, items in a scale can be based on a simple counting of events. But even if there is no good and meticulous log of events, then Eq. (3.1) can remain applicable. For example, items of the POEM scale have a one-week recall period. The first item, "How many days has your skin been itchy because of your eczema" asks a subject to count days, but without a meticulous log of events, the response will not be exact and should be considered as a measurement response represented by Eq. (3.1).

An observed scale score is a single numeric value based on the scores of the individual items constituting the scale. A value for a scale score may be the average, sum, or some other transformation on the set of item scores. Sum scores are quite common as they are conceptually understandable and computationally simple. By adding or averaging multiple items on the same scale, the effect of errors associated with each item gets attenuated, thereby leading to more accurate or reliable measurement.

If the sum score, or equivalently the average score, is taken across the seven symptom items on POEM, this summary or aggregated score would approach the true score of severe atopic dermatitis for a particular individual. Doing so implies that the items will correlate to some degree with each other and also the total score (or, equivalently, average score). In order for these claims to be realized, CTT is based on the theory of parallel tests that underpins the construction of simple summated scales, where the observed scale score is computed by adding together (or, equivalently, averaging) all of the item scores (Crocker and Algina 1986; DeVellis 2006, 2017; Furr 2018; Lord and Novick 1968; Nunnally and Bernstein 1994; Spector 1992).

Classical test theory has its foundational roots in the theory of parallel tests, where in the parlance of psychometrics, each item is viewed as a "test" that is a representative value of the latent variable (the theory of parallel items would be a more apt description, but we will go with CTT convention). This theory posits that each item, like every other item on the same scale, serves as an indicator of effect reflecting the same unidimensional construct of interest (i.e., a reflective model), as previously stated. In our example on dermatitis, all items are taken as reflective or indicative of the patient's severity of atopic eczema.

Building on Eq. (3.1), CTT starts with three assumptions grounded in the theory of parallel tests. Its most basic form is based on responses to items aggregated across a sufficiently large number of respondents. First, each item is assumed to give an unbiased estimate of the true (latent) score and, therefore, the error associated with individual items is taken to have a mean of zero in expectation, as the average of the errors for a subject over many repeated items of the same construct should in principle be zero (i.e., $E[e_{ij}] = 0$ for any item i on patient j). Second, error terms are statistically independent (i.e., $covar(e_{ij}, e_{kj}) = 0$ for items i and $k(i \neq k)$; also note that responses between subjects are assumed to be statistically independent). Third, error terms and true scores are also statistically independent (i.e., $covar(e_{ij}, F_j) = 0$ for any item i).

Furthermore, the parallel tests (or measurements) are not unique to CTT of educational or psychological phenomena. For example, if the very precise weight measurement of a physical object is desired, then the weight will be measured repeatedly and, likely, using different instruments. The results of their measurements then will be averaged to produce a more precise estimation of the weight. In this hypothetical example, it is clear that those instruments are playing the role of the items and it should be noted that the three aforementioned CTT assumptions are also applicable here.

3.2 Person-Item Maps

3.2.1 CTT Revisited

As stated in CTT, which applies to COAs generally, each item measuring a concept is viewed as a "test" to produce a score, which represents the value of the latent variable. Technically this means that it will be enough to develop one "special" item to measure a concept but, in reality, we generally have several items to describe a concept. Such is done because we recognize that one item cannot adequately describe a concept of interest (as outlined in Section 1.2). To illustrate this point outside the realm of COAs (or PROs), consider the measurement on the basic mathematical proficiency of students (represented by Overall Concept in Figure 1.3). Therefore, for example, they are needed to be tested in algebra, geometry, trigonometry, and calculus. These specialty areas will be the four domain-level concepts, and the problem exercises to solve will be the items.

And therein lies the issue: Those mathematical problems to solve (items) should have different or varying levels of difficulty; otherwise, it will be impossible to correctly assess the knowledge of every student. Suppose all problems have the same "moderate" difficulty. Then, on average, they will not be solved correctly by any student who has a weak knowledge in mathematics, but all those problems will be solved correctly by students with strong mathematical skills. As a way to resolve this situation, every problem (item) should have a different level of difficulty (with every problem being somehow assigned a "difficulty" score).

Now say we have 10 algebra problems with 10 different levels of difficulty from 1 to 10. If a student will solve correctly all 10 problems, this student will have a maximum score of 10 (assuming one point is assigned to a correct solution). But what about a student who answered correctly only the most difficult problem but answered incorrectly all other nine less difficult or more simple problems? Then this student will get a score of 1 (even if this problem is the most difficult one). The logic behind this assignment is that, most likely, it was simply a fluke or luck, not the real knowledge or skill of the individual (otherwise, other problems would also be correctly solved).

It should be evident that this description of a mathematical "test" is inconsistent with CTT. The main assumption of CTT is given by Eq. (3.1). Yet if we take the simplest problem, then every student will likely be able to solve it correctly, which means that Eq. (3.1) cannot be representative of the true score. Recall that each item (in CTT) is assumed to give an unbiased estimate of the true (latent) score for a subject. For COAs we resolve this situation by simply giving a subject a choice of selecting one response among a gradation of response options on, for example, a 5-category Likert scale or an 11-category numerical rating scale.

Now suppose we are developing a performance outcome scale and one of its items asks subjects to rate their ability to do push-ups. This item is "I can perform *one* push-up." The response options are from 1 ("strongly disagree") to 5 ("strongly agree"). Given that we anticipate that most of the subjects from a particular population will be able to perform at least one push-up, this situation will lead to most of the subjects responding with a score of 5. This result will be representative of a ceiling effect, and the development of this item and inclusion of it as a part of a scale should be questioned. The more constructive item formulation would be, for example, "I can perform *ten* push-ups." Using this item expression is less likely to lead to a ceiling effect. These two different item stems – one push-up versus ten push-ups – therefore affect the possibility to have or not have a ceiling effect. At the same time, though, they can also be compared with our example of the mathematical test. The first formulation, "I can perform *one* push-up" can be viewed as the "simple" problem, and "I can perform *ten* push-ups" can be viewed as the "moderate" problem. The point is that the COAs, given their context of use, should have items with varying levels of difficulty and response options reflective of the population of interest.

Let's continue with our mathematical test. The better the knowledge a student has, the more problems this student will be able to solve successfully. Suppose every student will be given problems in order of their difficulty. A student with excellent preparedness will solve them correctly one by one, from first to tenth. But a student with average skill will correctly solve, say, only the first five or six problems. Of course, an excellent student having a bad day will solve only a few problems, whereas an average student could be lucky and correctly answer all 10 of them, but, in the long run, they will perform exactly as described previously. We can think about those problems as a set of gates, which should be open one by one, with every next one being more difficult to open.

3.2.2 Note on IRT

The IRT represents a different paradigm on how we think about items (Embretson and Reise 2000). Now items are "forced" to have different difficulties as an essential part of a model. The following equation represents the relationship between algebra proficiency measured by 10 problems and the probability to correctly solve a problem using a type of IRT model referred to as a Rasch model:

$$P_{ij}(\theta_j) = \frac{1}{1 + e^{-(\theta_j - b_i)}} \tag{3.2}$$

where

θ_j represents the level of knowledge or skill for subject j ($j = 1, 2, \ldots, N$, where N is the total number of students participating in the exam);

b_i represents difficulty of problem i ($i = 1, 2, \ldots, 10$); and

$P_{ij}(\theta_j)$ represents the probability of correctly solving problem i by subject j (given his or her level of knowledge or skill, represented by θ_j).

In Eq. (3.2), θ_j represents the latent true score for subject j, which is generally referenced in IRT as a person's "ability." It is important to note that abilities of subjects (θ_j) and parameters defining difficulty of items (b_i) are estimated simultaneously or jointly. However, if difficulty parameters of a set of items were already established or predefined, then it is possible to estimated abilities of new subjects, which were not included in the original development dataset, without reevaluating difficulty of items. For example, the Patient-Reported Outcomes Measurement Information System (PROMIS) adult Physical Function item bank v2.0 (www.healthmeasures. net), which measures the outcome of patients with musculoskeletal disorders by assessing physical function through a grading scale of activities of daily living, contains 165 items for which difficulty parameters are already estimated and can be used in the estimations of the abilities (without re-estimation of difficulties, as is done, for example, in Figure 3.5 later in this chapter). And therein lies the most important complication of using IRT to assess and estimate true scores of subjects as a part of a COA in clinical studies. Sample estimates of difficulty parameters for a scale to be used in a clinical study should be independent of and estimated prior to this study.

To do this for any scale, we need to create a representative dataset and obtain consensus by a community of researchers who have used this scale; otherwise, results will not be uniformly and meaningfully interpretable when comparing results from one study to another one. It is difficult to imagine whether such a consensus can be possibly done for the majority of COA scales that are used in clinical studies now or in the foreseeable future. The PROMIS initiative, of course, moves forward in this direction (www.promishealth.org), but much more is needed to be done. An ancillary point is that, even with already defined values of item difficulties, the calculation of true scores (abilities) would require realistically the use of a computer.

A comparison between Eqs. (3.1) and (3.2) indicates that Eq. (3.2) represents a completely different relationship between observed measurements and latent true scores. Observed measurements in Eq. (3.2) do not have a simple and direct relationship with latent true scores (as defined by Eq. (3.1)). Instead, the relationship is now probabilistic. Note that the promise of IRT is to improve the accuracy of the measurements (i.e., producing more accurate assessments of the latent true scores), but in the current state, as related to COAs, this promise was not fulfilled. Many, if not most, COA scales in clinical studies continue to be based on CTT from scale development through calculation of the scores for multi-item domains. Then the question arises, what can we use IRT for?

Consider the use of IRT to augment development of a new scale or to enrich understanding of an existing scale and with the practical understanding that the final scale, if used in a subsequent clinical study, is not likely to have its assessment of true scores (θ_j) based on the IRT approach, which is typically the case (although what follows is also applicable if it were not the case and the IRT approach were used to estimate θ_j). Instead, eventual assessments of scores are usually based on CTT (i.e., calculated as a sum or a mean of items in a domain).

3.2.3 Implementation of Person-Item Maps

Items in a domain can be evaluated and portrayed from a complementary, supplementary modeling perspective using person-item (or Wright) maps via Rasch modeling, previously expressed in Eq. (3.2) for a binary response, a one-parameter non-linear model (with the one-parameter being the difficulty parameter of each item) in which the probability of a positive response by a patient to a particular item (question) is a function of the difference between the patient's level on the attribute and the difficulty of the item (Bond et al. 2021; Bushmakin et al. 2017; Cappelleri et al. 2014; Stelmack et al. 2004; Wilson 2005; Wright and Masters 1981). Person-item maps can be a useful adjunct in enriching the interpretation, understanding, and interrelation to a wide spectrum of multi-item scales. For example, a person-item map was applied to enhance the interpretation of the Erectile Dysfunction Inventory of Treatment Satisfaction questionnaire by quantifying barriers to improvement of satisfaction with treatment (Bushmakin et al. 2017). While person-item maps can be created for rating scales with ordered polytomous item responses (ordinal scales), we concentrate here on rating scales with binary item responses or with ordered polytomous item responses that are (justifiably) combined and categorized into dichotomized responses in order to directly target a particular research question (e.g., see Bushmakin et al. 2017).

To describe person-item maps, we continue with our math test and specifically on algebra proficiency measured by 10 problems. Every problem, if solved correctly, will be given a score of 1, with an incorrect solution being given a score of 0. Our simulated dataset will have a very simple structure with one observation per subject with 10 variables (items), and every item can have a value of 1 or 0. In the next chapter (Chapter 4), such a dataset is created for a different purpose, but it can also be used here to illustrate the patient-item maps. To simulate the dataset for analysis, we execute the SAS code, first, from Figure 4.64 ("Simulating a scale with 10 continuous items") and, second, from Figure 4.66 ("Simulating binary responses"). After running these codes, the dataset "_sim_ds1" will be created (see Figure 3.1 for the structure of the dataset). In this example the first student (correctly) solved all 10 problems, the second student solved 4 problems, the third solved 9 problems, and so on.

Figure 3.2 shows the implementation of the analyses. The first PRINT procedure simply prints out the data (presented by Figure 3.1). This implementation of the IRT procedure depicts the implementation of the Rasch model. The following two lines

```
var i1-i10;
```

and

```
model i1-i10 /RESFUNC=RASCH;
```

define the variables and the model. The code line

```
ods output ParameterEstimates=ParmEst;
```

requests that parameters (i.e., difficulties b_i) of the model should be outputted in the dataset "ParmEst" and the option "OUT=irt_out" will add estimated abilities (θ_j) for every subject to the original dataset (and create a new dataset with all information from dataset "_sim_ds1" with the additional column "_Factor1" representing estimated abilities). Figure 3.3 represents estimated difficulties for every problem (item). Figure 3.4 summarizes estimated abilities for the entire dataset. (Note that IRT generally requires a lot of data to produce stable estimations; in this example, data were simulated for 3000 subjects.)

i1	i2	i3	i4	i5	i6	i7	i8	i9	i10
1	1	1	1	1	1	1	1	1	1
0	1	0	1	0	0	1	1	0	0
1	1	1	1	1	0	1	1	1	1
0	1	0	0	0	0	1	1	0	0
1	1	0	0	1	1	1	1	1	1

Figure 3.1 Dataset "_sim_ds1" (data for the first five subjects are shown).

```
Proc Print data=_sim_ds1 NOOBS; Var i1-i10; Run;
Proc Irt data=_sim_ds1 itemfit SCOREMETHOD=ML TECHNIQUE=NRRIDG OUT=irt_out;
    var i1-i10;
    model i1-i10 /RESFUNC=RASCH;
    ods output ParameterEstimates=ParmEst;
Run;
Proc Print Data=ParmEst NOOBS; where Parameter="Difficulty"; Run;
Proc Freq Data=irt_out; Tables _Factor1; Run;
```

Figure 3.2 The implementation of the Rasch model.

```
Item     Parameter     Estimate      StdErr    Probt
i1       Difficulty    -0.08577      0.06330   0.0877
i2       Difficulty    -3.79433      0.09366   <.0001
i3       Difficulty     2.69122      0.07716   <.0001
i4       Difficulty    -0.05792      0.06329   0.1801
i5       Difficulty    -1.34724      0.06643   <.0001
i6       Difficulty    -0.58873      0.06390   <.0001
i7       Difficulty    -1.07666      0.06529   <.0001
i8       Difficulty    -2.29363      0.07283   <.0001
i9       Difficulty     0.49542      0.06365   <.0001
i10      Difficulty     0.99862      0.06490   <.0001
```

Figure 3.3 Estimated difficulties (b_i).

```
                                          Cumulative    Cumulative
  _Factor1    Frequency     Percent       Frequency      Percent

      -99        117         3.90            117          3.90
-3.692230768     186         6.20            303         10.10
-2.537739953     236         7.87            539         17.97
-1.73367562      285         9.50            824         27.47
-1.076190334     293         9.77           1117         37.23
-0.479622691     308        10.27           1425         47.50
0.1101519255     293         9.77           1718         57.27
0.7469272904     317        10.57           2035         67.83
1.5166204318     352        11.73           2387         79.57
2.6301882675     345        11.50           2732         91.07
       99        268         8.93           3000        100.00
```

Figure 3.4 Frequencies of the estimated abilities.

The model represented by Eq. (3.2) also implies a very interesting property (especially pertinent for patient-item maps) that the abilities of subjects (θ_j) and difficulties of items (b_i) are both measured in the same units. This property of being on the same metric is the consequence of having the term ($\theta_j - b_i$) in Eq. (3.2). Only when such values are measured in the same units can they be meaningfully subtracted from each other (or summed). If a scale in our example is measuring algebra proficiency, then the estimated values of θ_j and b_i can be contrasted on the same abstract algebra proficiency "ruler." For example, in Chapter 4 (specifically, Section 4.2.2), we discuss the Roland-Morris Disability Questionnaire with 24 binary items where the estimated values of θ_j and b_i will be measured on the same abstract disability "ruler."

In Figure 3.4, we find a somewhat odd estimation of abilities for subjects with the lowest ability (i.e., for students who were not able to correctly respond to any problems, with responses of 0 to all 10 items)) and the highest ability (i.e., for students who successfully solved all problems, with responses of 1 to all 10 items). These results stem from the inability to do estimation via maximization of likelihood (note the option "SCOREMETHOD=ML" in Figure 3.2) for subjects whose response to all items is at either the lowest level or the highest level (it is akin to doing binary logistic regression with the binary outcome with the same outcome for all subjects). For those subjects, abilities values are simply assigned large values (−99 and 99 in this case; note that those values technically should be minus infinity [−∞] and plus infinity [+∞]). There is no specific agreement among researchers on this point, and different software packages deal with it in different ways. This inability to estimate factor score on a domain level (or, to be exact, for a unidimensional construct) is an important shortcoming of IRT as a method for use in the measurement of COAs in clinical studies. It should be noted that the IRT procedure addresses this concern by using different methods to estimate latent factor scores. For example, "SCOREMETHOD= EAP" requests the expected a posteriori method and "SCOREMETHOD= MAP" requests the maximum a posteriori method. Readers are encouraged to run analyses with those options to observe differences in results.

If scale difficulty parameters have been estimated using a representative sample, then to use this scale (or a set of problems) as a part of a clinical study (or exam), we need to estimate the abilities of the subjects without re-estimation of difficulty parameters. Earlier it was noted that the relationship between the observed outcomes and the latent factor is probabilistic. To obtain the true latent score (ability) for a subject, we need to have responses to all items and then estimate ability via maximization of likelihood.

Figure 3.5 shows this implementation using the NLP procedure. The first data step ("**Data** b;...") creates a dataset with just one column with estimated difficulty parameters presented by Figure 3.3 (which, as noted previously, is generated from SAS code in Figure 3.2). The next data step ("**Data** Responses; ...") creates a dataset with also only one column but now representing responses of a particular subject to all 10 items (or in terms of the algebra problems which problems were solved correctly and which are not). In this example, we are estimating the ability of the third subject from Figure 3.1, who addressed all problems correctly except for problem number six (i.e., 9 of 10 problems were addressed correctly).

```
Data b; Set ParmEst;
b=Estimate;
where Parameter="Difficulty";
Keep b;
Run;
Data Responses;
input U @@;
datalines;
1 1 1 1 0 1 1 1 1
;
Run;
Data Theta; Merge b Responses; Run;
Proc Print data=Theta NOOBS; Run;
Proc NLP Data=Theta Random=100; Max LogL; parms Theta;
P=Log(1/(1+exp(-(Theta-b)))); Q=Log(1-1/(1+exp(-(Theta-b)))); LogL=U*P + (1-U)*Q;
Run;
```

Figure 3.5 Estimation procedure to obtain a particular subject's ability (subject 3 from Figure 3.1) based on responses to items with known difficulty parameters.

Figure 3.6 shows the input dataset for the NLP procedure to execute maximum log-likelihood estimation, and Figure 3.7 shows the estimated ability for subject 3. We can see that estimated value of the ability is 2.63 (value of 2.630188 in Figure 3.7), which corresponds exactly (as it should) to the value 2.6301882675 in Figure 3.4.

The core code from Figure 3.5 will produce exactly the same values of the abilities as in Figure 3.4 for all subjects with item responses of at least one 0 and 1. To do this, we change only the values in the data step representing the pattern of responses ("**Data** Responses;..."). But if we will try to use this exact code from Figure 3.5 for the subjects with the lowest ability (all responses of 0) or the highest ability (all responses of 1), the corresponding result will be different from −99 and 99 (which are just arbitrary numbers in the current implementation of the IRT procedure). If we replace the sole value of 0 in the dataset "Responses" with the value of 1 (i.e., all responses will be 1 in Figure 3.5), then the estimated ability will be 15.3 (value of 15.346596 in Figure 3.8), given the default settings for conversion in the NLP procedure. This highlight the fact that it is important to understand what kind of algorithms are implemented before interpreting results.

b	U
-0.08577	1
-3.79433	1
2.69122	1
-0.05792	1
-1.34724	1
-0.58873	0
-1.07666	1
-2.29363	1
0.49542	1
0.99862	1

Figure 3.6 Example of the input dataset for estimation procedure to obtain a subject's ability based on responses to items with known difficulty parameters.

```
PROC NLP: Nonlinear Maximization
              Parameter Estimates
                                   Gradient
                                   Objective
  N Parameter        Estimate      Function
  1 Theta            2.630188      0.000000354
```

Figure 3.7 Estimated ability for subject 3 (who answered 9 of 10 items correctly) using NLP procedure.

```
PROC NLP: Nonlinear Maximization
              Parameter Estimates
                                   Gradient
                                   Objective
  N Parameter        Estimate      Function
  1 Theta            15.346596     0.000004812
```

Figure 3.8 Estimated ability using NLP procedure for the highest ability.

Note also that the option "Random = 100" is not necessary and only used here to have the same estimated results every time. Without this option, the estimated abilities can be slightly different every time when the NLP procedure is run. By using this option, we force NLP procedure to use the same set of pseudorandom numbers to initialize the search.

A person-item map allows for a visual inspection between difficulties of items of a scale and a distribution of estimated latent factor scores of subjects in a study. As noted previously, the abstract measurement units for difficulty parameters and latent factor scores are the same and, as such, can be put alongside the same line representing the same latent dimension. And estimated values will simply represent a location of difficulties and abilities on this latent dimension (x-axis). The estimated difficulties have just one "dimension," but for estimated latent factor scores we can attach a frequency of how many subjects have a particular score. Doing so creates a second dimension for a person-item map – the y-axis will represent those frequencies (the number of subjects with the same estimated latent factor score). All the information needed to build our person-item map is already produced and can be found in Figures 3.3 and 3.4.

Figure 3.9 shows the construction of our person-item map. The first data step ("`Data Theta;...`") creates a dataset with values of the estimated abilities (x-axis; represented by the variable `Location_On_Latent_Dimension`) and the number of subjects with those abilities (y-axis; represented by variable `Freq`). We took the first two columns from Figure 3.4 but with one notable exception: the values of −99 and 99 are excluded; the reason for their exclusion will be discussed later in this chapter. The second data step ("`Data b;...`") creates a dataset with values of the estimated difficulties (x-axis; also represented by the variable `Location_On_Latent_Dimension`) from Figure 3.3, but there is no second dimension for the difficulties, and we simply add a column with zero values (y-axis; represented by variable `Y`). The third column `ItemName` labels items, which will be added to the map to facilitate its interpretation. The next data step combines both datasets into one dataset called `Person_Item_Map`.

The first TEMPLATE procedure ("`proc template; define style PIM;...`") mostly defines parameters related to the appearance of the person-item map. The second TEMPLATE procedure ("`proc template; define stat-graph PersonItemMap;...`") defines how the figure is to be drawn. We define that two different plots should be generated and overlayed as the parts of the same figure. First, a bar chart is requested to present results based on abilities and corresponding frequencies ("`barchart x=Location_On_Latent_Dimension y=Freq;`"). Second, a scatter plot is used to create black dots with accompanying item names alongside the latent dimension ("`scatterplot x=Location_On_Latent_Dimension y=Y / Datalabel= ItemName...`"). And finally, the SGRENDER procedure builds the person-item map represented by Figure 3.10.

```
Data Theta;
input Location_On_Latent_Dimension Freq ;
datalines;
-3.692230768          186
-2.537739953          236
 -1.73367562          285
-1.076190334          293
-0.479622691          308
0.1101519255          293
0.7469272904          317
1.5166204318          352
2.6301882675          345
;
Run;
Data b;
input Location_On_Latent_Dimension  Y  ItemName : $3.0;
datalines;
 -0.08577     0        i1
 -3.79433     0        i2
  2.69122     0        i3
 -0.05792     0        i4
 -1.34724     0        i5
 -0.58873     0        i6
 -1.07666     0        i7
 -2.29363     0        i8
  0.49542     0        i9
  0.99862     0        i10
;
Run;
Data Person_Item_Map; Set b Theta; Run;
Proc Sort Data=Person_Item_Map; By Location_On_Latent_Dimension; Run;
Proc Template;
  define style PIM; parent=styles.listing;
    style GraphFonts from GraphFonts /
      'GraphDataFont'=("<sans-serif>,<MTsans-serif>",20pt)
      'GraphUnicodeFont'=("<MTsans-serif-unicode>",10pt)
      'GraphValueFont'=("<sans-serif>,<MTsans-serif>",10pt)
      'GraphLabelFont'=("<sans-serif>,<MTsans-serif>",20pt)
      'GraphFootnoteFont'=("<sans-serif>,<MTsans-serif>",20pt)
      'GraphTitleFont'=("<sans-serif>,<MTsans-serif>",20pt,bold);
    style GraphReference   / LINETHICKNESS=1 ContrastColor=lightgray;
    style GraphGridLines   / LINETHICKNESS=1;
    style GraphDataDefault / LINETHICKNESS=5
    ContrastColor=black    linestyle =1;
    style GraphData1 /       ContrastColor=black  Linestyle=1 ;
    style GraphData2 /       ContrastColor=black  Linestyle=2 ;
  end;
Run;
Proc Template;
  define statgraph PersonItemMap;
  begingraph;
     entrytitle 'Person-Item Map';
     layout overlay / xaxisopts=(label="Location On Latent Dimension" type=linear);
    barchart    x=Location_On_Latent_Dimension y=Freq / INTERVALBARWIDTH=60PX;
    scatterplot x=Location_On_Latent_Dimension y=Y    / Datalabel= ItemName
markerattrs=(color=black size=20 symbol=circlefilled);
     endlayout;
   endgraph;
   end;
Run;
ods listing style=PIM; ods graphics on /HEIGHT=1200PX WIDTH=2400PX IMAGEFMT=BMP;
Proc Sgrender data=Person_Item_Map template=PersonItemMap; Run;
ods graphics off;
```

Figure 3.9 Construction of the patient-item map.

Now, after a person-item map has been built, what kind of features should we be looking at to interpret it? We should first check whether the item difficulties (location of item difficulties) on the latent dimension are "well" distributed.

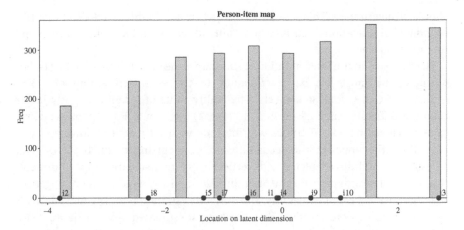

Figure 3.10 Person-item map.

Figure 3.10 depicts relatively sufficient spread for item difficulties. Nonetheless, in this simulated example, we see that items 1 and 4 have very close estimated difficulties (two dots practically overlap each other). If those results represent algebra problems, it means that one of those problems can be dropped. If those results represent a COA scale, however, the answer will not be that obvious. Although both items have practically the same estimated difficulty, they could be representative of two different and clinically relevant aspects of the measured latent factor; if so, the decision then the decision to delete (or not) one of them should be based on additional clinical insights and patient input.

Figure 3.10 also graphically emphasizes the ordering of items by difficulty. Item 2 is the most "simple to overcome," and item 3 is the most difficult. The ordered by difficulty items can be viewed as barriers to get better test results in the case of a math exam. In the case of a COA scale, if we assume that the response value of 1 to any of those 10 items means the presence of a particular symptom for an illness, then the interpretation of difficulties of items is not that straightforward.

What does it mean, specifically, that item 2 is the least difficult item and item 3 is the most difficult? For item 2 to be the least difficult means that it is chosen by many subjects (if item 2 is a mathematical problem, then it is likely be solved correctly by many students). For item 3 to be the most difficult means that it is selected or endorsed by a relatively small group of subjects (if item 3 is a mathematics problem, then it is expected to be solved successfully by only a small proportion of well-prepared students). In the case of this simulated COA symptom scale, the estimated "difficulty" parameter for an item is linked to the rarity of an event of having a particular symptom. Hence the interpretation of "difficulties" is connected to the context of this hypothetical symptom scale – as is every real-life COA scale, where a direct and clear interpretation on the "difficulties" of the scale should be determined. This contextual distinction also highlights the fact that IRT originated in educational setting where "difficulties" of problems have a clear and unambiguous meaning.

The next step in the interpretation of this map is the distribution of subjects. For example, the most left bar corresponds to the estimated ability of −3.69 (−3.692230768) for 186 subjects. The ability value of −3.69 is slightly larger than the difficulty value of −3.79 (−3.79433) for item 2. For a good scale, we expect that estimated difficulties will intermix with estimated abilities and will cover the entire range of estimated abilities on the latent dimension. In Figure 3.10, all estimated abilities (depicted with vertical bars) are inside the range of difficulties. Difficulty estimation for the least difficult item 2 is smaller (more negative) than the smallest estimated ability, and difficulty estimation for the most difficult item 3 is larger (more positive) than the biggest estimated ability (Figure 3.10). This gradation is not a strict rule. For example, the difficulty estimation for the most difficult item can be smaller than the largest estimated ability, and it is responsibility of a researcher to decide whether it is acceptable. The important point is that a representative sample of subjects should reflect heterogeneity on the concept of interest and include, in principle, all possible levels of the measured latent factor.

But what about the values of −99 and 99 from Figure 3.4? In this analysis, they are, respectively, the smallest and largest estimations of abilities. Earlier, we mentioned that in IRT modeling, the relationship between an item score (representing an observed measurement) and the latent factor score is probabilistic (as presented by Eq. (3.2)). This equation creates an interesting conundrum – we cannot unambiguously measure (or estimate) the latent factor score for subjects who responded to all items at the lowest level (0 in this simulated example) or the highest level (1). This probabilistic approach can produce an accurate and unambiguous solution only in the case when, in case of the mathematical test, the mixture of correctly and incorrectly solved problems are present for a student. If a student solved all problems correctly, this individual may be able to solve even more complicated problems, meaning that this measurement instrument (set of mathematical problems) is insufficient to gauge the ability of this student.

The best scenario (from a measurement standpoint) is when at least one problem is solved correctly or incorrectly by everyone during the exam (i.e., no one will have all problems answered correctly or all problems answered incorrectly). The IRT procedure is intelligent enough to recognize patterns of responses and does not even attempt to estimate abilities (latent factor scores) for those "extreme" subjects. But when we apply the NLP procedure to estimate the ability for a subject with all responses equal to 1 (by using maximum log-likelihood method), then the NLP procedure will simply produce the largest value that allowed for the NLP procedure to "think" that the process of estimation has converged (for a given convergence criteria). Any relatively large value for ability in Eq (3.2) will force the probability to be equal to 1. For example, say θ_j is much larger than and dominates b_i in Eq. (3.2), so that b_i can be safely ignored for all intents and purposes, then Eq. (3.2) reduces to

$$P_{ij}\left(\theta_j\right)=\frac{1}{1+e^{-\theta_j}}$$

If θ_j is even relatively large, say 10, then e^{-10} is approximately equal to 4.5E−05 and the $P_{ij}(\theta_j)\approx0.9999$. Thus, we do not even expect those extreme abilities to be covered by the range of estimated difficulties. Those estimated ability values, even if "SCOREMETHOD= EAP" or "SCOREMETHOD= MAP" is used, are expected to be smaller than the estimated smallest difficulty value and larger than the estimated largest difficulty value. As such, having them as a part of the person-item map can be considered optional.

Figure 3.10 was described as generally a "good" example of a person-item map (with some caveat about the redundancy regarding items 1 and 4). What would represent an inadequate person-item map? Let's consider several hypothetical examples. As previously noted, it is anticipated that the location of estimated values for difficulty parameters will be well distributed alongside of the latent dimension; that is, we should not see any obvious clustering of estimated difficulty values. But in Figure 3.11, for a hypothetical but realistic scale, we do see obvious clustering of difficulties. Besides items 1 and 4, items 5 and 10 have almost the same difficulty estimations and, moreover, items 7, 8, and 9 cluster tightly together.

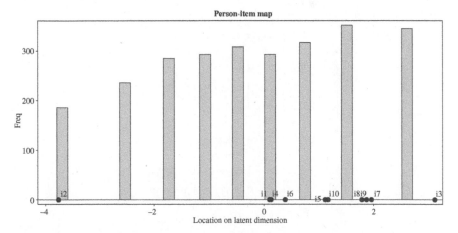

Figure 3.11 Inadequate hypothetical person-item map with example of clustered difficulties.

But what is even more suspect is that we have only one item (item 2) in the entire "negative" part on latent dimension, which can generally be interpreted in this example as not having items that are related to the ability of this scale to measure latent factor scores represented by negative values on latent dimension.

In Figure 3.10, a sizable number of subjects across all levels of the measured latent factor are present, which generally can be viewed as a representative sample. Nevertheless, Figure 3.12a shows a somewhat different distribution. Most subjects here have high latent factor scores, meaning (continuing with the example of a scale measuring symptoms) that most subjects have large number of symptoms (subjects with positive ability values on the latent dimension in this example). If a researcher is absolutely sure that the sample of subjects used in the

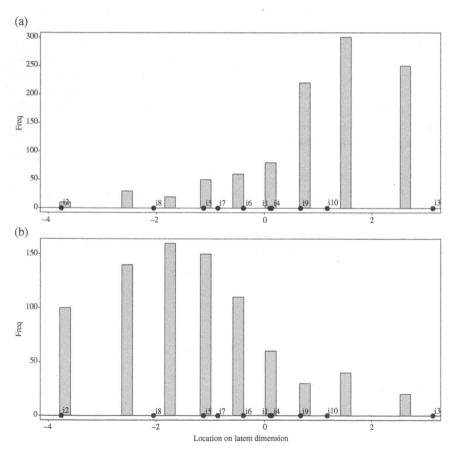

Figure 3.12 Person-item maps based on (a) baseline data and (b) end of treatment data from a hypothetical clinical study.

analysis is representative of the target population of interest, then Figure 3.12a can be an acceptable case of the person-item map.

However if Figure 3.12a is based on baseline data from a clinical study where it is expected, due to entry criteria, that most subjects will have a considerable number of symptoms, then the frequency of subject symptomology will be naturally skewed to right. When treatment data at the end of the study are used, then the opposite distribution is expected: It should tilt to the left (see Figure 3.12b, assuming that the active treatment is efficacious and therefore, overall, subjects will have appreciably smaller number of symptoms). It is important to note that, in both hypothetical analyses represented by Figure 3.12a and b, the estimated item difficulties should remain similar (at minimum the order of the item difficulties should stay the same) for a well-designed scale.

3.2.4 CTT-Based Scoring vs. IRT-Based Scoring

Generally, an advanced comprehensive theory should include a previous one as a limiting case (if the previous one was successful for describing the world around us at some level). For example, Newton's theory can be viewed as a limiting case of Einstein's theory of general relativity: "Einstein's theory of general relativity ... reduces to Newton's theory at large distances and small velocities." (Weinberg 1972).

The ultimate purpose of a COA scale, as a part of a clinical study, is to validly and reliably ***measure*** a specific outcome. With the introduction of IRT methodology, it is important to understand the relationship between CTT-based scores (typically simple averages or sum of an item's scores in a domain) and abilities scores based on IRT theory.

Let's begin our exposition by rerunning analyses from Figure 3.2 for the assessment of the Rasch model but using SCOREMETHOD = EAP, instead of SCOREMETHOD = ML, which will "generate" estimations of the abilities corresponding to the overall raw scores 0 to 10 (recall that abilities scores are −99 and 99 in analyses with SCOREMETHOD = ML). Figure 3.13 is analogous to the previously discussed Figure 3.4. In Figure 3.13, the estimated ability of −4.206916769 corresponds to the raw summed score of 0, −3.06960838 corresponds to the score of 1, −2.246129502 corresponds to the score of 2, and so on.

Figure 3.14 shows the relationship between the raw overall score from CTT for our simulated scale with 10 items and estimated abilities based on the Rasch model. This figure shows that the estimated abilities essentially align in mapping almost perfectly with raw summed scores from 1 to 9, where the relationship can be well approximated by a straight line. The only notable differences are at the extremes for raw summed scores of 0 and 10 points.

_Factor1	Frequency	Percent	Cumulative Frequency	Cumulative Percent
-4.206916769	117	3.90	117	3.90
-3.06960838	186	6.20	303	10.10
-2.246129502	236	7.87	539	17.97
-1.575223947	285	9.50	824	27.47
-0.984040812	293	9.77	1117	37.23
-0.428293786	308	10.27	1425	47.50
0.1269876912	293	9.77	1718	57.27
0.7181695822	317	10.57	2035	67.83
1.3949578408	352	11.73	2387	79.57
2.2453795025	345	11.50	2732	91.07
3.477133948	268	8.93	3000	100.00

Figure 3.13 Frequencies of the estimated abilities (using SCOREMETHOD = EAP).

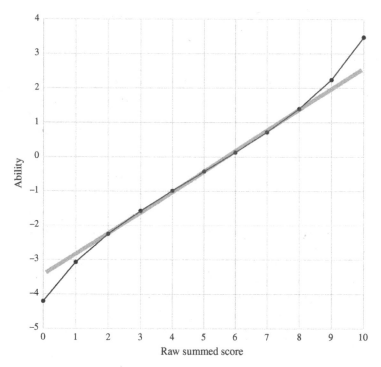

Figure 3.14 Relationship between CTT-based raw summed scores and IRT-based estimated abilities.

And that difference raises a couple of questions. Is this departure from linearity for extremely low and extremely high scores "real"? Or is it simply the artifact of the modeling relationships between abilities and difficulties using Eq. (3.2) (as was discussed in the previous section)? In the CTT framework, the "distance" between any adjacent scores is the same and equals 1 in our example. Yet in the

Rasch-based results, a "distance" between a raw score of 9 vs. a raw score of 10 (1.23 = 3.477133948-2.2453795025) is notably larger than the distance between, say, a raw score of 5 vs. 6 (0.56 = 0.1269876912-[-0.428293786]). If a researcher has supportive clinical evidence that a difference between a group of subjects with 9 out of 10 symptoms (i.e., score of 9) vs. a group of subjects with all 10 symptoms (i.e., score of 10) is meaningfully different from a difference between a group of subjects who has five symptoms from 10 (i.e., score of 5) vs. group of subjects who has six symptoms (i.e., score of 6), then an appropriate IRT model can be contemplated. Note that such evidence of similarity or dissimilarity of distances between adjacent pairs of raw scores *should not* be based on only the IRT model itself; knowledge of the scale and subject matter content need to be considered as well.

The results represented by Figure 3.14 are based on a simulated dataset. But what about real data? Let's revisit the PROMIS "Adult v2.0 – Physical Function 6b" scale (www.healthmeasures.net). Figure 3.15 represents a conversion table on this scale between raw scores and *T*-scores, which are linearly transformed IRT-based abilities having a mean of 50 and standard deviation of 10. Figure 3.16 represents the relationship between raw scores and *T*-scores (based on Figure 3.15; for all intents and purposes, the *T*-scores here can be considered as surrogate values for the abilities). As shown, the pattern of results is the same as that in Figure 3.14 with simulated data.

Figure 3.16 also shows that IRT-based *T*-scores are virtually perfectly aligned with raw scores from 8 to 28 (i.e., the relationship can be well approximated by a straight line for raw summed scores from 8 to 28). The only notable differences are for raw summed scores at the extremes: 6 and 7 points on one end, 29 and 30 points on the other. The difference between subjects with a raw summed score of 30 versus subjects with a raw summed score of 29 is 7.7 in T-score units. The difference between subjects with raw summed scores of 29 vs. subjects with raw summed scores of 28 is 2.4 in *T*-score units. The "distance" between subjects with raw scores of 29 and 30 is more than 3(7.7/2.4 = 3.2) times as large as the "distance" between subjects with raw scores of 28 and 29. As noted with the simulated data, whether such a difference between distances is justified depends in part on knowledge of the scale and subject matter content.

Any well-designed scale is likely to resemble a close relationship between raw overall scores (CTT-based summed or mean) and estimated abilities (based on an IRT model). For the middle part of scale scores, the extent of their correspondences will be essentially the same or display only small differences. Only for very low and very large values are noticeable (though not necessarily large) differences between raw overall scores and IRT-based scores (abilities) expected to be observed. This observation means that in clinical trials, the results for mean differences between treatment arms will likely be comparable in terms of the

Raw summed score	*T*-score
6	21
7	25
8	27.1
9	28.8
10	30.1
11	31.3
12	32.3
13	33.2
14	34.2
15	35
16	35.9
17	36.8
18	37.6
19	38.5
20	39.3
21	40.2
22	41.2
23	42.1
24	43.2
25	44.3
26	45.6
27	47.1
28	48.9
29	51.3
30	59

Figure 3.15 Conversion table for the "Adult v2.0 – Physical Function 6b" scale.

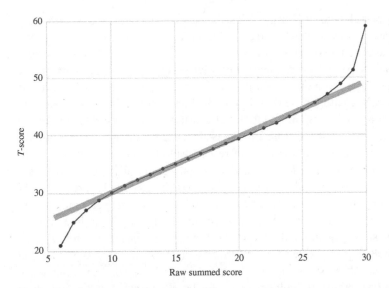

Figure 3.16 Relationship between raw summed scores and *T*-scores for the PROMIS "Adult v2.0 – Physical Function 6b" scale.

statistical significance and effect sizes using either scoring technique (CTT or IRT). Such a general conclusion can be made since, typically only a small proportion of subjects have extreme scores (be they low or high), and the differences in scoring for those extremes between the two methods should not considerably affect mean differences between treatments.

The relationships between CTT-based scoring and IRT-based scoring discussed above show that both theories are, in general, comparable in terms of the produced scores (which is an ultimate purpose of a measurement scale), as it should be. It is difficult to imagine a situation that we would have two different measurement theories that would produce radically different results while measuring the same latent outcomes.

Equation (3.1), which is the embodiment of CTT, is at the center of a vast majority of measurements in the physical world as well as the subjective realm, including educational testing and testing of COAs. However, IRT has a narrower field of empirical applicability that is generally related to educational testing and COA-based measurements. While it is hard to imagine IRT being a limiting case of CTT, we can posit CTT as a limiting case of IRT for the evaluation of COAs. One of the main assumptions in CTT is item equivalency, which gives justification to using the mean (or sum) of the items as a domain score.

Our simulated example in this chapter contains 10 items, which were described previously as representing 10 symptoms (yes, no) of an illness. The item equivalency postulate for this simulated scale means that (i) there is no difference between symptoms as relates to the contribution to the total score of a scale and (ii) the "distance" between any adjacent total scores is the same. For example, regarding the first part (i), every subject who selected any three symptoms (from 10) will have the same score of 3 in CTT. And, while it may not be obvious, it also holds in Rasch modeling. Note that only 11 distinct ability estimations were generated in Figure 3.4 corresponding to the 11 possible total scores, despite the fact that the same total raw score (from 1 to 9) based on the same number of symptoms chosen can come from a different set of responses to the same set of symptoms (items). But maybe this relation works only if abilities and difficulties were estimated simultaneously based on a dataset (as was the case in Figures 3.1–3.4). What if we generate a completely random set of difficulties and estimate abilities for subjects with the same raw summed score but based on different items?

Figure 3.17 shows the implementation of estimations of the abilities for two subjects. The first subject selected the first three symptoms, and the second subject selected the last three symptoms (represented by variable U). The same set of known item (symptom) difficulties is used for both subjects. For the first seven items, we defined difficulties (variable b) to be equal to 0, and for the last three items, difficulties are equal to 1. The implementation represented by Figure 3.17 is based on the earlier discussed Figure 3.5. For both subjects, exactly the same estimation of ability (-0.592267) is produced (see Figure 3.18), even though the first subject selected three symptoms with difficulty of 0 and the second subject selected three symptoms with a difficulty of 1. (Recall that difficulty values represent relative location on the latent dimension and absolute values of difficulties by themselves are irrelevant.) This finding illustrates the first part of the item equivalency postulate: there is no difference between items as it relates to the contribution of a domain score. And this part is fulfilled by both CTT and Rasch measurement.

But, paradoxically, items in IRT are not generally taken as equivalent, which in case of the Rasch model means that items have different difficulties. In this context, items with the same difficulty are considered an undesirable property for a scale. What if we set items to be the same (in terms of same difficulty) while estimating abilities? This situation will be as close as possible to creating a limiting case to see whether the Rasch model-based abilities (based on Eq. (3.2) but with the same predefined difficulties) will be close to CTT-based scores.

Figure 3.19 shows the implementation of the analyses to test the hypothesis that CTT is a limiting case of IRT. This example is built on the earlier analyses represented by Figures 3.5 and 3.17. Figure 3.19 shows the analyses just for one subject with raw score of 7 and with all difficulties equal to 0. As in Figure 3.17, a dataset with variable U and b is first generated, and then the NLP procedure is used to estimate ability. This analysis should be run 11 times for all possible raw scores from 0 to 10. Figure 3.20 provides four additional examples on how datasets should be created for subjects with different raw scores. Note that we already showed that

```
/*Subject 1*/
Data Theta1;
input U b;
datalines;
1    0
1    0
1    0
0    0
0    0
0    0
0    0
0    1
0    1
0    1
;
Run;
Proc NLP Data=Theta1 Random=100;
Max LogL; parms Theta;
P=Log(1/(1+exp(-(Theta-b)))); Q=Log(1-1/(1+exp(-(Theta-b)))); LogL=U*P + (1-U)*Q;
Run;
/*Subject 2*/
Data Theta2;
input U b;
datalines;
0    0
0    0
0    0
0    0
0    0
0    0
0    0
1    1
1    1
1    1
;
Run;
Proc NLP Data=Theta2 Random=100;
Max LogL; parms Theta;
P=Log(1/(1+exp(-(Theta-b)))); Q=Log(1-1/(1+exp(-(Theta-b)))); LogL=U*P + (1-U)*Q;
Run;
```

Figure 3.17 Estimation procedure to obtain abilities for two subjects with the same raw summed score of 3 (though based on different item responses) using the same set of known difficulty parameters.

```
Parameter Estimate for subject 1
                                     Gradient
                                     Objective
  N Parameter          Estimate      Function
  1 Theta             -0.592267     -1.413894E-8
Value of Objective Function = -5.414057338

Parameter Estimate for subject 2
                                     Gradient
                                     Objective
  N Parameter          Estimate      Function
  1 Theta             -0.592267     -1.413894E-8
Value of Objective Function = -8.414057338
```

Figure 3.18 Estimated abilities for two subjects with the same raw summed score of 3.

subjects with the same raw scores (independently of which items contributed to a total score) have the same estimated ability. Thus, any pattern of selected items with the same raw summed score will give the same estimated ability, which means that just one calculation needs to be performed for every possible total score.

```
Data Theta;
input U b;
datalines;
1    0
1    0
1    0
1    0
1    0
1    0
1    0
0    0
0    0
0    0
;
Run;
Proc NLP Data=Theta Random=100;
Max LogL; parms Theta;
P=Log(1/(1+exp(-(Theta-b)))); Q=Log(1-1/(1+exp(-(Theta-b)))); LogL=U*P + (1-U)*Q;
Run;
```

Figure 3.19 Estimation of the ability for a subject with raw total score of 7, with the same level of difficulty for every item.

Raw score of 0	Raw score of 2	Raw score of 8	Raw score of 10
`Data Theta;`	`Data Theta;`	`Data Theta;`	`Data Theta;`
`input U b;`	`input U b;`	`input U b;`	`input U b;`
`datalines;`	`datalines;`	`datalines;`	`datalines;`
`0    0`	`1    0`	`1    0`	`1    0`
`0    0`	`1    0`	`1    0`	`1    0`
`0    0`	`0    0`	`1    0`	`1    0`
`0    0`	`0    0`	`1    0`	`1    0`
`0    0`	`0    0`	`1    0`	`1    0`
`0    0`	`0    0`	`1    0`	`1    0`
`0    0`	`0    0`	`1    0`	`1    0`
`0    0`	`0    0`	`0    0`	`1    0`
`0    0`	`0    0`	`0    0`	`1    0`
`;`	`;`	`;`	`;`
`Run;`	`Run;`	`Run;`	`Run;`

Figure 3.20 Examples of the input datasets for the NLP procedure for estimation of the abilities.

After running the above-described analyses, we can obtain Figure 3.21 which represents raw total scores (from CTT) and their corresponding estimated abilities (from the Rasch model); Figure 3.22 represents those data graphically. Again, the relationship between raw summed scores from 1 to 9 can be well approximated by a straight line. This relationship illustrates the second part of the item equivalency postulate – that the "distance" between any adjacent total scores is the same – is largely maintained in both CTT and Rasch measurements. Overall, this finding means that a CTT approach to measure a latent concept by summation (or mean) of items can be considered as a limiting case of, in this particular example, Rasch modeling in the middle or intermediate range of scale scores. However, because this

```
PROC NLP: Nonlinear Maximization
              Parameter Estimates
                                          Gradient
                                         Objective
   N Parameter            Estimate        Function
Raw Score=0
   1 Theta               -14.322795     -0.000006021
Value of Objective Function = -6.021283E-6

Raw Score=1
   1 Theta                -2.197223     -0.000001639
Value of Objective Function = -3.250829734

Raw Score=2
   1 Theta                -1.386293     -0.000002587
Value of Objective Function = -5.004024235

Raw Score=3
   1 Theta                -0.847298     -5.415393E-9
Value of Objective Function = -6.108643021

Raw Score=4
   1 Theta                -0.405465     -7.203861E-9
Value of Objective Function = -6.73011667

Raw Score=5
   1 Theta                 0.000001462  -0.000003654
Value of Objective Function = -6.931471806

Raw Score=6
   1 Theta                 0.405465      0.000000216
Value of Objective Function = -6.73011667

Raw Score=7
   1 Theta                 0.847298      1.5812565E-9
Value of Objective Function = -6.108643021

Raw Score=8
   1 Theta                 1.386294      2.311773E-11
Value of Objective Function = -5.004024235

Raw Score=9
   1 Theta                 2.197221      0.000002938
Value of Objective Function = -3.250829734

Raw Score=10
   1 Theta                14.288643      0.000006230
Value of Objective Function = -6.230473E-6
```

Figure 3.21 Results on estimation of abilities corresponding to raw scores from 0 to 10 (difficulties of all items are set to 0).

virtual one-to-one mapping does not occur at the extreme levels of ability, we cannot conclude that this limiting case property holds for the entire range of the raw scores. As discussed previously in detail, the "distance" between estimated abilities corresponding to the raw minimal (or maximum) possible score and the next possible (or previously possible) raw score will be notably different from "distances" between adjacent scores for the remaining levels of ability.

The results represented in Figures 3.21 and 3.22 are produced using the same difficulty value of 0 for all items. It is important to note that the relative results for the relationship between raw scores and estimated abilities will be identical if a

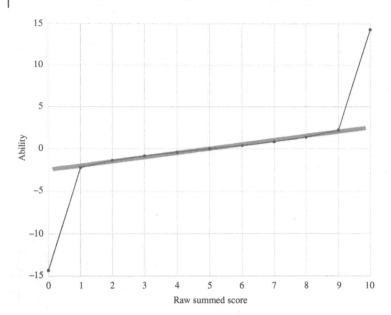

Figure 3.22 Relationship between CTT-based raw summed scores and IRT-based estimated abilities (difficulties of all items are set to 0).

different value is used for item difficulties. Using another value for item difficulty will change only the relative position of the line representing the relationship. For example, if all item difficulties are set to 1, then the entire line will simply move up by one point. Hence, in Figure 3.21 (when all item difficulties are 0), the raw score of 0 that corresponds to an ability score of 0.0 (`0.000001462`), and raw score of 2 that corresponds to an ability score of −1.4 (`−1.386293`) will now have estimated abilities of 1.0 and −0.4, respectively.

3.3 Summary

Measurement is at the heart of all science and of all applications of science. This is true for all areas of science, including the scientific attempt to understand or predict how humans behave, feel, and function. Psychometric theory, with its traditional infrastructure in the disciplines of education and psychology, provides a general modeling framework of measurement rules applicable across diverse fields, including health and medicine.

Scale items are necessary because many constructs cannot be assessed directly. Items that constitute a multi-item patient-reported outcome or COA are proxies for phenomena that cannot be directly observed (i.e., constructs). Historically, CTT has been a foundation to measure constructs that are not directly observable. Underpinning CTT, in turn, is the theory of parallel tests (and its variations), which posits that each item, like every other item on the same scale, serves as an indicator of effect reflecting the same unidimensional construct of interest (i.e., reflective model).

Classical test theory provides the groundwork for summated rating scales, where the observed scale score is computed by summing items scores together (or, equivalently, averaging) all of the item scores. Construction of summated rating scales requires that an item analysis be conducted. As discussed in Chapters 4 and 5, the purpose of item analysis is to find those items that form an internally valid and reliable scale and, in doing so, to discard those other items that do not. Some elements of classic test theory are illustrated with POEM, used in atopic dermatitis. In providing a short critique of CTT, we note that it applies more generally to any kind of measurement.

Item response theory is a statistical theory consisting of mathematical models expressing the probability of a particular response to a scale item as a function of the (latent or observed) attribute of a person and of certain characteristics of an item. The Rasch model is one type of IRT model that requires only a single difficulty parameter to describe an item. In the Rasch model, the probability of a positive response by a particular person to a specific item is a function of the difference between the amount of the person's latent attribute and the item's difficulty. The difficulty parameter in relation to the attribute parameter indicates the extent of a positive response to a particular item.

The Rasch model, which assumes equal item discrimination, corresponds exactly to (and is defined by) the order of item difficulties, and hence the order of the items is constant throughout levels of the attribute. This property enables person-item (or Wright) maps to be produced from a Rasch model to show the relationship between item difficulty and person attributes. These maps can illuminate the extent of item coverage or comprehensiveness, the amount of redundancy, and the range of the attribute in the sample. The visual appeal of this map enriches understanding and interpretation in suggesting to what extent the items cover the targeted range of the underlying scale and whether the items align with the target patient population.

While it is the beyond the scope of this chapter to cover CTT and IRT in much detail, a number of other sources provide in-depth coverage on CTT (e.g., Crocker and Algina 1986; DeVellis 2006, 2017; Furr 2018; Lord and Novick 1968; Nunnally and Bernstein 1994; Spector 1992) and IRT (e.g., Bartolucci et al. 2016; Bond et al. 2021; de Ayala 2022; DeMars 2010; Embretson and Reise 2000; Hambleton et al. 1991; Reeve 2003). We encourage the reader to consult them.

References

Bartolucci, F., Bacci, S., and Gnaldi, M. (2016). *Statistical Analysis of Questionnaires: A Unified Approach Based on R and Stata*. Boca Raton, FL: Chapman & Hall/ CRC Press.

Bond, T.G., Yan, Z., and Heene, M. (2021). *Applying the Rasch Model: Fundamental Measurement in the Human Sciences*, 4e. New York: Routledge/Taylor & Francis.

Bushmakin, A.G., Cappelleri, J.C., Stecher, V., and Lue, T.F. (2017). Quantifying barriers to improvement of treatment satisfaction in men with erectile dysfunction: use of person-item maps. *The Journal of Sexual Medicine* 14: 152–159.

Cappelleri, J.C., Lundy, J.J., and Hays, R.D. (2014). Overview of classical test theory and item response theory for quantitative assessment of items in developing patient-reported outcomes measures. *Clinical Therapeutics* 36: 648–662.

Charman, C.R., Venn, A.J., and Williams, H.C. (2004). The patient-oriented eczema measure: development and initial validation of a new tool for measuring atopic eczema severity from the patients' perspective. *Archives of Dermatology* 140: 1513–1519.

Crocker, L. and Algina, J. (1986). *Introduction to Classical and Modern Test Theory*. Belmont, CA: Wadsworth Group.

De Ayala, R.J. (2022). *The Theory and Practice of Item Response Theory*, 2e. New York: The Guilford Press.

DeMars, C. (2010). *Item Response Theory*. New York: Oxford University Press.

de Vet, H.C.W., Terwee, C.B., Mokkink, L.B., and Knol, D.L. (2011). *Measurement in Medicine*. Cambridge, UK: Cambridge University Press.

DeVellis, R.F. (2006). Classical test theory. *Medical Care* 44: S50–S59.

DeVellis, R.F. (2017). *Scale Development: Theory and Developments*, 4e. Los Angeles, CA: SAGE Publications, Inc.

Edwards, J.R. and Bagozzi, R.P. (2000). On the nature and direction of relationships between constructs and measures. *Psychological Methods* 5: 155–174.

Embretson, S.E. and Reise, S.P. (2000). *Item Response Theory for Psychologists*. Mahwah, NJ: Lawrence Erlbaum Associates.

Furr, R.M. (2018). *Psychometrics: An Introduction*, 3e. Thousand Oaks, CA: SAGE Publications, Inc.

Hambleton, R., Swaninathan, H.J., and Rogers, H.J. (1991). *Fundamentals of Item Response Theory*. Newbury Park, CA: Sage Publications.

Lord, F.M. and Novick, M.R. (1968). *Statistical Theories of Mental Test Scores*. Reading, MA: Addison-Wesley.

Nunnally, J.C. and Bernstein, I.H. (1994). *Psychometric Theory*, 3e. New York: McGraw-Hill.

Reeve, B.B. (2003). Item response theory modeling in health outcomes measurement. *Expert Review of Pharmacoeconomics & Outcomes Research* 3: 131–145.

Spector, P.E. (1992). *Summated Rating Scale Construction: An Introduction.* Newbury Park, CA: SAGE Publications, Inc.

Stelmack, J., Szlyk, J.P., Stelmack, T. et al. (2004). Use of person-item map in exploratory data analysis: a clinical perspective. *Journal of Rehabilitation Research and Development* 41: 233–242.

Weinberg, S. (1972). *Gravitation and Cosmology: Principles and Applications of the General Theory of Relativity.* New York: Wiley.

Wilson, M. (2005). *Constructing Measures: An Item Response Modeling Approach.* Mahwah, NJ: Lawrence Erlbaum Associates.

Wright, B.D. and Masters, G.N. (1981). *Rating Scale Analysis.* Chicago, IL: MESA Press.

4

Reliability

This chapter is an introduction to the concept and underpinning of reliability in the evaluation of a PRO instrument. While validity assesses the extent to which an instrument measures what it is meant to measure, reliability assesses how precise or stable the instrument measures what it measures on the same patient when the patient's condition does not materially change. Reliability, of a health measurement scale, therefore, is typically expressed in terms how well it yields reproducible and consistent results (Cappelleri et al. 2013; de Vet et al. 2011; Fayers and Machin 2016; Streiner et al. 2015).

An essential requirement of all measurements in clinical practice and research is that they be reliable. Reliability is defined as "the degree to which measurement is free from measurement error" (Mokkink et al. 2010). A measurement is never or seldom perfect. An observed score from a measurement reported by a patient has error associated with it and therefore does not equate to its true score. The true score is the limit that the mean score will be approaching if the measurements were hypothetically performed an infinite number of times. Reliability refers to the precision of the score observed, to its reproducibility, and not to its validity. Note that an instrument can be reliable but not valid, neither reliable nor valid, or both reliable and valid. Validity is limited by reliability. If responses are inconsistent, it necessarily implies invalidity as well (note that the converse is not true: consistent responses do not necessarily imply valid responses).

As part of scale validation, two types of reliability can be considered: *repeatability reliability* for single-item or multi-item scales and *internal reliability* for multi-item scales. Both types are conceptually and mathematically related. Repeatability reliability is based upon the analysis of correlations or variances between repeated measurements on the same set of subjects made over time

A Practical Approach to Quantitative Validation of Patient-Reported Outcomes: A Simulation-Based Guide Using SAS, First Edition. Andrew G. Bushmakin and Joseph C. Cappelleri.
© 2023 John Wiley & Sons, Inc. Published 2023 by John Wiley & Sons, Inc.

(*test–retest reliability*), made by different observers (*inter-rater reliability*), or involve different variants of the same attribute or construct (*equivalent-forms reliability*).

This chapter focuses on test–retest reliability. Any reliable single-item measure or multi-item summary score should yield reproducible or consistent values on different occasions for the same set of patients whose condition remains stable over the time period evaluated. Such test–retest reliability is a critical feature of measurement theory. If a patient is in a stable condition, an instrument should yield reproducible results when it is repeated on that patient. Under this assumption, when patients complete the same PRO questionnaire on multiple occasions (time points), the level of agreement between the PRO scores at multiple occasions is a measure of the reliability of the PRO measure.

The PRO instrument is measured at one time (test) and then at least at one other time (retest). Selecting the right period between test and retest, or between times or occasions, is crucial. Too long a period would increase the chance of a true change in the status of the patient; too short a period would allow subjects to recall their responses. Poor test–retest reliability may indicate a problem with the nature of construct, the items (or scales) themselves, or the nature of the target population. For example, the assessment of current pain may show low test–retest reliability because the intensity of pain may vary over time (values of the construct, or the concept of interest, are changing). In such a case, it would be more appropriate to take average values of pain across time. Even if a patient's underlying condition or disease is not fluctuating over time, test–retest reliability may be compromised when the items are poor or with special populations such as the very young, the very old, and patients with cognitive impairment (e.g., Alzheimer's disease).

This chapter also concentrates on internal reliability, also known as internal consistency, which is based on item-to-item correlations, as well as the number of items, in multi-item scales. It is assessed cross-sectionally, at a single time, and can be evaluated at different single time points in a given study. This form of reliability uses item correlations to assess the homogeneity or similarity of multiple items on a scale that are intended to measure complementary aspects of the same underlying concept of interest. Thus, like test–retest reliability, internal reliability quantifies the degree of correspondence between multiple measurements from the same patient.

Cronbach's coefficient alpha is the most widely used method to assess internal consistency (Cronbach 1951). In addition to test–retest reliability, it is also a main focus of this chapter. It is a function of the variances of items representing a domain, the variance of the domain score, and the number of items in this domain. Cronbach's alpha presumes that the multi-item domain of a scale reflects a single concept (latent variable) and, therefore, is unidimensional.

4.1 Reproducibility/Test–Retest

4.1.1 Measurement Error Model

The test–retest reliability property of every scale is deeply rooted in measurement theory (Crocker and Algina 1986). The measured variable y can be thought of as a mixture of two components: one component is the "true" score measure F, and the other is measurement error e. Both of these components are not observed (i.e., latent), but they sum up to yield y. That is,

$$y = F + e \tag{4.1}$$

The above equation can also be graphically represented as a causal model (Figure 4.1).

If variances of the "true" score of the measure F and the measurement error e were known, then one form of the intraclass correlation coefficient (ICC), defined here as the proportion of total variance that is due to true differences among subjects, can be calculated as:

$$ICC = Var(F)\big/\big[Var(F) + Var(e)\big] \tag{4.2}$$

As a way to illustrate the estimation of this ICC based on the aforementioned measurement error model, let us consider the following simulation. If the observed measurement is represented by response Y collected only once for every subject, then the model for the response for subject i can be expressed as

$$Y_i = F_i + e_i \tag{4.3}$$

where

Y_i is the observed value of the measured outcome for subject i ($i = 1, 2, \ldots, N$; N represents the number of subjects);
F_i is the "true" value of the measured outcome for subject i; and
e_i is the measurement error [assumed to be from a normal distribution with mean 0 and variance σ_e^2, i.e., $e_i \sim N(0, \sigma_e^2)$].

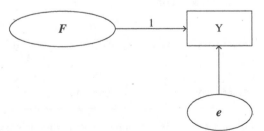

Figure 4.1 Measurement error model.

```
/* In this example there are 500 subjects (NumberOfSubjects) and every subject has
only 1 observation. To define variances for latent "true" score (VarF) and
measurement error (VarME) the following values are used: 1 and 0.2.*/
options nofmterr nocenter pagesize=2000 linesize=256;

%Let NumberOfSubjects=500; %Let a=5; %Let VarF =1; %Let VarME=0.2;
Data _icc_calis;
  Do ID=1 To &NumberOfSubjects;
    F= &a + rannor(1)*sqrt(&VarF) ;
    e= rannor(3)*sqrt(&VarME) ;
    y = F + e;
    output;
  End;
Run;
Proc Means Data=_icc_calis; Run;
Data _icc_calis; Set _icc_calis; Keep y ID; Run;
```

Figure 4.2 Simulating a dataset based on measurement error model.

Note that Eq. (4.3) clearly and directly corresponds to Eq. (4.1); the difference is that, in Eq. (4.1), *F* and *e* variables are unknown, but in the simulation, we will define them and then try to extract them through a modeling process. Figure 4.2 represents the SAS code to generate a simulated dataset. The following three SAS code lines produce the outcome for a subject (represented by Eq. (4.3)):

```
F= &a + rannor(1)*sqrt(&VarF) ;
e= rannor(3)*sqrt(&VarME) ;
y = F + e;
```

To simulate a real-life data, the final dataset _icc_calis keeps only two variables, one representing an ID of a subject (which is not used in the current analysis) and the other being a measured outcome represented by variable *y*.

Figure 4.3 represents the implementation of the analysis using the CALIS procedure. With only one observation for a subject, it is impossible to separate variability associated with every measurement into two components: one component representing measurement error for every subject and the second component representing variability of the "true" score between subjects. For the example below, therefore, we assume that the measurement error is known from prior studies ($e = 0.2$), and the CALIS procedure is used to estimate the variance of the unobserved "true" score.

```
Proc Calis cov data=_icc_calis G4=1000 GCONV=1E-10 Method=ML TECHNIQUE=LEVMAR ALL;
LINEQS
y = F + e;
Variance
F = varF, e = 0.2;
Testfunc ICC; ICC = varF/(varF + 0.2);
Run;
```

Figure 4.3 Implementation of the measurement error model.

```
                 Estimates for Variances of Exogenous Variables
Variable                                          Standard
Type         Variable     Parameter    Estimate      Error     t Value    Pr > |t|
Latent       F            varF          1.05914    0.07971     13.2866     <.0001
Error        e                          0.20000

                    Tests for Parametric Functions
Parametric                         Standard
Function        Estimate             Error      t Value    Pr > |t|
ICC             0.84116            0.01006      83.6485     <.0001
```

Figure 4.4 ICC estimation.

Figure 4.4 represents the corresponding partial output. The estimated variance for the latent variable F (which represents "true" score) is 1.06 (1.05914), and the estimated ICC is 0.84 (0.84116). The variance of the "true" score used to create the simulated dataset is 1.0, and the true ICC for this dataset is 0.83 (1.0/[1.0+0.2]), which is almost identical to the value of 0.84 estimated from the CALIS procedure.

The above analysis also points to the new possible approach for test–retest assessment. Note that in our simulation only one observation to estimate ICC was used; it was possible only because measurement error was assumed to be known. If, when publishing validation manuscripts, researchers will report not only ICCs but also both variances used in the estimation, it would enable an accurate assessment of test–retest reliability in the future using just one observation per subject.

4.1.2 Two Time Points

In the previous section, we were able to estimate ICC only because we assumed the variance of the measurement error to be known from previous experience with a PRO. In reality, however, this information is typically not available and should be estimated as a part of the test–retest assessment. For the model to be successful to estimate two unknown variances simultaneously, at least two observations for a subject are needed (this requirement will be relaxed later in the chapter).

To illustrate the estimation of the ICC in question based on the measurement error model with two observations per subject, let us consider the following simulation. The measurement is represented by response $Y1$ at the first occasion and by $Y2$ at the second occasion for every subject. Then the model for the response for subject i can be expressed by two following equations:

$$\begin{cases} Y1_i = F_i + e_{1i} \\ Y2_i = F_i + e_{2i} \end{cases} \tag{4.4}$$

where

$Y1_i$ and $Y2_i$ are the measured outcomes for subject i ($i = 1, 2, \ldots, N$; N represents the number of subjects) at the first and second occasions;

F_i is the "true" value of the measured outcome for subject i (*note that it is exactly the same value, but unknown, at both occasions*);

e_{1i} and e_{2i} are the measurement errors [both assumed to be from the same normal distribution with mean 0 and variance σ_e^2, i.e., $e_i \sim N(0, \sigma_e^2)$];

Figure 4.5 represents Eq. (4.4) graphically as a causal model.

The code to produce a simulated dataset for data collected at two time points is represented by Figure 4.6. Note that observed scores at both time points for a subject are represented by the sum of exactly the same "true" score (F) and different (but taken form the same normal distribution) error terms (MErr1 and MErr2). Note again that to imitate a real-life situation the final dataset only incorporates the ID of a subject and two observed scores. Figure 4.7 represents the structure of the dataset for analyses.

Figure 4.8 represents the implementation of the model to extract the variance associated with the true score and the variance associated with the measurement error. In this example, we do not need to know values for the measurement error variance a priori. The information provided by two measurements for a subject allows for the model to be estimable. For a causal model to be estimable, the number of parameters needed to be estimated should be less or equal to the number of

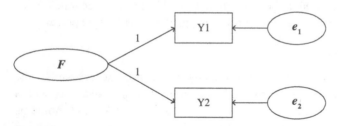

Figure 4.5 Measurement error model for two time points.

```
/* For this example, there are 500 subjects (NumberOfSubjects) and every subject
has 2 observations. To define variances for latent "true" score (VarF) and
measurement error (VarME), we used the values of 1 and 0.2, respectively. */
options nofmterr nocenter pagesize=2000 linesize=256;
%Let NumberOfSubjects = 500; %Let a  = 5; %Let VarF  = 1; %Let VarME = 0.2;
Data _icc_calis;
    Do ID=1 To &NumberOfSubjects;
              /* F represents true score */
              F  = &a + rannor(1)*sqrt(&VarF) ;
              /* MErr1 and MErr2 represent measurement errors */
              MErr1=rannor(3)*sqrt(&VarME); MErr2=rannor(5)*sqrt(&VarME);
              y1 = F  + MErr1 ; y2 = F  + MErr2 ;
              output;
    End;
Run;
Proc Means Data=_icc_calis; Run;
Data _icc_calis; Set _icc_calis;  Keep y1 y2 ID; Run;
Proc Print Data=_icc_calis NOOBS; Where ID <=10; Run;
```

Figure 4.6 Simulating a dataset based on measurement error model with two observations per subject.

```
ID       y1         y2
 1     6.76908    6.98218
 2     4.91768    3.63752
 3     5.47492    5.24793
 4     4.70194    4.92003
 5     5.32537    5.35215
 6     4.35687    4.07011
 7     3.84366    4.23409
 8     6.23918    7.14710
 9     3.51817    4.36876
10     5.35793    5.93783
```

Figure 4.7   Dataset structure with two observations per subject (first 10 subjects are shown).

```
Proc Calis cov data=_icc_calis  G4=1000 GCONV=1E-10 Method=ML TECHNIQUE=LEVMAR ALL;
LINEQS
y1 = F + e1, y2 = F + e2;
Variance
F=varF, e1=varMError, e2=varMError;
Parameters varF varMError;
Testfunc  ICC; ICC = varF/(varF+varMError);
Run;
```

Figure 4.8   Implementation of the measurement error model with two observations per subject.

variances and covariances between observed variables. When fitting a causal model, we try to define model parameters in a way that the variance–covariance matrix based on the modeled results is, as much as possible, close to the variance–covariance matrix based on the observed data. In our case, we have two observations and, as a result, two variances (for variables *Y1* and *Y2*) and one covariance between variables *Y1* and *Y2*, meaning that we have three observed or known elements in the variance–covariance matrix. Yet we only need to define two parameters (true score variance and measurement error variance), which make this model estimable. This also explains why the model with just one observation was not estimable (see previous Section 4.1.1) – one observation provides only one variance (i.e., the observed variance–covariance matrix contains only one element), but we still need to define the same two parameters: true score variance and measurement error variance.

Figure 4.9 represents the partial output corresponding to the model implementation represented by Figure 4.8. The estimated variance for the latent variable *F* is 1.02 (1.02217), and the estimated variance for the measurement error variance is 0.21 (0.21164) and, as a result, the estimated *ICC* is 0.83 (0.82847). In this simulation, the same values (as in Section 4.1.1) are used to define variances of the "true" score and measurement errors: 1.0 and 0.2. As mentioned in Section 4.1.1, the true *ICC* for this dataset is 0.83, which is almost exactly the same value (before rounding) generated by the CALIS procedure.

```
              Estimates for Variances of Exogenous Variables
Variable                                      Standard
Type        Variable    Parameter    Estimate    Error    t Value  Pr > |t|
Latent      F           varF         1.02217     0.07173  14.2512  <.0001
Error       e1          varMError    0.21164     0.01340  15.7956  <.0001
            e2          varMError    0.21164     0.01340  15.7956  <.0001

              Tests for Parametric Functions
Parametric                        Standard
Function       Estimate            Error    t Value    Pr > |t|
ICC            0.82847           0.01404    59.0056     <.0001
```

Figure 4.9 ICC estimation.

4.1.3   Random-Effects Model for ICC Estimation

In many real-life situations, the data to be used for test–retest analyses can be collected not just at two time points but more frequently. For example, if an outcome is assessed daily, it is advisable to examine the test–retest property of a particular scale by collecting data during, say, a week before the start of the treatment. In this situation, it is not expected that all data from every subject on every day will be obtained during the week. As a result, we will be facing two analytical challenges: first, presenting this model using causal framework can get complicated; and, second, and more important, we need to account for the possibility of the missing data. To overcome those issues, we can use a slightly different approach to represent a measurement error model, which, in turn, will allow the use of a random-effects model. Eq. (4.3) for the response of subject i for the data collected multiple (two or more) times can be rewritten as follows:

$$Y_{ij} = F_i + e_{ij} \tag{4.5}$$

where

Y_{ij} is the measured outcome for subject i ($i = 1, 2, \ldots, N$; N represents the number of subjects) at occasion j ($j = 1, 2, \ldots, K$; K represents the number of time points);
F_i is the "true" value of the measured outcome for subject i (note again that the value, though unknown, is fixed for a given subject at all occasions);
e_{ij} is measurement error [assumed, as before, to be from a normal distribution with mean 0 and variance σ_e^2, i.e., $e_i \sim N(0, \sigma_e^2)$];

Let us represent the "true" score F_i as the sum of two values: the overall unknown mean (m) and the difference between F_i and this overall mean

$$F_i = m + \left(F_i - m\right) \tag{4.6}$$

Now let us denote ($F_i - m$) as d_i, making Eq. (4.6) be rewritten as

$$Y_{ij} = m + d_i + e_{ij} \tag{4.7}$$

where

Y_{ij} and e_{ij} represent the same parameters described in Eq. (4.5);

m is the overall mean of the true (unknown) values of the measured outcome based on data from all subjects; and

d_i is the difference between "true" value of the measured outcome for subject i and m (*note that d_i is exactly the same, but unknown, at all occasions*); d_i often referenced and characterized as representing between-subjects variability.

This Eq. (4.7) represents one of the most basic random-effects models: a random intercept model. It is evident that the variance of the d is equal to the variance of the F; therefore, the *ICC* (see Eq. 4.2) can also be depicted as

$$ICC = Var(d)/\left[Var(d) + Var(e)\right] \qquad (4.8)$$

Before describing an implementation of the model to estimate ICC using the MIXED procedure, we need to restructure our simulated data into format conventional for the repeated measures framework. This new data structure also requires an additional parameter as part of the model: the *ID* of the subject to inform the model that a certain set of data belongs to the same subject. Figure 4.10 converts dataset "`_icc_calis`" (created by the code from Figure 4.6 and represented by Figure 4.7) into such a new dataset. Note again that to simulate real-life situation only variables *ID* and *y* are kept. Figure 4.11 represents the structure of the new dataset for a few subjects. The dataset has the same data (as in Figure 4.7), but now information for every subject is split into two rows.

```
Data _icc_mixed; Set _icc_calis;
y=y1; output;
y=y2; output;
Keep ID y;
Run;
Proc Print Data=_icc_mixed NOOBS; Where ID <=5; Run;
```

Figure 4.10 Creating vertical structure of the dataset for the MIXED procedure.

```
ID          y
 1       6.76908
 1       6.98218
 2       4.91768
 2       3.63752
 3       5.47492
 3       5.24793
 4       4.70194
 4       4.92003
 5       5.32537
 5       5.35215
```

Figure 4.11 The vertical structure of the dataset for the MIXED procedure (first five subjects are shown).

```
Proc Mixed data=_icc_mixed COVTEST;
Class ID ;
Model y= / solution;
Random Int / subject=ID solution;
Run;
```

Figure 4.12 Implementation of the model to assess between-patient and within-patient variances.

Covariance Parameter Estimates					
Cov Parm	Subject	Estimate	Standard Error	Z Value	Pr > Z
Intercept	ID	1.0223	0.07172	14.25	<.0001
Residual		0.2114	0.01337	15.81	<.0001

Figure 4.13 Covariance parameter estimates.

Figure 4.12 represents the implementation of the corresponding ICC estimation using the MIXED procedure. Figure 4.13 represents the estimations for the variances of the parameters d and e from Eq. (4.7) (represented by the section "Covariance Parameter Estimates" in the MIXED procedure output). The value of 1.0223 (which is labeled as "Intercept ID") represents the estimated variance of the parameter d, and the value of 0.2114 (which is labeled as "Residual") represents the estimated variance of the parameter e (measurement error). Comparing these results with the results using the CALIS procedure, we see that the MIXED procedure gives virtually the same values given in Section 4.1.2 with the CALIS procedure (compare Figures 4.12 and 4.9); even the standard errors for estimated variances are practically the same. This observation illustrates the virtual equivalence of the assessing ICC using causal modeling approach (CALIS procedure) versus random-effects model (MIXED procedure).

There are several other important outcomes from this implementation of the model which need to be discussed. Though they are not directly linked to ICC estimations, those outcomes can provide additional input for better understanding of the test–retest property of a scale. The "solution" option in the "Model" statement gives the overall mean of the "true" unobserved scores (m). In this example, the overall mean is 5.0303, which represents the intercept in the model (see Figure 4.14 and specifically "Solution for Fixed Effects").

Recall from Figure 4.6 the code line "%Let a = 5;", which was one of the parameters used to generate "true" scores (F) values and represented the mean of those values. But we can go beyond the overall mean and estimate the "true" score for every individual subject – the "solution" option in the "Random" statement will output a difference (d_i from Eq. 4.7) between overall mean and "true" score (see Figure 4.14 for partial output for the first 10 subjects under "Solution for Random Effects"). For example, the estimated "true" score for the first subject can be calculated as

$$5.0303 + 1.6724 = 6.7027.$$

```
                   Solution for Fixed Effects
                           Standard
Effect         Estimate      Error      DF    t Value    Pr > |t|
Intercept       5.0303      0.04750     499    105.91      <.0001

                   Solution for Random Effects
                              Std Err
Effect      ID    Estimate      Pred      DF    t Value    Pr > |t|
Intercept    1     1.6724      0.3125     500     5.35       <.0001
Intercept    2    -0.6822      0.3125     500    -2.18      0.0295
Intercept    3     0.3001      0.3125     500     0.96      0.3374
Intercept    4    -0.1988      0.3125     500    -0.64      0.5250
Intercept    5     0.2795      0.3125     500     0.89      0.3715
Intercept    6    -0.7403      0.3125     500    -2.37      0.0182
Intercept    7    -0.8985      0.3125     500    -2.88      0.0042
Intercept    8     1.5070      0.3125     500     4.82       <.0001
Intercept    9    -0.9850      0.3125     500    -3.15      0.0017
Intercept   10     0.5597      0.3125     500     1.79      0.0739
```

Figure 4.14 Estimating "true" scores.

From Figure 4.11, we know that in this simulated example, subject $ID = 1$ has two observations with outcomes 6.7690838668 and 6.9821775119. The usual way to increase the precision of the measurement is to calculate the mean of the observed values – in this case, the mean will be 6.8756. But the MIXED procedure gives 6.7027 – this value is an estimation of the "true" score for subject with $ID = 1$, also known as the Best Linear Unbiased Prediction (or BLUP). This result could have an important implication in estimation of the treatment effect in a clinical study.

Typically, the model for estimation of treatment effects has baseline values of an outcome (dependent) variable as a covariate. For this purpose, the standard practice is to use a value of an outcome before treatment has been given or to calculate a mean of the pretreatment values and then use it as covariate in a model. The approach described here can provide more accurate and, importantly, is rooted in the measurement theory estimations of the baseline values, which in turn can lead to more precise estimation of the treatment effects.

For the example in this section, we used the same simulated dataset from Section 4.1.2; in this section, we just needed to restructure it accordingly. If we had three or more observations for a subject, the same code represented by Figure 4.12 can be used, meaning this code is generic and does not need to be edited or changed in any way, provided that the dataset has the correct structure and the variables in the dataset are named accordingly. Another important advantage of this general implementation is that it encompasses all available data. We are not restricted to use subjects with only at least two or more observations collected – even if a subject has just one observation, his or her data will be used in the analysis, providing additional information to estimate the variance of the "true" score. More generally, subjects do not need to have *the same* number of observations if multiple observations are available for test–retest analysis.

With this introduction of the MIXED procedure for ICC estimation, we can go back to the beginning of this chapter and show how this approach can be applied

```
Proc Mixed data=_icc_calis COVTEST;
Class ID ;
Model y= / solution;
Random Int / subject=ID solution;
PARMS (0.5) (0.2) /hold=2;
Run;
```

Figure 4.15 Implementation of the model to estimate between-subjects variance (with fixed measurement error variance).

to the dataset with just one observation per subject. Let us recall the simulated dataset generated by Figure 4.2 ("Simulating a dataset based on measurement error model") in Section 4.1.1 ("Measurement Error Model"). In Section 4.1.1, when implementing the model (using the CALIS procedure), we needed to set measurement error variance to the predefined value of 0.2 for the model to be estimable. To do the same here, we just need to add one additional statement in the implementation represented by Figure 4.12.

Figure 4.15 represents the implementation of the model for the dataset with just one observation per subject. Note that, in this case, we need the additional variable *ID*, which we kept in the dataset but not used in Section 4.1.1. The additional statement is the PARMS statement, which specifies initial values for the covariance parameters. If more than two observations are available for a sufficient number of subjects, then both variances needed for ICC can be estimated (those two parameters can be found in the output under the umbrella of the "Covariance Parameter Estimates"; see Figure 4.13). When constructing the PARMS statement as a part of the MIXED procedure for the dataset, when just one observation per subject is available, we need to keep the order of variances as they appeared in the "Covariance Parameter Estimates." Hence the first estimated parameter represents variance between subjects ("Intercept ID ...") which we still want to estimate, but the second parameter, which represents the variance of the measurement error ("Residual ..."), is fixed to a predefined value (in our simulation this value is 0.2). In the following statement

"PARMS (.5) (0.2) /hold=2;"

the value of 0.5 is just the initial value for the between subjects variance; the value of 0.2 is also the initial value for the measurement error variance, but by adding ".../hold=2;" we instruct the MIXED procedure *to not estimate* the second parameter and just use value of 0.2 during the iteration process. Figure 4.16

Covariance Parameter Estimates					
Cov Parm	Subject	Estimate	Standard Error	Z Value	Pr > Z
Intercept	ID	1.0591	0.07971	13.29	<.0001
Residual		0.2000	0	.	.

Figure 4.16 Between-subjects variance estimation.

represents the results of the analyses (note that dataset "`_icc_calis`" produced by the code from Figure 4.2 was used). As we can see, the MIXED procedure produced the same estimation of the variance (`1.0591`) as shown in Figure 4.4 (note that even the standard error is the same).

It is interesting to also point out that this implementation of the model represented by Figure 4.13 is extremely close to the analysis of aggregated data or meta-analysis (Alemayehu et al. 2017). In the meta-regression, we also need to preserve variances of the individual observations.

4.1.4 Test–Retest Reliability Assessment in the Context of Clinical Studies

4.1.4.1 Pre-Treatment/Pre-Baseline Data

The 2009 FDA guidance states that test–retest assesses "stability of scores over time when no change is expected in the concept of interest." (FDA 2009). In most clinical studies, the period when we do not anticipate a "true" score to change is the pre-treatment or pre-baseline period. During this period, we usually have at least two opportunities to collect data on the PRO outcome, namely, at screening and at baseline. Keeping data on all screened subjects (even those who were later rejected for participation in the study) will allow for more precision in the estimation of an ICC.

If clinical study data are planned to be used for the validation of a scale, it is vital to collect data not only needed to establish active treatment superiority over a placebo but also data needed for the validation as, for example, data on PGIC and PGIS (described in Chapter 2). Regarding ICC estimation, let us consider the following hypothetical scenario. Let us say we have a PRO measure with a range of scores from 0 (a particular attribute of illness is not present) to 10 (a particular attribute of illness is extremely severe), and scores of subjects from 0 to 3 are regarded as "mild," score from 4 to 6 as "moderate," and from 7 to 10 as "severe." Although at screening, we possibly can have subjects with scores from 0 to 10, in reality, it will be difficult to find a reasonable number of subjects with very low or very high scores; most likely majority of subjects will be "moderate."

For the purpose of assessing test–retest reliability of a PRO scale, a clinical team should make an effort to find "mild" and "severe" subjects as well (even in the situation when a drug is developed for "moderate" subjects only and the clinical team is only interested to have only those "moderate" subjects at baseline). It is important to point out that, during the study, subjects will become "mild" (if the drug is beneficial) and, at the same time, we anticipate that subjects in the placebo arm could become worse, with some of them being eventually characterized as "severe."

The upshot is that test–retest reliability for a PRO scale should be established for all ranges (all possible scores, not only "moderate" subjects) and, for this purpose, we must have a variety of subjects at screening and baseline. Thus, in general, we recommend having the same (or reasonably close to) number of subjects at screening and baseline with all three levels of severity ("mild," "moderate," and "severe"). As such, data on subjects who were later rejected from participation in the study during the randomization phase should be collected at both time points (screening and baseline).

The attentive reader may have already noticed that we did not make a distribution assumption for the "true" unobserved score when characterizing the model earlier in this chapter. In the current simulations, we used a normal distribution to generate "true" score (F) values. Ideally, the optimal allocation is to have one-third of subjects who are mild, one-third moderate, and one-third severe in the concept of interest. Let us examine how the assumption of true scores following a uniform (instead of a normal) distribution will affect the results. Is the model suggested for ICC estimation robust enough to handle this type of data?

Figure 4.17 creates the simulated dataset with two observations per subject with "true" score distributed uniformly with values from 0 to 10. The below SAS code is practically the same as in Figure 4.6 – the key difference is that to generate F the *ranuni* function was used.

Now we can apply without any change the same code represented by Figures 4.8 (causal modeling approach using the CALIS procedure) and 4.12 (random-effects model using the MIXED procedure). Figures 4.18 and 4.19 show partial output with estimated variances. Note that variance of the uniformly distributed values from a to b is

$$Var(F) = (b - a)^2 / 12 \tag{4.9}$$

```
/* For this example, there are 500 subjects (NumberOfSubjects) and every
subject has 2 observations. The variance for measurement error (VarME) is
given as 1. The latent "true" score (F) is simulated to be uniformly
distributed with values from 0 to 10.*/
options nofmterr nocenter pagesize=2000 linesize=256;
%Let NumberOfSubjects = 500; %Let a = 0; %Let b  = 10; %Let VarME = 1;
Data _icc_calis;
    Do ID=1 To &NumberOfSubjects;
        /* F represents true score */
        F= &a + &b*ranuni(1) ;
        /* MErr1 and MErr2 represent measurement errors */
        MErr1=rannor(3)*sqrt(&VarME); MErr2=rannor(5)*sqrt(&VarME);
        y1 = F  + MErr1 ; y2 = F  + MErr2 ;
        output;
    End;
Run;
Proc Means Data=_icc_calis; Run;
Data _icc_calis; Set _icc_calis; Keep y1 y2 ID; Run;
Data _icc_mixed; Set _icc_calis;
y=y1; output;
y=y2; output;
Keep ID y;
Run;
```

Figure 4.17 Simulating a dataset based on measurement error model with two observations per subject ("true" score distributed uniformly with values from 0 to 10).

	Estimates for Variances of Exogenous Variables					
Variable				Standard		
Type	Variable	Parameter	Estimate	Error	t Value	Pr > |t|
Latent	F	varF	8.26423	0.55481	14.8957	<.0001
Error	e1	varMError	0.97158	0.06151	15.7956	<.0001
	e2	varMError	0.97158	0.06151	15.7956	<.0001

	Tests for Parametric Functions				
Parametric		Standard			
Function	Estimate	Error	t Value	Pr > |t|	
ICC	0.89480	0.00892	100.3	<.0001	

Figure 4.18   Estimated variances (CALIS procedure).

	Covariance Parameter Estimates				
			Standard	Z	
Cov Parm	Subject	Estimate	Error	Value	Pr > Z
Intercept	ID	8.2634	0.5548	14.89	<.0001
Residual		0.9732	0.06155	15.81	<.0001

Figure 4.19   Estimated variances (MIXED procedure).

Hence, for our simulation, it will be $(10 - 0)^2/12 = 8.33$. As shown in Figures 4.18 and 4.19, both approaches produced the same estimated value of 8.23 for this variance. Furthermore, the variance of the measurement error was estimated as 0.97, very close to the value of 1.00 defined in the simulation. The results of this simulation corroborate the fact that the models we use for ICC estimation are quite robust as relates to the distribution assumption for the "true" score.

4.1.4.2   Post-Baseline Data

Although the pre-treatment period is the best juncture to collect data for the assessment of test–retest reliability (when it is reasonable to assume that subjects are stable between screening and baseline and no intervention of the studied drug), these data are not always collected. In this case, the next best option will be to collect data using a separate, specifically designed non-interventional study. Non-interventional study can be as simple as collecting data on a PRO at two different occasions from representative samples of subjects. If the two above options are not feasible or practical, then post-baseline data can be used. It is important to note that those analyses based on post-baseline data can only serve as a surrogate for the valid test–retest analyses using pre-baseline data.

The cornerstone of test–retest reliability is the assumption that subjects do not change in the underlying concept of interest measured by a PRO and, therefore, all differences in this measured outcome for a subject are presumed to be explained by *only* measurement error; that is, subjects are considered to be stable. It is difficult to assume that post-baseline data for any subject are not contaminated by the effect of treatments in the study. To define those stable subjects, we need to have a different not related and preferably global measure which could be used to identify stable subjects. For example, PGIC and PGIS (see Chapter 2) could be good candidates to play this role. It is important to note the following weakness of this approach: The subjects we select based, say, on PGIC will be stable relative to the PGIC measurement, not relative to measurement scale we validate. We make the assumption that, if subjects do not change when measured by PGIC, they also do not change when measured by the target PRO scale.

Consider the following situation. Earlier in this section, a PRO measure was introduced with a range of scores from 0 (a particular attribute of illness, as measured by the PRO, is not present) to 10 (a particular attribute of illness is extremely severe). Let us continue with this example. The PRO and PGIS scales were collected at baseline. One week later, the PRO, PGIS, and PGIC scales were collected. To assess test–retest in this situation, we simply need to select subjects who did not change (i.e., who responded "no change" on PGIC at week one or who had the same score on PGIS at baseline and week later) and simply apply, for example, the implementation described in Figure 4.12 to the PRO data for those "stable" subjects. But are those subjects really stable?

If subjects are truly stable, it would mean that mean change from baseline on the PRO measure in question for those subjects should be zero (or close to zero). To investigate this, let us consider the following simulation (see Figure 4.20). In this simulation, change from baseline (ChgY) in this PRO can be from −10 to 10, and PGIC has values from 1 to 7 (value of 4 represents "no change," values more than 4 represent improvement and values less than 4 represent worsening). The first data step (**data** _corr_type = corr;...) generates a dataset (with the standard structure representing the correlation between two variables) with the parameters representing distributions of the outcome values. This dataset serves as the input information for the SIMNORMAL procedure, which generates the dataset "_sim_ds" with simulated data for both variables.

For example, the simulated variable ChgY is defined to have a mean of 0, a standard deviation of 3.5, and have a correlation of 0.70 with simulated variable PGIC. The simulated variable PGIC has a mean of 4 and standard deviation of 1. The chosen standard deviation of 3.5 for ChgY and 1 for PGIC will lead to the generation of normally distributed values from about −10 to 10 for ChgY and

```
data _corr_ (type=corr);
input
_TYPE_ $   _NAME_ $   ChgY      PGIC      ;
datalines;
  CORR       ChgY       1          0.7
  CORR       PGIC       0.7        1
  MEAN       .          0          4
  STD        .          3.5        1
  N          .          500        500
;
run;
proc simnormal data=_corr_ out=_sim_ds numreal=500 seed=10000; var ChgY PGIC; run;
proc corr data=_sim_ds ; Var ChgY PGIC; Run;
```

Figure 4.20 Simulating change from baseline in a PRO measure.

from about 1 to 7 for PGIC. Figure 4.21 shows the results of the CORR procedure applied to the simulated dataset. As can be seen, the means, standard deviations, and correlations are close to the values defined in the dataset "_corr_".

Figure 4.22 shows the implementation of the analysis. First, we represent PGIC by the integers from 1 to 7. The output of the FREQ procedure (see Figure 4.23) shows a somewhat typical distribution of the PGIC values in a clinical study (especially in earlier parts of the study). It is common in clinical research to have a relatively small number of subjects who characterized themselves as "Very Much Improved" (here, there are only 8 subjects with PGIC = 1) and "Very Much Worse" (there is only 1 subject with PGIC = 7). At the same time, 185 subjects stated that they did not change (PGIC = 4). Note that those 185 subjects represent a subset we should use in a subsequent test–retest analysis.

```
The CORR Procedure
   2  Variables:      ChgY      PGIC
                                Simple Statistics
Variable       N          Mean       Std Dev          Sum        Minimum        Maximum
ChgY         500       0.09229       3.47832     46.14448       -9.72764        9.30188
PGIC         500       4.04072       0.99379         2020        1.25621        7.18458

Pearson Correlation Coefficients, N = 500
         Prob > |r| under H0: Rho=0
                  ChgY             PGIC
ChgY          1.00000          0.66718
                                <.0001
PGIC          0.66718          1.00000
              <.0001
```

Figure 4.21   The CORR procedure output.

```
Data _mixed_; Set  _sim_ds;
PGIC=Int(PGIC); PID=_N_; Week=1;
Run;
Proc Freq data=_mixed_; Tables PGIC; Run;
Title "First attempt";
Proc mixed data=_mixed_;
    Class PGIC Week;
    Model ChgY = PGIC / ddfm=kr s;
    Repeated Week / subject=PID ;
    LSMeans PGIC /cl;
Run;
Title "Second attempt";
Data _mixed_; Set _mixed_; If PGIC=7 Then PGIC=6; Run;
Proc mixed data=_mixed_;
    Class PGIC Week;
    Model ChgY = PGIC / ddfm=kr s;
    Repeated Week / subject=PID ;
    LSMeans PGIC /cl;
Run;
```

Figure 4.22   Implementation of the model to investigate the relationship between change from baseline in a PRO and a PGIC.

```
The FREQ Procedure
                             Cumulative   Cumulative
PGIC     Frequency    Percent  Frequency    Percent
---------------------------------------------------
  1          8         1.60        8          1.60
  2         71        14.20       79         15.80
  3        158        31.60      237         47.40
  4        185        37.00      422         84.40
  5         65        13.00      487         97.40
  6         12         2.40      499         99.80
  7          1         0.20      500        100.00

First attempt
The Mixed Procedure

          Class Level Information
Class     Levels    Values
PGIC        7       1 2 3 4 5 6 7
Week        1       1

          Dimensions
Subjects                    500
Max Obs per Subject           1

          Number of Observations
Number of Observations Read        500
Number of Observations Used        500
Number of Observations Not Used      0

     WARNING: Stopped because of infinite likelihood.
------------------------------------------------------------------

Second attempt
The Mixed Procedure

          Class Level Information
Class     Levels    Values
PGIC        6       1 2 3 4 5 6
Week        1       1

          Dimensions
Subjects                    500
Max Obs per Subject           1

          Number of Observations
Number of Observations Read        500
Number of Observations Used        500
Number of Observations Not Used      0

                                  Least Squares Means
                     Standard
Effect  PGIC  Estimate   Error   DF   t Value  Pr > |t|  Alpha    Lower     Upper
PGIC     1    -4.8916  0.9543   494   -5.13    <.0001    0.05   -6.7666   -3.0166
PGIC     2    -3.4375  0.3203   494  -10.73    <.0001    0.05   -4.0669   -2.8081
PGIC     3    -1.0003  0.2147   494   -4.66    <.0001    0.05   -1.4222   -0.5784
PGIC     4     1.1662  0.1984   494    5.88    <.0001    0.05    0.7763    1.5562
PGIC     5     3.1026  0.3348   494    9.27    <.0001    0.05    2.4448    3.7604
PGIC     6     5.3822  0.7486   494    7.19    <.0001    0.05    3.9113    6.8531
```

Figure 4.23 Relationship between change from baseline in a PRO and a PGIC.

If we try to run first Mixed procedure (under Title "`First attempt`"), it will not converge. The issue is that we only have one subject with PGIC = 7. The small number of responses in this type of modeling almost always will lead to convergence problems. To escape this issue, we can simply pool responses of PGIC = 6 with PGIC = 7 (see line "If PGIC = 7 then PGIC = 6;"). Now the model converges (see partial output under "Second attempt") – note that we now have only six categories representing PGIC (see output under "`Class    Level Information`").

The results of the analysis show that the "no change" category (PGIC = 4) corresponds to the estimated mean value of approximately 1.17 on the change score in the PRO measure (ChgY). The next step is to try to understand or interpret what this value of 1.17 (1.1662) signifies. Is this a big change and therefore cannot be ignored or it is just trivial change? To gauge the magnitude of this value of 1.17, we can reinterpret this change in terms of the effect sizes.

For example, earlier in this section, we considered that values on the PRO scale are distributed uniformly (with values from 0 to 10) at baseline, and theoretical variance for this sample of subjects is 8.33. Hence the standard deviation is 2.87 (square root of 8.33) and, as a result, the estimated mean difference of 1.17 corresponds to a standardized effect size of 0.41 (1.17/2.87), which is tangible and not trivial. Note that we should use the standard deviation at baseline for the entire sample of subjects (all 500 subjects in our simulation), not the standard deviation of the subsample of subjects (i.e., 185 subjects with PGIC = "no change" at week 1) and not the standard deviation of the change from baseline in these 185 subjects.

A standardized effect size of 0.2 may be considered small (i.e., the estimated change from baseline being 0.2 standard deviation unit), 0.5 medium, and 0.8 large; a value of approximately 0.1 is trivial (McLeod et al. 2016). The value of 0.41 can be interpreted as a "small-to-medium" effect size, closer to medium. This interpretation of the estimated mean change means that the anchor-based approach does not produce a sufficiently "stable" subsample of subjects. If the effect size of the estimated mean change could have been interpreted as, at least, "small," or even better "trivial," then this subsample of subjects would be acceptable to use for ICC estimation (with understanding that it still remains a surrogate assessment).

Based on the results of this simulation, Figure 4.24 depicts the relationship between PGIC and ChgY (the change in the PRO measure of interest). As noted, for this relationship, the "no change" category of PGIC corresponds to a positive mean value (line denoted as ChgY in Figure 4.24). As a matter of fact, there could also be other scenarios: the PGIC "no change" category can correspond to a negative mean value for a PRO measurement (line "Example 1" in Figure 4.24) or even very close to zero mean value (line "Example 2" in Figure 4.24). In practice, though, it is more likely to have the PGIC "no change" category correspond to a positive mean value or to a negative mean value for a PRO measurement and not to zero (or close to zero) mean value. It is not expected that *no change* on a global measure (or, in fact, any other measure) will map exactly to a *no change* on the other measure, except in situations when they measure essentially the same outcome (and even then, it may not happen because of measurement error).

4.1.4.3 Time Period Between Observations

Another important detail when assessing test–retest reliability is to consider the time period between observations. From this standpoint, we can differentiate target PRO measures into the three distinct categories: (i) the scales that measure a patient-reported concept "right now" (e.g., a subject is asked to assess his or her

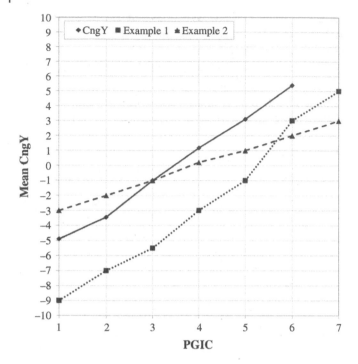

Figure 4.24 Relationship between patient global impression of change (PGIC) and estimated change in a PRO measure (ChgY).

pain severity right now); (ii) the scales that ask a patient to assess a concept over some period of time (e.g., over the last week); and (iii) scales that assess a concept since a predefined point in past, such as relative to baseline (PGIC is a good example of this type of scales).

Let us consider a scale that requests a subject to assess a concept "right now," the simplest mental task for a subject. In this situation, for the purpose of ICC estimation, the data could be collected during the pretreatment period, say, daily during a week. As a result, using all data from all subjects, we will be able to estimate ICC for *a single measurement* of a concept. For this type of recall, the period between observations should be driven by two factors.

First, the period between observations should be clinically and statistically relevant. It is typically not a good idea to ask about severity of the pain only few minutes apart; every 12 hours would be a better approach, for instance. It is very important to note that, mathematically, the modeling takes the measurements as statistically independent. This assumption means that a time period between observations should be such that we can assert that the measured concept does not change (true score for a subject is exactly the same at all occasions), but, simultaneously, we also can consider those observations as independent observations (basically assuming that covariance between measurement errors is zero; note that it was one of the assumption in our simulations in this chapter).

The second factor concerns the question, what if the ICC value for a single measurements will be less than desirable (say, less than 0.7)? Then to have reliable measurement of a concept during the treatment period of a study would require collection of those data more often and calculation of a mean from several observations to reliably assess the concept of interest (see the section "Spearman-Brown prophecy formula" later in this chapter).

As pointed out previously, the counterpart to "right now" is asking a patient to assess a concept over some period of time such as over the last 24 hours, last week, last month, and so forth. In this case, those scales can also be generally divided into at least two different categories. For example, a patient could be asked to assess pain severity during the last 24 hours (in this case, this patient is asked to recall the last 24 hours and mentally average pain severity over this period). A patient could be asked to assess *worst* pain severity during the last 24 hours (in this case, this patient was asked to recall the last 24 hours, go back to a moment when the pain was the worst, and report the severity of this pain hours later).

Regarding these two approaches (averaged vs. worst), researchers should be aware of their fundamental difference. Because we have a recall period (24 hours, a week, etc.), then outcomes collected at time points separated by the recall period can be treated as independent observations for a given subject – they cover distinct, not overlapping periods of time. This is a very important detail as measurements should be distinct and not collected during overlapping periods.

Let us say that a scale has a recall period of 24 hours, then we can collect just two observations at least 24 hours apart, and we will be able to estimate ICC. But in a study, subjects, likely to be asked to respond to a questionnaire, say, at night. Then for a scale when we ask to average experience, it will not be the big issue, even if measurements were not exactly 24 hours apart, say only 20 hours apart, the response will still cover the two mostly distinct periods of time. But if a scale when a patient is asked about worst experience is used, then if the measurements are separated in time less than a recall period, a patient could, in fact, recall the same worst event and report it as the two separate measurements. And, as a result, it would lead to an inflated ICC estimation. Therefore, it is important to design data collection so that the recall periods will not overlap. For example, if a recall period is 24 hours, then data can be collected 48 hours apart. In this situation, we will be assured that when a patient reports severity of worst symptoms, he or she is actually referencing two distinct events.

Another approach is when a patient is asked to assess a concept since the same a priori defined point in past, for example, from the beginning of the study to the

---

Overall, how satisfied are you with the drug that you received since you entered this trial?

Please check (X) ONE only:

□ (5) Extremely satisfied

□ (4) Satisfied

□ (3) Neither satisfied nor dissatisfied

□ (2) Dissatisfied

□ (1) Extremely dissatisfied

Figure 4.25 Patient-reported treatment satisfaction assessment.

current moment in time. For instance, Figure 4.25 illustrates an assessment on patient-reported treatment satisfaction when a patient evaluates current satisfaction with a drug relative to the beginning of the study.

Let us examine this type of recall period as it relates to the test–retest assessment. As it was pointed out earlier, we assume that observations used for ICC estimation should be independent (even if they are coming from the same person). And a tactic to ensure this is to collect data that are separated in time more than (or equal to) a recall period. Obviously, in this case, we cannot separate data. Every consecutive (after the first) observation will include all previous recall periods and, as such, those observations cannot be considered independent. As a result, for a scale with this type of recall period, the test–retest property cannot methodologically be established. It does not mean, however, that this type of scale cannot or should not be used in practice.

For example, PGIC is a good example of this type and we use it in analyses to establish Meaningful Within-Patient Change (see Chapter 7). We just do not recommend using this type of recall period for the measurement of the particular concept. Basically, if a recall period is "since the beginning of the study" or "since you entered this trial," then the test–retest property cannot be established and subsequently this scale cannot be fully validated.

4.1.5 Spearman-Brown Prophecy Formula

It is possible that in some cases, especially with a single-item scale, the test–retest reliability of an ICC could be substantially less than 0.7. A researcher is then faced with two possibilities. First, he can just use the scale "as is" with the understanding that the results (e.g., for comparison between experimental drug and placebo) could be erroneous and unpredictable – not because the intervention does not work, but simply because measurements based on this scale do not have acceptable test–retest reliability.

The second approach is to improve the reliability of the measurements through averaging multiple measurements and using an average value of scales scores for an individual in the modeling of the treatment effects. The averaging of the several measurements to improve test–retest reliability is rooted in the Spearman-Brown prophecy formula (DeVellis 2017):

$$R_m = \frac{mR}{1+(m-1)R} \tag{4.10}$$

where

m is the number of measurements to be averaged;
R_m is the reliability of the mean of the m measurements; and
R is the reliability of the single measurement;

When ICC is used as the measure of reliability to evaluate test–retest property of a scale, then Eq. (4.10) can be rewritten as

$$ICC_m = \frac{mICC}{1+(m-1)ICC} \tag{4.11}$$

Replacing *ICC* by *Var(F)/[Var(F) + Var(e)]* (see Eq. 4.2) will give

$$ICC_m = \frac{mVar(F)/[Var(F)+Var(e)]}{1+((m-1)Var(F)/(Var(F)+Var(e)))}$$

$$ICC_m = \frac{mVar(F)/[Var(F)+Var(e)]}{([Var(F)+Var(e)]+(m-1)Var(F))/(Var(F)+Var(e))}$$

$$ICC_m = \frac{mVar(F)}{[Var(F)+Var(e)+(m-1)Var(F)]}$$

$$ICC_m = \frac{mVar(F)}{Var(e)+mVar(F)}$$

$$ICC_m = \frac{Var(F)}{Var(F)+Var(e)/m}. \tag{4.12}$$

A comparison of Eq. (4.12) with the original definition of the *ICC* from Eq. (4.2) shows that measurement error is reduced by a factor of m, where m represents the number of averaged observations. This formula can also be rewritten to calculate the number of observations needed to be averaged to achieve a certain ICC level. For example, if we want to achieve ICC_m to be equal to 0.7, then Eq. 4.12 is transformed into the following:

$$m = \frac{0.7\,Var(e)}{0.3\,Var(F)}$$

or, more generally,

$$m = \frac{R\,Var(e)}{(1-R)\,Var(F)},$$

(4.13)

where R is the desired or required test–retest reliability.

Eq. (4.12) can be illustrated using the same model from Section 4.1.2 to estimate ICC. Recall the system of Eq. (4.4). If we sum those two equations, and divide left and right portion by two, we will get

$$\frac{Y1_i + Y2_i}{2} = F_i + \left[(e_{1i} + e_{2i})/2\right].$$

The elements in above equation can be interpreted as follows. The mean of two observations for the measured variable y is represented as a mixture of two components: one component is the "true" score measure F, and the other one is the measurement error e, which in this equation is $(e_1 + e_2)/2$. As previously stated, both of these components are not observed, but they sum up to yield the mean y based on two observations. With this interpretation in mind, Eq. (4.2) can be rewritten in this case as

$$ICC_2 = Var(F)\big/\left[Var(F) + Var\big((e_1 + e_2)/2\big)\right].$$

(4.14)

Here, ICC_2 represents the test–retest reliability for the mean of two observations. Recall that e_1 and e_2 are the measurement errors for a single measurement; both are assumed to be from the same normal distribution with mean 0 and variance σ_e^2, i.e., $e_i \sim N(0, \sigma_e^2)$, which means that $Var(e_1) = Var(e_2)$. Then Eq. (4.14) can be modified as

$$ICC_2 = Var(F)\big/\left[Var(F) + (1/4)\times Var(e_1 + e_2)\right]$$

$$ICC_2 = Var(F)\big/\left[Var(F) + (1/4)\times 2\times Var(e)\right]$$

$$ICC_2 = Var(F)\big/\left[Var(F) + Var(e)/2\right].$$

(4.15)

Eq. (4.12) also implies that, if we use averaged data vs. observed individual data, then the estimated "true" score parameters (i.e., mean and variance) will be the same whether the individual observations or the average of several observations are used. But their estimated measurement error will be different and, moreover, dependent on the number of averaged observations we use.

To illustrate this interpretation, let us consider the following simulation. Say we collected data during two pretreatment weeks, and we want to estimate test–retest reliability for the weekly averages ($ICC_7 = Var(F)/[Var(F) + Var(e)/7]$). We will use the same approach as represented by Figure 4.6 earlier in this chapter, but now 14 observations for every subject will be simulated (see Figure 4.26). First, we simulate observations for every subject and then convert dataset "_icc_" into dataset "_icc_mixed" with an appropriate structure for ICC estimation using the MIXED procedure. Note that, when creating vertical structure, we also added two additional observations representing the mean of the first seven observations ("y = (y1 + y2 + y3 + y4 + y5 + y6 + y7)/7;") and mean of the second seven observations ("y = (y8 + y9 + y10 + y11 + y12 + y13 + y14)/7;"). To distinguish between what in real life would be observed data and averaged data, the additional variable Record was added.

Figure 4.27 represents the implementation of the model needed to estimate variance parameters. Sorting dataset "_icc_mixed" by type of the data (based on the variable Record) will create the dataset represented by Figure 4.28

```
/* For this example, there ae 500 subjects (NumberOfSubjects) and every subject has
14 observations. To define variances for latent "true" score (VarF) and measurement
error (VarME) the following values are used: 1 and 0.2.*/
options nofmterr nocenter pagesize=2000 linesize=256;
%Let NumberOfSubjects = 500; %Let a  = 5; %Let VarF  = 1; %Let VarME = 0.2;
Data _icc_;
array v[14] v1-v14;
    Do ID=1 To &NumberOfSubjects;
                /* F represents true score */
                F  = &a + rannor(1)*sqrt(&VarF) ;
                Do i=1 to 14;
                v[i] = F  + rannor(i)*sqrt(&VarME) ;
                End;
                output;
    End;
Run;

Data _icc_mixed; Set _icc_;
array v[14] v1-v14;
Do i=1 to 14;
    y=v[i]; Record="Observed"; output;
End;
y=(v1+v2+v3 +v4 +v5 +v6 +v7 )/7; Record="Mean"; output;
y=(v8+v9+v10+v11+v12+v13+v14)/7; Record="Mean"; output;
Keep ID Record y;
Run;
```

Figure 4.26 Simulating a dataset based on measurement error model with 14 observations per subject.

```
Proc Sort Data=_icc_mixed; By Record ID; Run;
Proc Print Data=_icc_mixed NOOBS; Where ID In (1 2 499 500); Run;
Proc Mixed data=_icc_mixed COVTEST;
Class ID ;
Model y= / solution;
Random Int / subject=ID solution;
By Record;
Run;
```

Figure 4.27 Estimating variances using observed and averaged scores.

("**Proc Print** Data=_icc_mixed NOOBS;..."). In Figure 4.28, observations corresponding to Record = Mean represent weekly averages (two such observations per subject) and observations corresponding to Record = Observed represent single daily measurements (14 observations per subject). As a result, we can run two separate analyses by using the same SAS code (MIXED procedure) by just adding "By Record" statement.

Figures 4.29 and 4.30 show the results of estimations of the variances for both models. As expected, the estimations of the variance of the "true" score was almost exactly the same (1.0209 vs 1.0206; note that value of 1.0 was used in

```
ID       y       Record
  1   6.88624    Mean
  1   6.65062    Mean
  2   4.29637    Mean
  2   4.33856    Mean
...
499   3.91456    Mean
499   3.83830    Mean
500   5.00238    Mean
500   4.90086    Mean
  1   6.76908    Observed
  1   6.98218    Observed
  1   6.32035    Observed
  1   7.80582    Observed
  1   6.52566    Observed
  1   7.03454    Observed
  1   6.76609    Observed
  1   6.53910    Observed
  1   6.81908    Observed
  1   6.47487    Observed
  1   6.69296    Observed
  1   7.11117    Observed
  1   6.44519    Observed
  1   6.47197    Observed
  2   4.35687    Observed
  2   4.07011    Observed
  2   3.60083    Observed
  2   4.39801    Observed
  2   4.78843    Observed
  2   4.84183    Observed
  2   4.01855    Observed
  2   4.92647    Observed
  2   3.73147    Observed
  2   3.78039    Observed
  2   4.63098    Observed
  2   4.37980    Observed
  2   4.17045    Observed
  2   4.75035    Observed
```

Figure 4.28 Example of the dataset structure used in implementation represented by Figure 4.27.

```
...
499    4.72135    Observed
499    3.88280    Observed
499    4.17540    Observed
499    3.42202    Observed
499    3.89058    Observed
499    2.98256    Observed
499    4.32725    Observed
499    4.32587    Observed
499    4.02570    Observed
499    4.01877    Observed
499    3.98406    Observed
499    4.26575    Observed
499    3.00621    Observed
499    3.24173    Observed
500    4.57008    Observed
500    5.13064    Observed
500    4.84730    Observed
500    5.34259    Observed
500    4.62906    Observed
500    5.18555    Observed
500    5.31141    Observed
500    4.89456    Observed
500    4.77440    Observed
500    4.80386    Observed
500    5.09487    Observed
500    5.04970    Observed
500    5.03850    Observed
500    4.65015    Observed
```

Figure 4.28 (Continued).

```
Record=Mean
                   Covariance Parameter Estimates
                                   Standard        Z
Cov Parm    Subject    Estimate    Error      Value    Pr > Z
Intercept   ID          1.0209     0.06551    15.58    <.0001
Residual                0.02763    0.001747   15.81    <.0001
```

Figure 4.29 Covariance parameter estimates using mean scores.

```
Record=Observed
                   Covariance Parameter Estimates
                                   Standard        Z
Cov Parm    Subject    Estimate    Error      Value    Pr > Z
Intercept   ID          1.0206     0.06551    15.58    <.0001
Residual                0.1977     0.003468   57.01    <.0001
```

Figure 4.30 Covariance parameter estimates using observed single scores.

simulation), and estimation of the measurement error using dataset with observed data was close to the value we used to simulate data (0.1977; note that value of 0.2 was used in simulation), but estimation of the measurement error using mean scores was almost exactly seven times less (0.02763) compared with value of 0.2 from a single measurement.

4.1.6 Domain Score Test–Retest vs. Item Test–Retest

When assessing test–retest reliability, we generally center on the reliability of the domain scores, not the individual items constituting this domain. For example, if a domain is represented by k items and reliability for this domain score is R_d, then we can use Spearman-Brown formula (Eq. 4.10) to estimate reliability R_i of a single item:

$$R_d = \frac{kR_i}{1+(k-1)R_i}$$

$$R_d\left[1+(k-1)R_i\right] = kR_i$$

$$R_d + (k-1)R_i R_d = kR_i$$

$$R_d = kR_i - (k-1)R_i R_d$$

$$R_d = R_i\left[k-(k-1)R_d\right]$$

$$R_i = \frac{R_d}{k+(1-k)R_d}. \qquad (4.16)$$

Equation (4.16) represents the "reversed" Spearman-Brown prophecy formula. Let us say that the ICC for a domain score is 0.7, and this domain is represented by five items. Then reliability of a single item will be

$$R_i = \frac{0.7}{5+(1-5)0.7} = 0.32.$$

The above exemplifies the important fact that individual items in a multi-item domain generally have low reliability. Even if this domain has reliability of 0.9, then the individual item reliability would be only 0.64, which is less than 0.7 value (recall that 0.7 is generally considered the lowest boundary of acceptable reliability).

It is important to note two assumptions we employed in this example. One assumption is that every item in a domain measures the same underlying construct. This assumption is well grounded as the items in a domain should represent the same construct; otherwise, they should not be part of the same domain. The second assumption is not as simple as the first one: the measurement error for every item is the same (to be exact, it is represented by the same distribution). Although this assumption may not be exactly accurate, measurement errors for individual items generally will be close to each other. If items have drastically different measurement errors, it would mean that their corresponding multi-item scale is not well developed. Yet, even if individual item measurement errors are relatively close, estimation of item reliability based on Eq. (4.16) is approximate and represents an "average" item in a domain.

We should also mention another interesting and noteworthy point about the Spearman-Brown prophecy formula. To develop formula (4.16), we started with formula (4.10), assuming that an item's reliability R_i is unknown, but R_i was in a place where a generally known reliability value should be entered. In fact, we could directly use Spearman-Brown formula as presented by Eq. (4.10), but (what is somewhat counterintuitive) now replace m by $1/k$. Let us start with formula (4.10) by replacing R_m by item reliability R_i, R by R_d, and m by $1/k$:

$$R_i = \frac{(1/k)R_d}{1+\big((1/k)-1\big)R_d}$$

$$R_i = \frac{R_d}{k\Big[1+\big((1/k)-1\big)R_d\Big]}$$

$$R_i = \frac{R_d}{k+(1-k)R_d}.$$

As we can see, this last equation is exactly the same as Eq. (4.16).

4.1.7 Observer-Based and Interviewer-Based Scales

In addition to patient-reported measurements – the central topic of this book – there are two additional types of scales: (i) observer-based and (ii) interviewer-based. Those two types are very close and sometimes even intermixed together. The main difference is that an observer-based scale (sometimes called proxy-based) is when a subject-related measurement is assessed by a non-healthcare individual observer (such as a parent or caregiver who is not trained in the healthcare specialty under consideration) but, unlike an interviewer-based scale, the subject is not probed or questioned by anyone; therefore, the entire measurement of a construct stems solely from observation of subject's behavior, performance, or actions. This type of scale can be found in measurements designed, for example, for very small children who have not yet developed enough or adults with some specific illnesses (e.g., Alzheimer's disease) that affect thinking abilities or cause memory decline. Examples of observer rating scales include the proxy version of POEM (Charman et al. 2004), which is a seven-item PRO measure used to assess the impact of atopic dermatitis recalled over the past week.

Another example is when a subject state is rated by a clinician, a clinician-rated scale, who is specifically trained in the disease or condition under consideration (Powers et al. 2017). Clinician-rated outcomes are especially pertinent in studies that include children and adults because these clinicians can assess both children and adults; however, the same PRO measure can rarely be applied to both children and adults.

Rather than simply observing, the interviewer is actively seeking answers about a measured outcome, for example, about the severity of a particular symptom. For instance, a parent can discuss with a child a particular symptom and, based on this discussion, assign a severity of this symptom. And in some scales, both approaches (observer and interviewer) could be used. For example, the Alzheimer's Disease Assessment Scale (Mohs et al. 1983) is scored on the basis of patient observation and an interview of an informant. A hybrid type of scale is the Cornell Scale for Depression in Dementia (Alexopoulos et al. 1988), where the clinician interviews the patient's caregiver on each item on the scale and then briefly interviewers the patient.

Generally, when the observer or interviewer scales are used in a study, we need to assess not only test–retest reliability but also inter-observer or inter-interviewer reliability. It is important to emphasize the word "generally" in the previous sentence. In certain circumstances, there is no need to assess inter-observer or inter-interviewer reliability, as the study design makes it unnecessary. For example, if for a subject, all measurement for a scale based on a same observer, then there is no need to assess between-observer reliability (the same for interviewer-based scales). Or, the study protocol may require the same parent to rate a child during the entire study. If it is anticipated that a study will involve different observers (or raters or interviewers), then we need to assess between-observer or inter-interviewer reliability and test–retest reliability. In this case, care should be taken in assessing both reliabilities.

First, let us consider between-observer or inter-interviewer reliability. To assess this, we can simply apply the methods discussed earlier in this chapter, especially in Sections 4.1.2 and 4.1.3. In order to estimate ICC, we need to have at least two measurements performed, for example, by a set of different observers (or interviewers) evaluating the same set of subjects. The critical difference is that now those two assessments should be performed at the same time or two time points that realistically can be considered as done simultaneously. For example, if a recall period is "in the last 24 hours," then assessments by two observers should be done, say, no more than one or two hours apart.

Another subtle point here is that both observers should also *observe* the same subject during the same 24 hours. This example shows that if multiple observers will rate the same subject and we need to assess between-observer reliability, then a measurement scale should not have a lengthy recall period; otherwise it will, almost certainly, lead to a logistical nightmare. The best-case scenario is when an observer rates the current state of a subject (i.e., recall period is "right now").

From the standpoint of the recall period, interviewer-based scales provide a notable advantage over observer-based scales. Let us again consider the scenario with recall period "in last 24 hours." Now we do not need two interviewers following a subject during the last 24 hours; it is sufficient for two (or more) interviewers to *interview* the same subject about his or her experience during the last 24 hours. This example shows that if multiple interviewers will rate the same subject, and we need to assess inter-reviewer reliability, then a measurement scale could have lengthy recall period.

When assessing between-observer or inter-reviewer reliability, the best approach will be that all repeated (and occurred reasonably simultaneous) measurements should be performed by different observers or reviewers. If, for some subjects, data will include observations when the same observer will rate a subject two or more times, then it will lead to inflating of the ICC assessment, because it will lower measurement error.

In the situation with multiple observers or interviewers for test–retest reliability assessment, we also need to pay special attention to the scheme on how data should be collected. Although during the study, it is possible that a subject could be rated by the same rater, in ICC calculations, we should (in an ideal world) always have two different raters for every subject who contributed two observations, three different raters for every subject who contributed three observations, and so on. By doing so, we will not inflate ICC estimation and will have most conservative test–retest reliability assessment. From the logistical standpoint, the most workable approach would be to have just two observations per subject with every observation rated by a different observer or interviewer.

4.1.8 Uncovering True Relationship Between Measurements

4.1.8.1 Accounting for Measurement Error

In some studies, assessments can be collected and evaluated at one of the local medical centers or at a global central location. For example, at a local medical center, a clinician can assess hair loss for a subject and, at the same time, pictures of this subject can be sent to a central location, where all pictures for all subjects will be evaluated by the same rater. To assess the reliability of these measurements, we can apply the same approach described at length in Section 4.1.7.

But examining the ICC will not answer the most important question: Is there a difference, and if so by how much, between those locally appraised outcomes and centrally appraised outcomes? A straightforward approach is to examine the relationship between central and local data using ordinary linear regression with, for instance, centrally evaluated values as an anchor and locally evaluated values as an outcome. In this case, though, we would assume that centrally evaluated data are "perfect" and thus measured without any measurement error, which, of course, is not true or accurate. What is really of interest is uncovering and quantifying the true (error-free) relationship between central and local measurements and, as such, uncover their underlying agreement. A similar problem arises if we would like to understand, say, relationship between measurements of severity of illness assessed by a subject and simultaneously by a physician.

Another example is the measurement of disease activity in ulcerative colitis. One of the four components of the Mayo score (Schroeder et al. 1987) is the finding of flexible proctosigmoidoscopy or colonoscopy (also referenced as endoscopic findings). Results of the endoscopy are interpreted by a clinician who assigns a score from 0 ("Normal or inactive disease") to 3 ("Severe disease [spontaneous bleeding, ulceration]") to this component. To increase the reliability of results, a governing body could request that all endoscopy samples be assessed at one "central" facility, which can significantly complicate the study logistics and increase the cost of the study.

If a developer of a drug would like to use "local" centers to assess endoscopy, it would not be merely enough to show that the estimated ICC is reasonable. Ideally, it is needed to show that we either have the perfect relationship between "central" and "local" interpretation of the endoscopy results, that is,

$$F_l = F_c$$

where

F_c is the "true" endoscopy scores assigned centrally;
F_l is the endoscopy scores assigned locally (see also Figure 4.31a) or, at least that
$\quad F_c$ and F_l differ by only a constant d

$$F_l = d + F_c$$

(see Figure 4.31b).

In real life, however, it is more likely that neither of the two above relations will be present, and a relationship will be more general, which can be represented by following equation:

$$F_l = d + aF_c, \tag{4.17}$$

where F_c and F_l are the same "true" central and local endoscopy scores (as given previously) and d and a represent intercept and slope, respectively. If a is reasonably close to the value of one, then the line representing the relationship will be parallel to the perfect line (see Figure 4.31b) and, in this case, results for the treatment differences should be the same, whichever type of measurement

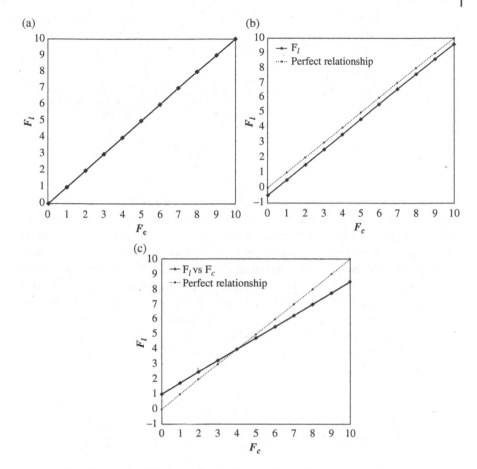

Figure 4.31 Examples of the relationship between F_l and F_c.

(local or central) is used. But if a is noticeably different from one (see also Figure 4.31c), then treatment differences results based on locally assessed endoscopy are not expected to be equivalent to the treatment differences based on centrally-assessed endoscopy. We should stress that above we discussed relationships between "true" unobserved (latent) endoscopy scores; that is, we acknowledge that both measurements (local and central) are not perfect and include a measurement error.

Let us consider the following simulated example where the local and central measurements represented by the scale with values from 0 to 10 with higher score indicating more severity in a measured trait. Figure 4.32 depicts the relationships between true and observed local and central measurements.

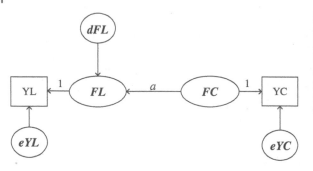

Figure 4.32 Model to estimate relationship between "true" central and local measurements by accounting for measurement errors (see text for description of variables).

In Figure 4.32, the unobserved variables *FL* and *FC* represent "true" central and local scores, variables *YL* and *YC* represent observed scores, unobserved variables *eYL* and *eYC* are the measurement errors, and *dFL* is the error term in linear regression representing relationship between *FL* and *FC* (generally an error term associated with latent variable is referred as disturbance). This model logically can be partitioned into three overlapping segments: (i) two segments represent measurement error parts of the model (see Figure 4.33a and b), which are methodologically identical to the Figure 4.1 (the first figure in this chapter) and (ii) a central segment (Figure 4.33c) that represents regression model to assess the relationship between the "true" scores (the main interest in this analysis).

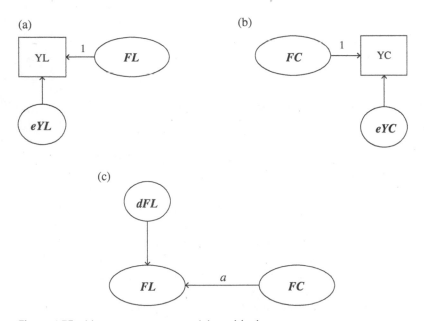

Figure 4.33 Measurement error model partitioning.

The first step in simulating the data is to create "true" local and central scores. The "true" measurements are represented by variables *FL* and *FC*, and the equation for the relationship between true measurements for subject *i* can be expressed as

$$FL_i = d + a \times FC_i + dFL_i \tag{4.18}$$

where

FL_i is the "true" value of the measured locally outcome for subject *i* ($i = 1, 2, \ldots,$
   N; *N* represents the number of subjects);
FC_i is the "true" value of the measured centrally outcome for subject *i*;
d is the intercept;
a is the slope;
dFL_i is the error [assumed to be from a normal distribution with mean 0 and variance σ_{fl}^2, i.e., $dFL_i \sim N(0, \sigma_{fl}^2)$].

The below data step (see Figure 4.34) creates a dataset with two variables *FC* (central) and *FL* (local). Note that, in our simulation, the relationship between those two outcomes is postulated as follows (with intercept of −0.1 and slope of 1.1):

$$FL = -0.1 + 1.1 * FC + \text{rannor}(1) * \text{sqrt}(0.2). \tag{4.19}$$

The next step is to create observed local and central scores. This step (see Figure 4.35) is the same as in Sections 4.1.1 and 4.1.2 for modeling observed data (see, for example, the SAS code in Figure 4.2). Note that we keep only the observed values in the dataset (Keep ID YC YL;). Although subject ID is not used in any analyses in this section, it is advisable to have a subject identification variable to

```
/*Create "true" central (FC) and local (FL) scores for 1000 subjects.*/
Data _tmp_1;
Do ID=1 to 1000;
FC = 5+rannor(1)*sqrt(1.2); FL =-0.1 + 1.1*FC + rannor(1)*sqrt(.2); Output;
End;
Run;
```

Figure 4.34   Simulating "true" central and local measurements.

```
/*Create "observed" central (YC) and local (YL) scores by adding
measurement error to "true" scores */
Data _tmp_2; Set _tmp_1;
YC = FC + rannor(2)*sqrt(0.05);    YL = FL + rannor(2)*sqrt(0.10);
Keep ID YC YL;
Run;
Proc Means Data=_tmp_2; Run;
```

Figure 4.35   Simulating local and central observed values.

```
Proc Calis cov data = _tmp_2 method = ML technique = LEVMAR all;
Lineqs
FL = 0 intercept + a FC+ dFL,
YC = b intercept + FC  + eYC,
YL = c intercept + FL  + eYL;
Variance
FC   =  VarFC , dFL  =   vardFL,
eYC  =  0.05  , eYL  =   0.10;
Cov
eYC eYL = 0;
Testfunc interceptFL ; interceptFL = c - a*b;
Run;
```

Figure 4.36 Examining relationship between "true" scores with the measurement error model.

highlight some data or understand outliers. The structure of the dataset will be analogous to the structure of the dataset represented by Figure 4.7, but instead of variables *Y*1 and *Y*2, we now have variables *YC* and *YL*.

The next step is to model the relationships between variables (see Figure 4.36). We are fitting the "Mean and Covariance Structures" model, meaning that we not only estimate effects of one variable onto another variable but also fit the mean structure of the variables.

Let us examine the implementation of the model in more details. The two lines of SAS code

```
YC = b intercept + FC + eYC,
YL = c intercept + FL + eYL,
```

represent the relationship between true and observed scores. These two lines of code are almost identical to the implementation in Section 4.1.1 (see Figure 4.3) with the exception of the additional term for the modeling mean structure. The term "b intercept" in the above first SAS code line directs CALIS procedure to estimate the mean of the *YC* outcome (parameter *b*; note that it also represents the intercept in this equation, i.e., *YC* = *b* when latent variable *FC* = 0).

The last equation under "Lineqs" statement models the relationship between unobserved true scores. This equation corresponds to Eq. (4.19), which represented simulated relationship between true scores. Parameter *a* corresponds to the slope (which was 1.1 in simulation). But because in the modeling (i) the latent variables metric is not defined and (ii) for model identification purposes, we specified the mean of the *FL* to be zero ("0 intercept"). We should stress that it does not mean that we assigned zero to the intercept in Eq. (4.17), we will return later to this matter.

Under "Variance" statement we direct CALIS procedure to estimate the variance of the latent true score *FC* (FC =VarFC; it is technically the same as we had in Section 4.1 in Figure 4.3) and the variance of the disturbance (dFL =vardFL).

We do not request to estimate variance of the latent true score FL as it will be defined by the two above variances. By now it should be clear that the model is not estimable if we treat variances of the measurement errors as free parameters (i.e., needed to be estimated). We use the same values we used in the simulation (0.05 and 0.10) to predefine variances of the measurement errors (eYC =0.05 and eYL =0.10). Under "Cov" statement we postulate that measurement errors are independent (covariance between eYC and eYL is zero).

The last statement "Testfunc" needs additional explanation. The relationship between true scores is defined by two parameters: intercept and slope. The slope is represented by the parameter a, yet there is no parameter representing the intercept. From Eq. (4.17), it can be concluded that

$$mean(F_l) = d + a \times mean(F_c).$$
(4.20)

Hence, the observed variable Y_l and the true (latent) variable F_l differ only by measurement error. This means that the population mean of the variable Y_l and mean of true value F_l will be equal. As such, Eq. (4.20) can be rewritten as

$$mean(Y_l) = d + a \times mean(Y_c).$$
(4.21)

Recall that in the modeling the parameter b represents the estimation of $mean(Y_c)$ and c represents the estimation of $mean(Y_l)$. As a result, Eq. (4.21) will be simplified to

$$c = d + a \times b$$

and intercept can be calculated as

$$d = c - a \times b.$$
(4.22)

The statement "Testfunc" provides the ability to estimate additional functions based on the estimated values of the parameters in the model. In our case, we want to estimate the intercept based on the estimated model parameters. Note that statement "interceptFL = c - a*b" corresponds exactly to the above Eq. (4.22).

After executing SAS code represented by Figures 4.34 and 4.35, the dataset "_tmp_2" for the analysis will be produced. The Means procedure shows (see Figure 4.37) that we simulated data for 1000 subjects and, for every subject in this dataset, we have one observation with two outcomes representing observed local and central measurements.

Variable	N	Mean	Std Dev	Minimum	Maximum
ID	1000	500.5000000	288.8194361	1.0000000	1000.00
YC	1000	4.9633896	1.0951641	1.9188325	8.6937043
YL	1000	5.3517554	1.3080215	0.9920521	9.0833845

Figure 4.37 Results of the MEANS procedure.

```
Mean and Covariance Structures: Maximum Likelihood Estimation

                     Linear Equations
FL =           0     intercept  +   1.1052(**) FC  +   1.0000 dFL
YC =    4.9634(**) intercept  +   1.0000     FC  +   1.0000 eYC
YL =    5.3518(**) intercept  +   1.0000     FL  +   1.0000 eYL

                  Effects in Linear Equations
                                              Standard
Variable      Predictor     Parameter   Estimate     Error       t Value     Pr > |t|
FL            intercept                       0
FL            FC            a            1.10515      0.01836     60.2099     <.0001
YC            intercept     b            4.96339      0.03465     143.2       <.0001
YC            FC                         1.00000
YL            intercept     c            5.35176      0.04138     129.3       <.0001
YL            FL                         1.00000

              Estimates for Variances of Exogenous Variables
Variable                                         Standard
Type          Variable    Parameter   Estimate    Error       t Value    Pr > |t|
Latent        FC          VarFC       1.14938     0.05366     21.4178    <.0001
Disturbance   dFL         vardFL      0.20711     0.01647     12.5721    <.0001
Error         eYC                     0.05000
              eYL                     0.10000

              Tests for Parametric Functions
Parametric                      Standard
Function      Estimate          Error       t Value    Pr > |t|
interceptFL   -0.13355          0.09310     -1.4344     0.1515
```

Figure 4.38 Partial output of the CALIS procedure (from Figure 4.36).

The next step is to run a model represented by Figure 4.36 (the partial output represented by Figure 4.38). Here the estimation of the slope between true local and central measurements is 1.1052 ("...1.1052(**) FC ..."), which is practically equal to the value of 1.1 used in the simulation. The estimated value of the intercept is −0.13355 ("interceptFL -0.13355 ..."; in the simulation the value of intercept is −0.1). Other estimated parameters in the model are also close to values we used to simulate data. For example, the variance of the disturbance term in the regression for true scores is estimated as 0.20711 ("Disturbance dFL vardFL 0.20711...") versus 0.2 in the simulation. The CALIS procedure estimates the means of the observed variables *YC* and *YL* as 4.96339 ("YC intercept b 4.96339...") and 5.35176 ("YL intercept c 5.35176..."). Note that those estimated means are virtually the same as the mean values of those variables in Figure 4.37.

To highlight the differences between the aforementioned measurement error model and ordinary regression with observed variables, let us model the relationship between variables *YC* and *YL* using the REG procedure. Figure 4.39 represents the implementation of the analyses, with the same dataset "_tmp_2" being used by the model represented by Figure 4.36. Figure 4.40 represents the partial output of the REG procedure. As anticipated, the results for intercept and slope are different from those estimations using the measurement error model.

But an interesting question is how this regression model with observed outcomes can be implemented as a measurement error model and how this model

```
Proc Reg data=_tmp_2;
Model YL=YC;
Run; Quit;
```

Figure 4.39 Modeling relationship between observed outcomes with REG procedure.

```
The REG Procedure
Dependent Variable: YL
                        Parameter Estimates
                        Parameter       Standard
Variable        DF      Estimate          Error   t Value   Pr > |t|
Intercept        1       0.09513        0.08883      1.07     0.2845
YC               1       1.05908        0.01748     60.60    <.0001
```

Figure 4.40 Relationship between observed outcomes: intercept and slope.

```
proc calis cov data = _tmp_2 method = ML technique = LEVMAR all;
Lineqs
YC = b intercept + FC  + eYC,
YL = c intercept + FL  + eYL,
FL = 0 intercept + a FC+ dFL;
Variance
FC   = VarFC ,      dFL  =   vardFL,
eYC  = 0.0000001, eYL  =  0.0000001;
Cov
eYC eYL = 0;
Testfunc interceptFL ; interceptFL = c - a*b;
run;
```

Figure 4.41 Measurement error model equivalent to the ordinary regression.

will be different from the model represented by Figure 4.36. To implement the model using the CALIS procedure, which will resemble the measurement error model and at the same time will also be equivalent to ordinary regression (represented by Figures 4.39), we start with the same implementation given by Figure 4.36. Figure 4.41 represents this new implementation. Note that the only difference from the Figure 4.36 is that now predefined values of 0.05 and 0.10 for variances of the measurement errors are postulated to equal to zero (Actually, we set those variances to be equal to very small values, otherwise the CALIS procedure will produce several "WARNING" messages; readers are encouraged to set those values to zeros to investigate the consequences.)

Figure 4.42 represents partial output for the corresponding CALIS procedure. As we can see, the estimated slope and intercept for the "true" measurements are exactly the same ("...1.0591(**) FC ...";"interceptFL 0.09513...") as found from the REG procedure. This finding highlights the important fact that when an analysis is based on observed outcomes, as is done with ordinary regression, we disregard the existence of the measurement errors and treat those outcomes as true measurements, which is typically not true. It is also important to note that, even if we will have more observations, the ordinary regression will not be converging to the relationship between true unobserved measurements.

```
The CALIS Procedure
Mean and Covariance Structures: Maximum Likelihood Estimation

                         Linear Equations
YC =      4.9634(**) intercept  +   1.0000      FC  +   1.0000 eYC
YL =      5.3518(**) intercept  +   1.0000      FL  +   1.0000 eYL
FL =      0          intercept  +   1.0591(**) FC  +   1.0000 dFL

                 Tests for Parametric Functions
Parametric                          Standard
Function            Estimate          Error    t Value    Pr > |t|
interceptFL         0.09513         0.08879     1.0714      0.2840
```

Figure 4.42 Partial output of the CALIS procedure (from Figure 4.41).

4.1.8.2 Measurement Error Model with Two Observations

In the previous section, the measurement errors were taken as known, but, in fact, this is usually not a case. In Section 4.1.2, we showed that at least two observations per subject are needed to estimate measurement error. In assessing relationship between true scores when measurement errors are unknown, we also need to have at least two observations for every subject.

The relationships between "true" local and central and observed local and central measurements collected two times are represented by Figure 4.43. In Figure 4.43, the variables $YL1$, $YC1$, $YL2$ and $YC2$ represent observed scores collected at occasion one ($YL1$ and $YC1$) and at occasion two ($YL2$ and $YC2$), unobserved variables FL and FC represent "true" central and "true" local measurements, and unobserved variables eYL and eYC are the measurement errors associated with the observed scores locally and centrally. Note that it is assumed that true scores and measurement errors are the same at both time points (as we had in Section 4.1.2).

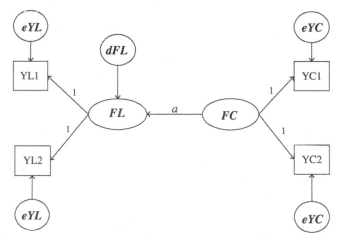

Figure 4.43 Model to estimate the relationship between "true" central and local measurements accounting for measurement errors with two observations.

We should highlight again that true scores are assumed to be *numerically* the same at both time points. But when we describe measurement errors as the same at both time points, we mean that they could be *numerically different* but taken from the *same distribution*. The variable *dFL* (disturbance) is the error term in the linear regression representing the relationship between *FL* and *FC*.

To simulate data, we first will create "true" local and "true" central scores. The "true" measurements are represented by variables *FL* and *FC*. The equations for relationship between true measurements for subject *i* can be expressed as

$$FL_i = d + aFC_i + dFL_i \qquad\qquad (4.23)$$

where

FL_i is the "true" value of the measured locally outcome for subject i ($i = 1, 2, \ldots,$ N; N represents the number of subjects) at both time points;

FC_i is the "true" value of the measured centrally outcome for subject i at both time points;

d is the intercept;

a is the slope;

dFL_i is the error [assumed to be from a normal distribution with mean 0 and variance σ_{fl}^2, i.e., $dFL_i \sim N(0, \sigma_{fl}^2)$].

Note that this equation is practically the same as Eq. (4.18) discussed earlier. But there are distinct important differences and theoretical assumptions made when we describe relationships between true scores in this case. We postulate not only that at both time points, the relationship between "true" scores is exactly the same, but also that the "true" local score at first occasion is the same as "true" local score at second occasion (the same for "true" central score). Hence, we only need one equation to describe such a relationship. In fact, we assume that the "true" score is the same at any time point between occasion one and occasion two, with no change in the patient's underlying health state on the concept of interest, which is the same assumption given in Section 4.1.2.

Figure 4.44 represents the simulation of the "true" scores. We simulate data for 1000 subjects (the mean of the "true" central score is 5 and the variance is 1.2). Slope and intercept for the relationship between "true" local score and "true"

```
options nocenter linesize=256;
/*Create "true" central (FC) and local (FL) scores. */
Data _tmp_1;
   Do ID=1 to 1000;
      FC = 5+rannor(1)*sqrt(1.2);  FL  =-0.1 + 1.1*FC + rannor(1)*sqrt(.2);
      Output;
   End;
Run;
Proc Means Data=_tmp_1; Run;
```

Figure 4.44 Simulating "true" scores at two time points.

central score are represented by values of 1.1 and -0.1, respectively, and the error term is represented by following snippets of SAS code: "`rannor(1)*sqrt(.2)`".

The next step is to simulate the observed data. The following four equations represent relationships between true and observed scores at both time points (compare these equations with those in Eq. 4.1):

$$YL1_i = FL_i + eYL1_i$$

$$YL2_i = FL_i + eYL2_i$$

$$YC1_i = FC_i + eYC1_i$$

$$YC2_i = FC_i + eYC2_i$$

where

$YL1_i$ is the observed value of the measured locally outcome for subject i at the first time point ($i = 1, 2, \ldots, N$; N represents the number of subjects);

$YC1_i$ is the observed value of the measured centrally outcome for subject i at the first time point;

$YL2_i$ is the observed value of the measured locally outcome for subject i at the second time point;

$YC2_i$ is the observed value of the measured centrally outcome for subject i at the second time point;

$eYL1_i$ is the measurement error at the first time point for local measurements [assumed to be from a normal distribution with mean 0 and variance σ_l^2, i.e., $eYL1_i \sim N(0, \sigma_l^2)$];

$eYL2_i$ is the measurement error at the second for local measurements [assumed to be from a normal distribution with mean 0 and variance σ_l^2, i.e., $eYL2_i \sim N(0, \sigma_l^2)$];

$eYC1_i$ is the measurement error at the first time point for central measurements [assumed to be from a normal distribution with mean 0 and variance σ_c^2, i.e., $eYC1_i \sim N(0, \sigma_c^2)$];

$eYC2_i$ is the measurement error at the second time point for central measurements [assumed to be from a normal distribution with mean 0 and variance σ_c^2, i.e., $eYC2_i \sim N(0, \sigma_c^2)$].

It is important to emphasize again that measurement errors are the "same" for local measurements at both time points (to be exact, they are taken from the same normal distribution with variance σ_l^2). The same is true for the centrally obtained measurements: The measurement errors are the "same" at both time points meaning that they are taken from the same normal distribution with variance σ_c^2. Figure 4.45 shows the implementation for this portion of the simulation. Note that the variance of the measurement errors for local measurements is 0.10 at both time points and the variance of the measurement errors for central measurements is 0.05, also at both time points. We assume that the simulated variance is

```
/*Create "observed" central (YC) and local (YL) scores by adding measurement error
to true scores */
Data _tmp_2; Set _tmp_1;
YC1  = FC  + rannor(3)*sqrt(0.05);     YL1  = FL  + rannor(4)*sqrt(0.10);
YC2  = FC  + rannor(5)*sqrt(0.05);     YL2  = FL  + rannor(6)*sqrt(0.10);
Keep ID YC1 YL1 YC2 YL2;
Run;
Proc Means Data=_tmp_2; Run;
```

Figure 4.45 Simulating observed values.

smaller for central location, which reflects the likely operational reality that central location assessments will be conducted by the same set of machines and/or evaluators. Note that we retain, as in real life, only observed data in the dataset "_tmp_2".

Figure 4.46 depicts the implementation of the corresponding model. Under the "Lineqs" statement there are now five equations (compared with three equations in Figure 4.36), representing now two time points. Under "Variance" statement there is an analogous set of variables and parameters, the exception being the measurement errors which are now free parameters that need to be estimated. To inform this model that, for example, variances of the measurement errors for local measurements should be the same and thus we used the same parameter "vareYL" assigned to both error terms "eYL1" and "eYL2".

Figure 4.36 includes only one line of code under "Cov" statement, informing the model that local measurement errors and central measurement errors are independent (the covariance between variables representing those errors is zero). The current model includes four measurement errors with the assumption that all of them are independent from each other: the set of six pair-wise statements ("eYC1 eYL1 = 0,... eYC2 eYL2 = 0") declares the independence of the

```
proc calis cov data = _tmp_2 method = ML technique = LEVMAR MEANSTR all;
Lineqs
FL = 0 intercept  + a FC + dFL,
YC1 = b intercept + FC  + eYC1,    YL1 = c intercept + FL  + eYL1,
YC2 = b intercept + FC  + eYC2,    YL2 = c intercept + FL  + eYL2;
Variance
FC   = varFC   , dFL  = vardFL  ,
eYC1 =  vareYC , eYC2 =  vareYC ,
eYL1 =  vareYL , eYL2 =  vareYL ;
Cov
eYC1 eYL1 = 0 , eYC1 eYC2 = 0 , eYC1 eYL2 = 0 ,
eYL1 eYC2 = 0 , eYL1 eYL2 = 0 ,
eYC2 eYL2 = 0 ;
Testfunc interceptFL1 ; interceptFL1  = c - a*b;
run;
```

Figure 4.46 Modeling relationship between true scores with two observations per subject.

variables representing measurement errors. The "Testfunc" statement is the same as we had in model with just one observation (from Figure 4.36).

After execution of the SAS code from Figures 4.44–4.46, Figure 4.47 shows partial output from the CALIS procedure. The estimated value of the slope between true local and central measurements is 1.1039 ("...+ 1.1039(**) FC +..."), which is practically equal to the value of the 1.1 used in the simulation. The estimated value of the intercept is −0.13117 ("interceptFL1 −0.13117..."; in simulation the value of intercept was defined as −0.1). Other estimated parameters in the model are also close to values used to simulate data. For example, variance of the disturbance term in the regression for true scores is

```
                        Linear Equations
FL  =          0       intercept  +   1.1039(**) FC  +   1.0000 dFL
YC1 =   4.9647(**) intercept  +   1.0000     FC  +   1.0000 eYC1
YL1 =   5.3496(**) intercept  +   1.0000     FL  +   1.0000 eYL1
YC2 =   4.9647(**) intercept  +   1.0000     FC  +   1.0000 eYC2
YL2 =   5.3496(**) intercept  +   1.0000     FL  +   1.0000 eYL2
```

Effects in Linear Equations

Variable	Predictor	Parameter	Estimate	Standard Error	t Value	Pr > |t|
FL	intercept		0			
FL	FC	a	1.10393	0.01606	68.7501	<.0001
YC1	intercept	b	4.96473	0.03462	143.4	<.0001
YC1	FC		1.00000			
YL1	intercept	c	5.34957	0.04114	130.0	<.0001
YL1	FL		1.00000			
YC2	intercept	b	4.96473	0.03462	143.4	<.0001
YC2	FC		1.00000			
YL2	intercept	c	5.34957	0.04114	130.0	<.0001
YL2	FL		1.00000			

Estimates for Variances of Exogenous Variables

Variable Type	Variable	Parameter	Estimate	Standard Error	t Value	Pr > |t|
Latent	FC	varFC	1.17199	0.05358	21.8735	<.0001
Disturbance	dFL	vardFL	0.20970	0.01342	15.6267	<.0001
Error	eYC1	vareYC	0.05048	0.00226	22.3495	<.0001
	eYC2	vareYC	0.05048	0.00226	22.3495	<.0001
	eYL1	vareYL	0.10622	0.00475	22.3495	<.0001
	eYL2	vareYL	0.10622	0.00475	22.3495	<.0001

Covariances Among Exogenous Variables

Var1	Var2	Estimate	Standard Error	t Value	Pr > |t|
eYC1	eYL1	0			
eYC1	eYC2	0			
eYC1	eYL2	0			
eYL1	eYC2	0			
eYL1	eYL2	0			
eYC2	eYL2	0			

Tests for Parametric Functions

Parametric Function	Estimate	Standard Error	t Value	Pr > |t|
interceptFL1	−0.13117	0.08154	−1.6086	0.1077

Figure 4.47 Partial output for the estimation of the parameters of the relationship between true scores with two observations per subjects.

estimated as 0.20970 ("Disturbance dFL vardFL 0.20970...") versus 0.2 used in simulation. The variance of the "true" central score is estimated as 1.17199 ("Latent FC varFC 1.17199...") versus 1.2 in simulations ("...+rannor(1)*sqrt(1.2);" in Figure 4.44). The estimated variances of the measurement errors ("Error eYC1 vareYC 0.05048..." and "... eYL1 vareYL 0.10622...") are also practically the same compared with values used to simulate data ("...+ rannor(3)*sqrt(0.05);" and "...+ rannor(4)*sqrt(0.10);" in Figure 4.45).

When discussing the same model with just one observation per subject, we also showed what would happen if observed measurements are assumed to be "perfect." We demonstrated that, in this case, results based on the CALIS procedure will be equivalent to the results of simple regression using the REG procedure. In case of two observations, the situation is almost the same.

Let us start with modification of the model implementation using the CALIS procedure (see Figure 4.48) by simply replacing the following four lines (which specify variance of the measurement errors as free parameters needed to be estimated; from Figure 4.46)

```
eYC1 = vareYC ,
eYC2 = vareYC ,
eYL1 = vareYL ,
eYL2 = vareYL ;
```

by a small value of 0.00001:

```
eYC1 = 0.00001 ,
eYC2 = 0.00001 ,
eYL1 = 0.00001 ,
eYL2 = 0.00001 ;
```

```
proc calis cov data = _tmp_2 method = ML technique = LEVMAR MEANSTR all;
Lineqs
FL = 0 intercept  + a FC + dFL,
YC1 = b intercept + FC + eYC1,    YL1 = c intercept + FL  + eYL1,
YC2 = b intercept + FC  + eYC2,   YL2 = c intercept + FL  + eYL2;
Variance
FC   = varFC    , dFL  =   vardFL  ,
eYC1  =  0.00001, eYC2  =   0.00001,
eYL1  =  0.00001, eYL2  =   0.00001;
Cov
eYC1 eYL1 = 0 , eYC1 eYC2 = 0 , eYC1 eYL2 = 0 ,
eYL1 eYC2 = 0 , eYL1 eYL2 = 0 ,
eYC2 eYL2 = 0 ;
Testfunc interceptFL1 ; interceptFL1  = c - a*b;
run;
```

Figure 4.48 Modeling relationship between true scores with two observations per subject, assuming no measurement errors in observed measurements.

```
                         Linear Equations
FL   =          0      intercept  +  ·1.0807(**) FC  +   1.0000 dFL
YC1  =    4.9647(**) intercept    +   1.0000     FC  +   1.0000 eYC1
YL1  =    5.3496(**) intercept    +   1.0000     FL  +   1.0000 eYL1
YC2  =    4.9647(**) intercept    +   1.0000     FC  +   1.0000 eYC2
YL2  =    5.3496(**) intercept    +   1.0000     FL  +   1.0000 eYL2

              Estimates for Variances of Exogenous Variables
Variable                                       Standard
Type          Variable   Parameter   Estimate    Error     t Value   Pr > |t|
Latent        FC         varFC       1.19723     0.05357   22.3494   <.0001
Disturbance   dFL        vardFL      0.29304     0.01311   22.3487   <.0001
Error         eYC1                   0.0000100
              eYC2                   0.0000100
              eYL1                   0.0000100
              eYL2                   0.0000100

              Tests for Parametric Functions
Parametric                    Standard
Function       Estimate         Error      t Value    Pr > |t|
interceptFL1   -0.01564        0.07958     -0.1966     0.8441
```

Figure 4.49 Partial output for the estimation of the parameters of the relationship between true scores with two observations per subjects (assuming no measurement errors).

Figure 4.49 represents partial output based on the model with no measurement errors. The estimated slope (1.0807) and intercept (−0.01564) are, as expected, different from values used to simulate data. We also expect the same estimated values for intercept and slope using simple linear regression. Earlier, we considered the following two equations

$$YL1_i = FL_i + eYL1_i$$

$$YL2_i = FL_i + eYL2_i.$$

If the measurement errors are postulated as zero, then these equations will be reduced to

$$YL1_i = FL_i$$

$$YL2_i = FL_i.$$

And from these two equations the following relationship between local true and local observed measurements emerges:

$$FL_i = \left(YL1_i + YL2_i\right)/2.$$

The same relationship will also be true between central true and central observed measurements in the absence of measurement errors. Figure 4.50 shows the creation of the new observations representing local and central measurements as the means of the observed measurements and using those

```
Data _reg_;  Set _tmp_2;
YC=(YC1+YC2)/2;  YL=(YL1+YL2)/2;
Run;
Proc Reg data=_reg_ ;
Model YL=YC;
Run; Quit;
```

Figure 4.50 Modeling relationship between observed outcomes with the REG procedure with two observations per subject.

		Parameter Estimates			
		Parameter	Standard		
Variable	DF	Estimate	Error	t Value	Pr > |t|
Intercept	1	-0.01562	0.07960	-0.20	0.8444
YC	1	1.08066	0.01566	69.02	<.0001

Figure 4.51 Intercept and slope (REG procedure).

new variables in the regression. Figure 4.51 shows the estimated intercept and slope (by REG procedure) with the results matching the earlier results from Figure 4.49.

4.2 Cronbach's Alpha

4.2.1 Likert-Type Scales

Internal consistency reliability is the property of a multi-item scale and assesses the extent of inter-item relationships. The main assumption is that all individual items in a domain are affected by a single latent construct and, as such, should behave in concert. Cronbach's coefficient alpha is the most widely used method to assess internal consistency (Cronbach 1951). For a domain represented by n items, Cronbach's coefficient alpha is represented by the following formula:

$$\alpha = \frac{n}{n-1}\left(1 - \frac{\sum_{i=1}^{n} Var(X_i)}{Var\left(\sum_{i=1}^{n} X_i\right)}\right) \tag{4.24}$$

where $Var(X_i)$ is the variance of the ith item, $\sum$ represents the summation over the n items, and $Var\left(\sum_{i=1}^{n} X_i\right)$ can be viewed as the variance of a domain score (domain score is calculated as a sum of n items). Note that $Var\left(\sum_{i=1}^{n} X_i\right)$ in Eq. (4.24) is equal to the sum of all elements in the variance–covariance matrix associated with the set of n variables X_i (see Figure 4.52) and $\sum_{i=1}^{n} Var(X_i)$ is equal to the sum of the diagonal elements of the same variance–covariance matrix.

$$\begin{bmatrix} var(X_1) & covar(X_2, X_1) & \dots & covar(X_n, X_1) \\ covar(X_1, X_2) & var(X_2) & \dots & covar(X_n, X_2) \\ \dots & \dots & \dots & \dots \\ covar(X_1, X_n) & covar(X_2, X_n) & \dots & var(X_n) \end{bmatrix}$$

Figure 4.52 Variance–covariance matrix associated with the set of variables X_i ($i = 1, 2, \dots, n$).

$$\begin{bmatrix} 3.0 & 1.4 & 3.5 \\ 1.4 & 1.2 & 1.5 \\ 3.5 & 1.5 & 6.5 \end{bmatrix}$$

Figure 4.53 Variance–covariance matrix example for a domain with three items.

Consider a domain with three items (Figure 4.53 represents an example of the variance–covariance matrix for those three items).

Note that variance–covariance matrix is always square and symmetric. The symmetry property is the consequence of the symmetry property of the covariance; that is, for any i and j, $covar(X_i, X_j) = covar(X_j, X_i)$. To estimate Cronbach's coefficient alpha (as stated by formula 4.24), we only need variances and covariances of those three items:

$$\alpha = \frac{3}{3-1}\left(1 - \frac{(3.0+1.2+6.5)}{(3.0+1.2+6.5+2\times1.4+2\times3.5+2\times1.5)}\right) = 0.817.$$

Figure 4.54 creates the simulated dataset with three items ($X1$, $X2$, and $X3$) per subject ($n = 100$) based on the variance–covariance matrix represented by Figure 4.53. Then the CORR procedure is used to estimate Cronbach's coefficient alpha (see Figure 4.55 for partial output). First, let us compare this variance–covariance matrix (see Figure 4.53 and values under the "datalines" statement in the data step in Figure 4.54) with data generated from a matrix based on simulated data (see Figure 4.55 under "Covariance Matrix, DF = 99"). We can see that the two sets of values are close; for example, the variance of the item

```
options nocenter;
data _cov_ (type=cov);
input
_TYPE_ $   _NAME_ $   X1       X2       X3;
datalines;
 COV        X1        3        1.4      3.5
 COV        X2        1.4      1.2      1.5
 COV        X3        3.5      1.5      6.5
 N          .         100      100      100
;
run;
proc simnormal data=_cov_ out=_sim_ds numreal=100 seed=700; var X1 X2 X3; run;
proc corr data=_sim_ds alpha nomiss Cov; Var X1 X2 X3; run;
```

Figure 4.54 Simulating a dataset and estimating Cronbach's coefficient alpha.

```
The CORR Procedure
   3  Variables:     X1         X2         X3

                 Covariance Matrix, DF = 99
                     X1                  X2                 X3
X1          3.242708788          1.442906269        3.681151721
X2          1.442906269          1.241491003        1.579724553
X3          3.681151721          1.579724553        6.406721696


   Cronbach Coefficient Alpha
Variables                    Alpha
Raw                       0.827679
```

Figure 4.55 Cronbach's coefficient alpha: CORR procedure partial output.

X3 was defined as 6.5, and, in simulated dataset, this variance was calculated to be 6.4 (6.406721696). Note that the estimated Cronbach's coefficient alpha value of 0.828 ("Raw 0.827679"; see Figure 4.55) is also close to the value of 0.817, which was calculated based on the initial variance–covariance matrix.

If items are independent, then all off-diagonal elements in the variance–covariance matrix (Figure 4.52) will be zero, with $Var\left(\sum_{i=1}^{n} X_i\right)$ being reduced to the sum of only diagonal elements (i.e., $\sum_{i=1}^{n} Var(X_i)$) and hence

$$\alpha = \frac{n}{n-1}\left(1 - \frac{\sum_{i=1}^{n} Var(X_i)}{Var\left(\sum_{i=1}^{n} X_i\right)}\right) = \frac{n}{n-1}\left(1 - \frac{\sum_{i=1}^{n} Var(X_i)}{\sum_{i=1}^{n} Var(X_i)}\right),$$

$$\alpha = \frac{n}{n-1}\left(1 - \frac{\sum_{i=1}^{n} Var(X_i)}{\sum_{i=1}^{n} Var(X_i)}\right) = \frac{n}{n-1}(1-1) = 0$$

As a result, Cronbach's coefficient alpha for such a domain will be zero. To illustrate this outcome, we only need to replace the data step from Figure 4.54 by the data step represented by Figure 4.56, where all off-diagonal covariances are replaced by zeros (Figure 4.57 represents partial output).

```
data _cov_ (type=cov);
input
_TYPE_ $  _NAME_ $   X1      X2      X3;
datalines;
COV        X1        3       0       0
COV        X2        0       1.2     0
COV        X3        0       0       6.5
N           .        100     100     100
;
run;
proc simnormal data=_cov_ out=_sim_ds numreal=100 seed=700; var X1 X2 X3; run;
proc corr data=_sim_ds alpha nomiss Cov; Var X1 X2 X3; run;
```

Figure 4.56 Simulating a dataset with independent items and estimating Cronbach's coefficient alpha.

```
                Covariance Matrix, DF = 99
                  X1              X2              X3
X1        3.242708788     -0.104241769    -0.196767533
X2       -0.104241769      1.319198924     0.221433193
X3       -0.196767533      0.221433193     6.105529772


                        Simple Statistics
Variable      N       Mean    Std Dev       Sum     Minimum     Maximum
X1          100   -0.14151    1.80075  -14.15050    -4.64632     3.84692
X2          100   -0.07376    1.14856   -7.37601    -2.61402     2.64764
X3          100    0.14061    2.47094   14.06144    -5.22804     6.54136


 Cronbach Coefficient Alpha
Variables                Alpha
Raw                  -.022718
```

Figure 4.57 Partial output with results of the simulation with independent items.

First, we note that, although very close to zero, the estimated Cronbach's coefficient alpha is represented by a negative estimate of -0.022718. It demonstrates the noteworthy fact that Cronbach's coefficient alpha could be less than zero. Recall that $Var\left(\sum_{i=1}^{n} X_i\right)$ is equal to the sum of all elements of the variance–covariance matrix. If the sum of off-diagonal covariance elements is negative, then

$$\sum_{i=1}^{n} Var\left(X_i\right) > Var\left(\sum_{i=1}^{n} X_i\right),$$

$$\frac{\sum_{i=1}^{n} Var\left(X_i\right)}{Var\left(\sum_{i=1}^{n} X_i\right)} > 1,$$

$$\left(1 - \frac{\sum_{i=1}^{n} Var\left(X_i\right)}{Var\left(\sum_{i=1}^{n} X_i\right)}\right) < 0.$$

Let us demonstrate above with a simulated example (see Figures 4.58 for simulation and Figure 4.59 for partial output). Note that, for this simulation, the

```
data _cov_ (type=cov);
input
_TYPE_ $  _NAME_ $   X1       X2       X3;
datalines;
COV       X1          3      -0.8     -2.7
COV       X2       -0.8       1.2      0.6
COV       X3       -2.7       0.6      6.5
N          .        100       100      100
;
run;
proc simnormal data=_cov_ out=_sim_ds numreal=100 seed=700; var X1 X2 X3; run;
proc corr data=_sim_ds alpha nomiss Cov; Var X1 X2 X3; run;
```

Figure 4.58 The simulation to generate negative Cronbach's coefficient alpha.

```
            Covariance Matrix, DF = 99
                 X1              X2              X3
X1        3.242708788    -0.959245100    -3.062364401
X2       -0.959245100     1.365679432     0.928379125
X3       -3.062364401     0.928379125     6.672420284

  Cronbach Coefficient Alpha
Variables              Alpha
Raw                 -1.82157
```

Figure 4.59 Partial output with results of the simulation with negative Cronbach's coefficient alpha.

Cronbach's coefficient alpha value of −1.82 ("Raw −1.82157") is notably less than zero.

The good news is that for a vast majority of the scales, this type of result will occur if a mistake was done in recording item values. For example, a reverse scoring transformation should have been applied, but, for some reason, it was not. Another possible situation is when the initial validation was performed, and it could have been discovered that some items do not belong to a domain they were initially assigned to.

There is, of course, also a completely different type of scale with causal items (indicator variables). For this type of scale, we do not anticipate that items will march together (or have a substantial positive correlations). Instead, we anticipate that most items for this type of scale will not have tangible positive correlations. It should be noted that for this type of scales, it is not recommended to assess Cronbach's coefficient alpha (Fayers et al. 1997; Streiner 2003).

The maximum value of one for Cronbach's coefficient alpha can be reached when a variance for any item and covariance for any two items in a domain are numerically *identical*. If we posit that all elements in the matrix represented by Figure 4.52 are the same, then the following is true:

$$Var(X_i) = Var(X_j) = covar(X_i, X_j) = Var(X).$$

Then in Eq. (4.24), we can simply replace $Var\left(\sum_{i=1}^{n} X_i\right)$ by $n^2 Var(X)$ (where value of n^2 represents a number of elements in the square matrix) and $\sum_{i=1}^{n} Var(X_i)$ by $nVar(X)$ (which is simply a sum of the diagonal elements). Consequently, Eq. (4.24) can be simplified as shown below

$$\alpha = \frac{n}{n-1}\left(1 - \frac{nVar(X)}{Var(nX)}\right),$$

$$\alpha = \frac{n}{n-1}\left(1 - \frac{nVar(X)}{n^2 Var(X)}\right),$$

$$\alpha = \frac{n}{n-1}\left(1 - \frac{n}{n^2}\right) = 1.$$

It is worth mentioning again that to achieve a value of one for Cronbach's coefficient alpha, we assume that the variances and covariances of items in a domain should be identical. Yet, the means for every item still can be different, which indicates that, technically, there is no requirement that responses to items be identical. If that were the case, it would mean that all items are redundant, and we can pick any one item from this domain to get the same information. To simulate this, we can simply replace the data step in Figure 4.58 by the following SAS code that sets values of the variances for every item and their covariances to the same value, which here is the arbitrary value of 1:

```
data _cov_ (type=cov);
input
_TYPE_ $ _NAME_ $ X1 X2 X3;
datalines;
 COV X1 1 1 1
 COV X2 1 1 1
 COV X3 1 1 1
 N  .  100 100 100
;
run;
```

Another worthwhile point is that items can share a perfect correlation of one yet still have different variances. In this case, Cronbach's coefficient alpha will not achieve its maximum possible value of one. For simplicity (and without loss of generality), consider a domain with just two items (represented by variables X_1 and X_2):

$$\alpha = \frac{2}{2-1}\left(1 - \frac{Var(X_1) + Var(X_2)}{Var(X_1 + X_2)}\right)$$

$$\alpha = \frac{2}{1}\left(1 - \frac{Var(X_1) + Var(X_2)}{Var(X_1) + Var(X_2) + 2\,cov(X_1, X_2)}\right),$$

$$\alpha = \frac{2}{1}\left(1 - \frac{Var(X_1) + Var(X_2)}{Var(X_1) + Var(X_2) + 2Corr(X_1, X_2)\sqrt{Var(X_1)Var(X_2)}}\right).$$

If $Corr(X_1, X_2) = 1$, but $Var(X_1) \neq Var(X_2)$, the above equation will generate a value less than one.

To illustrate the above points, we will slightly change the way data are being simulated. In previous simulations, we first defined a variance–covariance matrix and then used this matrix as the input for the SIMNORMAL procedure. For the current simulation, though, we will use the more conventional approach to define parameters of the simulated dataset through defining the means and variances for every item and the correlations between items. Note that we do not need to change anything in the SIMNORMAL procedure – the procedure is "intelligent" enough to recognize the structure and type of the input data set to use it correctly.

The simulation (see Figure 4.60) has three items $X1$, $X2$, and $X3$, which perfectly correlated, but have different variances (2^2, 3^2, and 1.5^2) and different means (5, 8, and 6). Figure 4.61 represents partial output of the CORR

```
options nocenter;
data _corr_(type=corr);
input
_TYPE_ $  _NAME_ $  X1       X2       X3;
datalines;
  CORR     X1         1        1        1
  CORR     X2         1        1        1
  CORR     X3         1        1        1
  MEAN     .          5        8        6
  STD      .          2        3        1.5
  N        .          100      100      100
;
run;

proc simnormal data=_corr_ out=_sim_ds numreal=100 seed=100; var X1 X2 X3; run;
proc corr data=_sim_ds alpha nomiss Cov; Var X1 X2 X3; run;
```

Figure 4.60 Estimating Cronbach's coefficient alpha for a domain with perfectly correlated items.

```
                    Covariance Matrix, DF = 99
                  X1                  X2                  X3
X1          4.53219088          6.79828632          3.39914316
X2          6.79828632         10.19742947          5.09871474
X3          3.39914316          5.09871474          2.54935737

                            Simple Statistics
Variable       N        Mean        Std Dev         Sum       Minimum       Maximum
X1            100     5.09801        2.12889     509.80055    -2.84830       9.36792
X2            100     8.14701        3.19334     814.70083    -3.77244      14.55188
X3            100     6.07350        1.59667     607.35041     0.11378       9.27594

  Cronbach Coefficient Alpha
Variables            Alpha
Raw                0.958580
Standardized       1.000000

             Cronbach Coefficient Alpha with Deleted Variable
                    Raw Variables              Standardized Variables
Deleted        Correlation                  Correlation
Variable       with Total        Alpha      with Total        Alpha
X1              1.000000       0.888889       1.000000       1.000000
X2              1.000000       0.979592       1.000000       1.000000
X3              1.000000       0.960000       1.000000       1.000000
```

Figure 4.61 The CORR Procedure output: Cronbach's coefficient alpha for a domain with perfectly correlated items.

procedure. As anticipated the value of the Cronbach's coefficient alpha, which is 0.96 ("Raw 0.958580"), is less than 1. The CORR procedure also provides results for the same set of variables but standardizes them first to have the same variance. In this simulation, standardized Cronbach's coefficient alpha obviously is equal to 1. Note that we almost always should use raw Cronbach's coefficient alpha.

Then do we even need standardized Cronbach's coefficient alpha? To answer this, let us consider a domain represented by only two items with extremely different range: say, the first item is represented by a Likert-type scale from 1 to 5 and the second item is represented by the Visual Analogue Scale from 0 to 10. If we use raw scores for those items for assessment of Cronbach's coefficient alpha, then standardized Cronbach's coefficient alpha will be the appropriate choice. But for a domain like this, to calculate a domain score, we will not simply sum those two items (if someone does then there is something very wrong with this scale). The proper approach will be to transform, for example, the score for the first item to be also from 0 to 10. And after scores for the first item are transformed, only then should we assess Cronbach's coefficient alpha. Generally speaking, if scores for some items in a domain should be reversed scored and/or transformed to be used in summation to calculate a domain score, then those scores should be used in calculation of Cronbach's coefficient alpha for this domain. Going back to the question of whether there is even a need for a standardized Cronbach's coefficient alpha as a part of the quantitative validation of a scale, then the answer is clear: not really.

Cronbach's coefficient alpha of 0.7 may be considered a minimum threshold for measurement scales (Fayers and Machin 2016; Reeve et al. 2013). Generally, values above 0.8 would be desired (de Vet et al. 2011; Fayers and Machin 2016; Nunnally and Bernstein 1994; Streiner et al. 2015). A consensus for the value of Cronbach's coefficient alpha is between 0.70 and 0.90 (de Vet et al. 2011), but values between 0.90 and 0.95 are also acceptable (Cappelleri et al. 2013).

It should be stressed that very high values for Cronbach's coefficient alpha do not necessarily imply that the scale is well designed. After all, having a lot of items in a scale whose items barely correlate with each other will produce a decent Cronbach's coefficient alpha. Let us simulate data for a domain with 12 items with a predefined pairwise correlation of only 0.2 (see Figure 4.62 for simulation and Figure 4.63 for partial output). As we can see the Cronbach's coefficient alpha is more than 0.7 (0.753707), which should indicate that this domain has an acceptable internal consistency reliability. But we know that this is not a well-behaved domain, because correlations between items are very small. This highlights an important point: calculating and considering Cronbach's coefficient alpha is generally not enough to assess internal consistency reliability in its entirety. There are three additional sets of outcomes that should also be evaluated.

```
data _corr_(type=corr);
input
_TYPE_ $ _NAME_ $ i1   i2   i3   i4   i5   i6   i7   i8   i9   i10  i11  i12  ;
datalines;
CORR     i1      1    .2   .2   .2   .2   .2   .2   .2   .2   .2   .2   .2
CORR     i2      .2   1    .2   .2   .2   .2   .2   .2   .2   .2   .2   .2
CORR     i3      .2   .2   1    .2   .2   .2   .2   .2   .2   .2   .2   .2
CORR     i4      .2   .2   .2   1    .2   .2   .2   .2   .2   .2   .2   .2
CORR     i5      .2   .2   .2   .2   1    .2   .2   .2   .2   .2   .2   .2
CORR     i6      .2   .2   .2   .2   .2   1    .2   .2   .2   .2   .2   .2
CORR     i7      .2   .2   .2   .2   .2   .2   1    .2   .2   .2   .2   .2
CORR     i8      .2   .2   .2   .2   .2   .2   .2   1    .2   .2   .2   .2
CORR     i9      .2   .2   .2   .2   .2   .2   .2   .2   1    .2   .2   .2
CORR     i10     .2   .2   .2   .2   .2   .2   .2   .2   .2   1    .2   .2
CORR     i11     .2   .2   .2   .2   .2   .2   .2   .2   .2   .2   1    .2
CORR     i12     .2   .2   .2   .2   .2   .2   .2   .2   .2   .2   .2   1
MEAN     .       5    8    6    7    5.5  7.1  8    8.5  6.3  6.8  9    5.8
STD      .       .5   .5   .5   .5   .5   .5   .5   .5   .5   .5   .5   .5
N        .       100  100  100  100  100  100  100  100  100  100  100  100
;
run;
proc simnormal data=_corr_ out=_sim_ds numreal=100 seed=100; var i1-i12; run;
proc corr data=_sim_ds alpha nomiss Cov; Var i1-i12; run;
```

Figure 4.62 Simulating a domain with low correlated items and estimating Cronbach's coefficient alpha.

```
Cronbach Coefficient Alpha

Variables             Alpha
Raw                   0.753707
Standardized          0.754134

          Cronbach Coefficient Alpha with Deleted Variable
                Raw Variables              Standardized Variables
Deleted    Correlation                 Correlation
Variable   with Total       Alpha      with Total       Alpha
i1         0.482837      0.725167      0.489134      0.725511
i2         0.308769      0.746174      0.304987      0.747221
i3         0.348122      0.742170      0.343488      0.742785
i4         0.304307      0.746091      0.306726      0.747021
i5         0.375815      0.738571      0.374777      0.739140
i6         0.443332      0.730952      0.446918      0.730599
i7         0.301351      0.748209      0.301693      0.747598
i8         0.370388      0.739122      0.368408      0.739885
i9         0.503614      0.723721      0.504352      0.723660
i10        0.411050      0.734339      0.412010      0.734756
i11        0.506375      0.722097      0.508745      0.723124
i12        0.305657      0.746973      0.301128      0.747662
```

Figure 4.63 Partial output for simulation of a domain with low correlated items.

The first one, as we have just mentioned, is that the correlations between items should not be too low (say, <0.20) or too high (say, >0.80). Our empirical experience suggests that inter-item correlations between 0.4 and 0.7 are most likely for most reliable measures. But those thresholds should be applied only if data are representative of the entire population of interest – that is, as we discussed earlier in this chapter, there should be a representative number of "mild," "moderate," and "severe" subjects as differentiated by the scale.

Consider a domain with a score range from 0 to 10. We should have a substantial number of subjects for all levels of scores. But, for instance, such is not likely to be met at the baseline when there are a relatively small number of "mild" subjects (if any), a considerable number of "moderate" subjects and a moderate number of "severe" subjects. This composition, as well as other imbalanced composition with regard to severity, could lead to unstable and low pairwise correlations. As such, provided that treatments are beneficial, post-baseline data are usually more suitable for internal consistency reliability assessments. Note also that when using post-baseline data for this type of analysis, the data should be pooled from all treatment arms (assuming that treatment is beneficial, and a study also has a placebo or control arm). This approach is more likely to provide considerable range of scores for a domain, from low to high, across the breadth of measurement spectrum.

The second set of outcomes, which should also be evaluated, is the corrected item-to-total correlations. If we want to assess how an item relates to a domain, we cannot simply calculate correlation between a domain score and this item score, because this score for this item is the part of the domain score, and as a result the relationship will be overstated. To escape this issue, when corrected item-to-total correlations are computed, a domain score is recalculated every time to exclude the item we investigate. In the CORR procedure output (see Figure 4.63), the results are given under "`Correlation with Total`" (for "`Raw Variables`" part of the output). For example, for item 1 the corrected item-to-total correlation is 0.48 (`0.482837`). For good scale, it is an expectation that all those corrected item-to-total correlations should be at least 0.3 (Nunnally and Bernstein 1994; Squires et al. 2011) and, based on our years of empirical experience, preferably at least 0.4 or larger.

For this simulated example (see Figure 4.63), we have item-to-total correlations for seven items (from 12) with values less than 0.4, which, if it were a real scale, would indicate that more than half of the items do not sufficiently correlate with corrected total score and those items could be the candidates for removal. In practice, we anticipate that for a well-designed scale with data coming from a representative sample, the corrected item-to-total correlations will be larger than 0.4 for all items (again, with some reservations for baseline data given the restriction on the range of data). The previously stated recommendation, that items in a domain should be reversed scored and/or transformed for use in Cronbach's coefficient alpha calculations, is even more profound for calculations of the corrected item-to-total correlations – failing to do so will lead to unpredictable results for this second part of the analyses.

The third (and final) part of additional analyses (beyond Cronbach's coefficient), which is an equally important part, involve computing Cronbach's coefficient alpha with each variable (item) deleted. This formulation is a set of Cronbach's coefficient alpha using all but one item (referenced as the deleted item). Let us say a scale has 12 items. Then there will be 12 different Cronbach's coefficient alphas calculated, with every one of them based on only the remaining

11 items. For example, if item 1 is excluded (deleted item) from the calculation, then Cronbach's coefficient alpha based on the remaining results will be 0.73 ("i1 ... 0.725167 ..."; see Figure 4.63 under "Raw Variables" and then under "Alpha").

For a well-designed scale, all those values should be smaller than the value of the Cronbach's coefficient alpha when all items were used, as it is assumed that all items are needed to cover different facets of the same concept. If, suddenly, the value of Cronbach's coefficient alpha increases when an item was deleted (relative to the value when all items were used), then the item is a decrement to internal consistency of the underlying concept. In our simulation (see Figure 4.63), the overall Cronbach's coefficient alpha based on all 12 items was 0.75 ("Raw 0.753707") and, as we can see, all values of Cronbach's coefficient alpha with deleted variables are smaller than 0.75, meaning that all items are "good" from this particular perspective and no item should be deleted from the scale. In addition to Cronbach's coefficient alpha, this added evaluation regarding item deletion and the two other criteria noted here should be evaluated in tandem.

Let us summarize this example. Overall, Cronbach's coefficient alpha value was acceptable (larger than 0.7). Yet between item correlations were small (they were only about 0.2). And the item-to-total correlations for more than a half of items were also smaller than 0.4. But values of Cronbach's coefficient alphas with deleted variables were smaller than overall Cronbach's coefficient alpha, meaning that all items are needed. These results emphasize the importance of investigating those additional set of outcomes to support internal consistency – only calculating and reporting Cronbach's coefficient alpha is just not enough. Additional critiques of Cronbach's alpha appear elsewhere, including the use of coefficient omega as an alternative estimate of reliability (DeVellis 2017).

4.2.2 Dichotomous Items

Generally, items in a PRO scale are designed in a way that allows patients to select or pick a response from the range of the values. For example, for the concept of pain, it could be 11 categories rating scale (values of 0, 1, 2, . . ., 9, 10). Another often used scale is the five-category Likert or Likert-like scale. A common property of this type of responses is that they are often considered or treated as continuous responses. When summing responses from all items in a domain, we not only assume that distances between response categories are the same but also assume that a subject can have an underlying level of pain equal to, a non-integer, say, 8.7 (i.e., between categories). Because a subject is given an opportunity to select from a predefined set of discrete values, this particular subject would most likely select a value of 9 (i.e., closest integer to 8.7). From this reason, visual analog scales were introduced, where a subject selects a point across a continuum of values representing his or her response on a scale, often represented by a straight horizontal line 100 mm in length.

In many cases, when a scale has items with dichotomous responses, the continuous approximation can still hold. It is atypical that we would have a true binary item (as, for example, employed vs. unemployed, alive vs. dead) as a part of a measurement sale. Typically, those binary items could be considered as taken from a continuum of possibilities, and then we force a subject to make a choice.

Consider, for instance, the Roland-Morris Disability Questionnaire (Roland and Morris 1983), which has 24 items with all of them binary. For example, the first item is "I stay at home most of the time because of the pain in my back." It is easy to see that instead of "Yes/No" option for the response, the better approach would be reformulate item as "I stay at home because of the pain in my back" (i.e., exclude "most of the time") and have the following Likert scale response options: Never (0), Almost Never (1), Occasionally/Sometimes (2), Most of the time (3), Every time (4). This item (in its original yes/no form) simply forces a subject to (first) decide what the response would be on the continuous scale (Never, Almost Never, Occasionally/Sometimes, Most of the time, Every time) and (second) dichotomize the answer using "Most of the time" as a cut-off category (note that those words "Most of the time" are the part of the item).

Let us take a look at item 16 from the Roland-Morris Disability Questionnaire. This item is formulated as "I have trouble putting on my socks (or stockings) because of the pain in my back." Instead of the binary response for this item, the following response options would be more informative and appropriate: Not at all difficult (0), Mildly difficult (1), Moderately difficult (2), Extremely difficult (3). Again, a subject would probably think in terms of different levels of difficulty and then somehow dichotomize his or her response. But, in this example, the wording of the item does not even provide a clue for the cutoff, so every subject must decide which category should be used as the cutoff. For one subject, a "yes" answer will be selected only if it was extremely difficult "putting on . . . socks . . . because of the pain in . . . back." But for another subject, if it is only mildly difficult, he or she will respond "yes."

Response to binary items of this type is akin to the response to an item measuring change. When asking about the change from baseline, for instance, we are in fact asking the subject to perform a set of mental gymnastics: (i) recall what the measured outcome was at baseline, (ii) assess what the measured outcome is now, and (iii) subtract the baseline value from the current value. The point is that people do not think in binary terms; if they were, the vast majority of domains in measurement scales would be represented only by binary items. If we make the assumption that responses for a binary item can be considered to be representative of an underlying continuous distribution, then Pearson correlations between those

```
data _corr_(type=corr);
input
_TYPE_ $  _NAME_ $  i1    i2    i3    i4    i5    i6    i7    i8    i9    i10;
datalines;
  CORR      i1        1    .4    .5    .6    .6    .6    .6    .6    .6    .8
  CORR      i2       .4     1    .6    .6    .6    .6    .6    .6    .6    .6
  CORR      i3       .5    .6     1    .6    .6    .6    .6    .6    .6    .6
  CORR      i4       .6    .6    .6     1    .6    .6    .6    .6    .6    .6
  CORR      i5       .6    .6    .6    .6     1    .6    .6    .6    .6    .6
  CORR      i6       .6    .6    .6    .6    .6     1    .6    .6    .6    .6
  CORR      i7       .6    .6    .6    .6    .6    .6     1    .6    .6    .6
  CORR      i8       .6    .6    .6    .6    .6    .6    .6     1    .6    .6
  CORR      i9       .6    .6    .6    .6    .6    .6    .6    .6     1    .6
  CORR      i10      .8    .6    .6    .6    .6    .6    .6    .6    .6     1
  MEAN      .         7   7.8   6.5     7   7.4   7.1   7.2   7.4   6.9   6.8
  STD       .        .5    .6    .5    .5    .8    .5    .5    .5    .5    .5
  N         .      3000  3000  3000  3000  3000  3000  3000  3000  3000  3000
;
run;
proc simnormal data=_corr_ out=_sim_ds numreal=3000 seed=100; var i1-i10; run;
proc corr data=_sim_ds alpha nomiss Cov; Var i1-i10; Run;
```

Figure 4.64 Simulating a scale with 10 continuous items.

binary items will be "artificially" attenuated, being lower than they should be. We need to somehow account for the fact that those binary items represent dichotomized responses based on the more thorough and more comprehensive range of possible, though unspecified and hidden, response options.

To simulate a scale with binary responses, let us first simulate continuous items. Figure 4.64 represents a simulation for a hypothetical measurement scale represented by 10 items. We define the simulation so that most pairwise item correlations are equal to 0.6, except for correlations between items 1 and 2, 1 and 3, and 1 and 10, which are 0.4, 0.5, and 0.8. Figure 4.65 represents the partial output. Note that the simulated sample correlations are very close to the predefined values. Cronbach's coefficient alpha for this scale is 0.93, corrected item-to-total correlations are between 0.72 and 0.78, and values for Cronbach's coefficient alphas with deleted variables are all smaller than the overall Cronbach's coefficient alpha of 0.93, all of which indicate that every item in this scale should be kept.

Now, let's convert those continuous responses into binary responses (see Figure 4.66). To do so, we simply use the value of 7 as a cut-off score, which is near the mean value for all 10 items (mean range is from 6.5 to 7.8; see Figure 4.65). In the new dataset "_sim_ds1", items i1-i10 now have only two responses: 0 or 1. Figure 4.67 displays the output of the Cronbach's coefficient alpha analyses using binary items. Though we used a value of 7 as the cut-off to create binary responses, the means of the binary items differ a great deal, ranging from 0.17 to 0.91. For example, for item 2, about 91% of responses are equal to one, and only 9% of responses are equal to zero (giving a mean value of 0.91).

As expected, correlations between binary items using the Pearson correlation coefficient are notably smaller, and the majority of correlations are less than 0.4. But, even for those data, Cronbach's coefficient alpha, which in the case of binary

Simple Statistics

Variable	N	Mean	Std Dev	Sum	Minimum	Maximum
i1	3000	7.00495	0.49733	21015	5.03793	8.951165
i2	3000	7.81148	0.60203	23434	5.68761	10.12132
i3	3000	6.50797	0.49962	19524	4.57110	8.26737
i4	3000	7.00992	0.49911	21030	5.10844	8.93693
i5	3000	7.40094	0.79769	22203	4.65238	10.34704
i6	3000	7.11149	0.49936	21334	5.34016	8.79067
i7	3000	7.19859	0.49777	21596	5.60226	8.79644
i8	3000	7.40412	0.50191	22212	5.63837	9.10284
i9	3000	6.90732	0.50548	20722	5.07365	8.87907
i10	3000	6.81796	0.49882	20454	4.97059	8.73301

	Alpha
Variables	
Raw	0.932336
Standardized	0.937080

Cronbach Coefficient Alpha with Deleted Variable

Deleted Variable	Raw Variables		Standardized Variables	
	Correlation with Total	Alpha	Correlation with Total	Alpha
i1	0.720447	0.926112	0.724617	0.931623
i2	0.724878	0.926024	0.724377	0.931635
i3	0.732818	0.925526	0.733999	0.931313
i4	0.750947	0.924689	0.752275	0.930275
i5	0.748132	0.929577	0.747980	0.930485
i6	0.750897	0.924689	0.750447	0.930364
i7	0.739182	0.925246	0.740220	0.930864
i8	0.755471	0.924453	0.755895	0.930098
i9	0.753041	0.924536	0.753758	0.930202
i10	0.777914	0.923436	0.781323	0.928849

Pearson Correlation Coefficients, N = 3000
Prob > |r| under H0: Rho=0

	i1	i2	i3	i4	i5	i6	i7	i8	i9	i10
i1	1.00000	0.39660	0.48820	0.60492	0.60036	0.59473	0.57820	0.59214	0.59643	0.79171
		<.0001	<.0001	<.0001	<.0001	<.0001	<.0001	<.0001	<.0001	<.0001
i2	0.39660	1.00000	0.60110	0.59744	0.59522	0.61401	0.59979	0.61897	0.60892	0.60965
	<.0001		<.0001	<.0001	<.0001	<.0001	<.0001	<.0001	<.0001	<.0001
i3	0.48820	0.60110	1.00000	0.59595	0.60831	0.59549	0.59034	0.59721	0.60509	0.60353
	<.0001	<.0001		<.0001	<.0001	<.0001	<.0001	<.0001	<.0001	<.0001
i4	0.60492	0.59744	0.59595	1.00000	0.59527	0.59846	0.59367	0.61505	0.61518	0.60860
	<.0001	<.0001	<.0001		<.0001	<.0001	<.0001	<.0001	<.0001	<.0001
i5	0.60036	0.59522	0.60831	0.59527	1.00000	0.60931	0.58485	0.60292	0.60056	0.59968
	<.0001	<.0001	<.0001	<.0001		<.0001	<.0001	<.0001	<.0001	<.0001
i6	0.59473	0.61401	0.59549	0.59846	0.60931	1.00000	0.59499	0.60691	0.59758	0.60112
	<.0001	<.0001	<.0001	<.0001	<.0001		<.0001	<.0001	<.0001	<.0001
i7	0.57820	0.59979	0.59034	0.59367	0.58485	0.59499	1.00000	0.60598	0.60328	0.59460
	<.0001	<.0001	<.0001	<.0001	<.0001	<.0001		<.0001	<.0001	<.0001
i8	0.59214	0.61897	0.59721	0.61505	0.60292	0.60691	0.60598	1.00000	0.60579	0.60320
	<.0001	<.0001	<.0001	<.0001	<.0001	<.0001	<.0001		<.0001	<.0001
i9	0.59643	0.60892	0.60509	0.61518	0.60056	0.59758	0.60328	0.60579	1.00000	0.60139
	<.0001	<.0001	<.0001	<.0001	<.0001	<.0001	<.0001	<.0001		<.0001
i10	0.79171	0.60965	0.60353	0.60860	0.59968	0.60112	0.59460	0.60320	0.60139	1.00000
	<.0001	<.0001	<.0001	<.0001	<.0001	<.0001	<.0001	<.0001	<.0001	

Figure 4.65 Partial output for a scale with 10 continuous items: Cronbach's coefficient alpha.

```
Data _sim_ds1; Set  _sim_ds;
array v{10} i1-i10;
Do k=1 to 10;
If v[k]>=7 Then
    Do;   v[k]=1;    End;
Else
    Do;   v[k]=0;    End;
End;
Run;
Proc Corr data=_sim_ds1 alpha nomiss Cov; Var i1-i10; Run;
```

Figure 4.66   Simulating binary responses.

data is referred to as Kuder–Richardson 20 (KR-20), continues to be relatively high with a value of 0.84. Comparing the output from Figure 4.67 with output from Figure 4.65, we also see that corrected item-to-total correlations and Cronbach coefficient alpha (KR-20) with deleted variables are also lower for binary data (versus continuous data).

Knowing that origin of the binary data in this simulation was the dataset with continuous responses, we can "correct" between items' correlations and corrected item-to-total correlations analyses using polychoric correlations. To estimate polychoric correlations between items, we simply need to add the "POLYCHORIC" option in the CORR procedure (see Figure 4.68). When estimating polychoric correlations, we also need to define additional parameter representing the number of possible states a variable can have; for a binary variable it will be 2. This information is specified by keyword "NGROUPS".

Figure 4.69 shows the results of the estimations of the polychoric correlations. We see drastic differences between Pearson correlation estimations and polychoric correlation estimations for binary items. First, recall that originally we defined that most correlations between continuous items to be 0.6 (see Figures 4.64 and 4.65), and most polychoric correlations between binary items are also now very close to 0.6 (see Figure 4.69), but Pearson correlations between binary items are notably smaller than 0.6 (see Figure 4.67).

Second, to illustrate robustness of the polychoric assessments, the correlations between continuous items 1 and 2, 1 and 3, and 1 and 10 were predefined to be 0.4, 0.5, and 0.8 (see Figure 4.64). Pearson correlations between the same binary items are 0.17, 0.27, and 0.54 (see Figure 4.67). But polychoric correlations between the same binary items are 0.38, 0.50, and 0.78 (see Figure 4.69). These values are remarkably close to the predefined values for the correlations between those four items, when they were simulated as continuous outcomes. It shows that calculating polychoric correlations between binary items (as the replacement for Pearson) allows us to improve the accuracy of the strength of relationships between items.

The next step is to recalculate corrected item-to-total correlations using polychoric correlations. Figure 4.70 demonstrates the estimation of the corrected item-to-total

Simple Statistics

Variable	N	Mean	Std Dev	Sum	Minimum	Maximum
i1	3000	0.51167	0.49995	1535	0	1.00000
i2	3000	0.91167	0.28383	2735	0	1.00000
i3	3000	0.16800	0.37393	504.00000	0	1.00000
i4	3000	0.50767	0.50002	1523	0	1.00000
i5	3000	0.68567	0.46433	2057	0	1.00000
i6	3000	0.58333	0.49309	1750	0	1.00000
i7	3000	0.65033	0.47694	1951	0	1.00000
i8	3000	0.79467	0.40401	2384	0	1.00000
i9	3000	0.42867	0.49497	1286	0	1.00000
i10	3000	0.35933	0.47989	1078	0	1.00000

Cronbach Coefficient Alpha

Variables	Alpha
Raw	0.842007
Standardized	0.839172

Cronbach Coefficient Alpha with Deleted Variable

Deleted Variable	Raw Variables Correlation with Total	Alpha	Standardized Variables Correlation with Total	Alpha
i1	0.592931	0.821932	0.580892	0.819735
i2	0.364473	0.841150	0.365686	0.839798
i3	0.425695	0.836752	0.418581	0.834988
i4	0.587083	0.822548	0.584794	0.819360
i5	0.568105	0.824442	0.563771	0.820805
i6	0.574209	0.823856	0.572798	0.820514
i7	0.571301	0.824110	0.572167	0.820575
i8	0.507776	0.830193	0.511192	0.826377
i9	0.587502	0.822486	0.584488	0.819389
i10	0.572112	0.824031	0.565483	0.821216

Pearson Correlation Coefficients, N = 3000
Prob > |r| under H0: Rho=0

	i1	i2	i3	i4	i5	i6	i7	i8	i9	i10
i1	1.00000	0.16823	0.26776	0.41047	0.41297	0.39440	0.40237	0.33708	0.41232	0.53984
		<.0001	<.0001	<.0001	<.0001	<.0001	<.0001	<.0001	<.0001	<.0001
i2	0.16823	1.00000	0.13673	0.25735	0.30033	0.26347	0.29149	0.31866	0.23640	0.20619
	<.0001		<.0001	<.0001	<.0001	<.0001	<.0001	<.0001	<.0001	<.0001
i3	0.26776	0.13673	1.00000	0.32125	0.26968	0.29840	0.26219	0.20414	0.36023	0.35287
	<.0001	<.0001		<.0001	<.0001	<.0001	<.0001	<.0001	<.0001	<.0001
i4	0.41047	0.25735	0.32125	1.00000	0.38451	0.40651	0.38246	0.35442	0.44209	0.40679
	<.0001	<.0001	<.0001		<.0001	<.0001	<.0001	<.0001	<.0001	<.0001
i5	0.41297	0.30033	0.26968	0.38451	1.00000	0.41519	0.40693	0.38637	0.37321	0.33798
	<.0001	<.0001	<.0001	<.0001		<.0001	<.0001	<.0001	<.0001	<.0001
i6	0.39440	0.26347	0.29840	0.40651	0.41519	1.00000	0.40113	0.35038	0.40554	0.36803
	<.0001	<.0001	<.0001	<.0001	<.0001		<.0001	<.0001	<.0001	<.0001
i7	0.40237	0.29149	0.26219	0.38246	0.40693	0.40113	1.00000	0.39559	0.39926	0.35830
	<.0001	<.0001	<.0001	<.0001	<.0001	<.0001		<.0001	<.0001	<.0001
i8	0.33708	0.31866	0.20414	0.35442	0.38637	0.35038	0.39559	1.00000	0.33525	0.29470
	<.0001	<.0001	<.0001	<.0001	<.0001	<.0001	<.0001		<.0001	<.0001
i9	0.41232	0.23640	0.36023	0.44209	0.37321	0.40554	0.39926	0.33525	1.00000	0.39994
	<.0001	<.0001	<.0001	<.0001	<.0001	<.0001	<.0001	<.0001		<.0001
i10	0.53984	0.20619	0.35287	0.40679	0.33798	0.36803	0.35830	0.29470	0.39994	1.00000
	<.0001	<.0001	<.0001	<.0001	<.0001	<.0001	<.0001	<.0001	<.0001	

Figure 4.67 Partial output: KR-20 coefficient for simulated dataset with binary responses.

```
Proc Corr Data=_sim_ds1 POLYCHORIC(NGROUPS=2) nomiss ;
Var i1-i10;
run;
```

Figure 4.68 Estimating polychoric correlations: CORR procedure.

Figure 4.69 Polychoric correlations estimations results.

```
/* Calculate the total score for every subject using "Sum" function */
Data _corr_; Set _sim_ds1; TotalScore=Sum(of i1-i10); Run;
/* Calculate corrected total score by subtracting value of the item 1 from the
total score */
Data _corr_deleted_item; Set _corr_; TotalScoreDel=TotalScore - i1; Run;
/* Estimate polychoric corrected item-to-total correlation between item 1 and
corrected total score */
Proc Corr Data=_corr_deleted_item Pearson POLYCHORIC(NGROUPS=10) nomiss ;
Var i1 TotalScoreDel ;
Run;
```

Figure 4.70 Calculating corrected item-to-total polychoric correlation for item 1.

correlation for binary item 1. The first step is to calculate the total score for every subject (observation) using "Sum" function and creating dataset "_corr_". The next step is to calculate corrected total score by subtracting the value of item 1 from the total score (see code line "TotalScoreDel=TotalScore - i1;") and creating variable "TotalScoreDel" as a part of the dataset "_corr_ deleted_item".

The last segment illustrates how the CORR procedure is used to estimate the polychoric corrected item-to-total correlation. One important difference from the estimation of the polychoric correlations between binary items from Figure 4.68 and Figure 4.70 is the parameter "NGROUPS".

As it was pointed out, this parameter should represent maximum number of possible states for both variables – the item 1 has 2 states, and variable "TotalScoreDel" can be represented by values 0, 1, 2, . . ., 9 or 10 different states (note that variable "TotalScore" is represented by values 0, 1, 2,. . .10 or 11 different states). Figure 4.71 shows the results of the estimations. Note that the Pearson correlation value of 0.59293 is exactly the same as in Figure 4.67 ("i1 0.592931. . ."), which shows that the procedure we used to calculate corrected item-to-total correlations produce the same results. The last part of the output shows the results of the polychoric correlations – the value of 0.71866, which is very close to the value of 0.720447 (Pearson based corrected item-to-total correlations for item 1 from Figure 4.65).

Snippet of code from Figure 4.70 shows how polychoric corrected item-to-total correlation can be calculated for just one item. This step can be reworked to calculate all 10 correlations automatically. To do this, we will use the LUA procedure, which is the SAS implementation of the modern scripting language. In this chapter, for this example (see Figure 4.72), we use only a few elements of the LUA. Figure 4.73 summarizes results from all analyses for corrected item-to-total correlation we performed in this section. The results clearly indicate that if we can

```
                                     Simple Statistics
Variable              N          Mean        Std Dev         Median        Minimum        Maximum
i1                 3000       0.51167        0.49995        1.00000              0        1.00000
TotalScoreDel      3000       5.08933        2.58139        5.00000              0        9.00000

Pearson Correlation Coefficients, N = 3000
        Prob > |r| under H0: Rho=0
                                     Total
                         i1        ScoreDel
i1                  1.00000         0.59293
                                    <.0001
TotalScoreDel       0.59293         1.00000
                    <.0001


                             Polychoric Correlations
                                                 -------------Wald Test------------
                                                 Standard                       Pr >
Variable        With Variable         N     Correlation      Error   Chi-Square  ChiSq
i1              TotalScoreDel       3000       0.71866      0.01327   2932.3192  <.0001
```

Figure 4.71 Results of the estimation of the polychoric correlations between item 1 and corrected total score.

```
Proc Lua restart;
Submit;
for ItemNumber=1, 10 do
sas.submit[[
Data _corr_deleted_item; Set  _corr_; TotalScoreDel=TotalScore - i@ItemNumber@;Run;


Proc Corr Data=_corr_deleted_item POLYCHORIC(NGROUPS=10) nomiss OUTPLC=PlcCorr
out=PrsCorr;
Var i@ItemNumber@ TotalScoreDel ;
Run;

Data PrsCorr1; Set  PrsCorr;
Pearson_Correlation=i@ItemNumber@;
Where _TYPE_="CORR" And _NAME_="TotalScoreDel";
Keep Pearson_Correlation;
Run;

Data PlcCorr1; Set  PlcCorr;
Polychoric_Correlation=i@ItemNumber@;
Where _TYPE_="CORR" And _NAME_="TotalScoreDel";
Keep Polychoric_Correlation;
Run;

Data _Corr_Corrected_@ItemNumber@;
Merge PrsCorr1 PlcCorr1;
Item="Item xx"; Item="Item @ItemNumber@";
Run;
]]
end
Endsubmit;
Run;

Data _Corr_Results;
Set
_Corr_Corrected_1 _Corr_Corrected_2 _Corr_Corrected_3 _Corr_Corrected_4
_Corr_Corrected_5 _Corr_Corrected_6 _Corr_Corrected_7 _Corr_Corrected_8
_Corr_Corrected_9 _Corr_Corrected_10;
Run;

Proc Print Data=_Corr_Results NOOBS;
Var Item Pearson_Correlation Polychoric_Correlation;
Run;
```

Figure 4.72 Using LUA to estimate polychoric corrected item-to-total correlations for the set of items.

Continuous items (Pearson based) (from figure 4.65)		Binary items (Pearson based) (from figure 4.67)		Binary items (Polychoric based) (based on the results produced by code from figure 4.72)	
i1	0.720447	i1	0.592931	Item 1	0.71866
i2	0.724878	i2	0.364473	Item 2	0.68068
i3	0.732818	i3	0.425695	Item 3	0.70269
i4	0.750947	i4	0.587083	Item 4	0.72298
i5	0.748132	i5	0.568105	Item 5	0.73421
i6	0.750897	i6	0.574209	Item 6	0.71332
i7	0.739182	i7	0.571301	Item 7	0.71868
i8	0.755471	i8	0.507776	Item 8	0.71866
i9	0.753041	i9	0.587502	Item 9	0.73342
i10	0.777914	i10	0.572112	Item 10	0.73875

Figure 4.73 Summary for corrected item-to-total correlations.

assume that binary items are representative of the continuum of responses, then polychoric-based corrected item-to-total correlations much more accurately represent relationships between items and corrected total scores.

It should be pointed out that to have stable estimate polychoric correlations we usually need to have a lot of data. In the simulation featured in this section, we had data simulated for 3000 subjects.

4.3 Summary

In this chapter, two major sections are covered: test–retest reliability and internal reliability (Cronbach's alpha). Test–retest reliability is portrayed from multiple perspectives. First, the measurement error model for a single score is formulated (Section 4.1.1) and then illustrated with two time points (Section 4.1.2). Estimation of reliability (through an ICC) follows from a random-effects model (Section 4.1.3). Then test–retest reliability assessment is given in the context of a clinical study (Section 4.1.4). Next, the Spearman-Brown prophecy formula is invoked to obtain the reliability for an average score based on the reliability of a single score (Section 4.1.5). A comparison follows between test–retest for a multi-item domain score and a single-item score (Section 4.1.6). Observer and interviewer-based scales are highlighted and described (Section 4.1.7). Uncovering the true relationship between measurements, which accounts for measurement error, is modeled and featured (Section 4.1.8). The other major section includes the methodology of Cronbach's alpha for Likert-type scales (Section 4.2.1) and then dichotomous items (Section 4.2.2).

References

Alemayehu, D., Bushmakin, A.G., and Cappelleri, J.C. (2017). Analysis of aggregate data. In: *Statistical Topics in Health Economics and Outcomes Research* (ed. D. Alemayehu, J.C. Cappelleri, B. Emir and K.H. Zou), 123–149. Boca Raton, FL: Chapman & Hall/CRC Press.

Alexopoulos, G.S., Abrams, R.C., Young, R.C., and Shamoian, C.A. (1988). Cornell scale for depression in dementia. *Biological Psychiatry* 23: 271–284.

Cappelleri, J.C., Zou, K.H., Bushmakin, A.G. et al. (2013). *Patient-Reported Outcomes: Measurement, Implementation and Interpretation*. Boca Raton, FL: Chapman & Hall/CRC Press.

Charman, C.R., Venn, A.J., and Williams, H.C. (2004). The patient-oriented eczema measure: development and initial validation of a new tool for measuring atopic eczema severity from the patients' perspective. *Archives of Dermatology* 140: 1513–1519.

Crocker, L. and Algina, J. (1986). *Introduction to Classical and Modern Test Theory*. Belmont, CA: Wadsworth Publishing.

Cronbach, L.J. (1951). Coefficient alpha and the internal structure of tests. *Psychometrika* 16: 297–334.

DeVellis, R.F. (2017). *Scale Development: Theory and Applications*, 4e. Thousand Oaks, CA: SAGE Publications, Inc.

de Vet, H.C.W., Terwee, C.B., Mokkink, L.B., and Knol, D.L. (2011). *Measurement in Medicine: A Practical Guide*. New York: Cambridge University Press.

Fayers, F.M. and Machin, D. (2016). *Quality of Life: The Assessment, Analysis and Reporting of Patient-Reported Outcomes*, 3e. Chichester, United Kingdom: Wiley.

Fayers, P.M., Hand, D.J., Bjordl, K., and Gronvold, M. (1997). Causal indicators in quality of life research. *Quality of Life Research* 6: 393–406.

Food and Drug Administration (FDA) (2009). Guidance for industry on patient-reported outcome measures: use in medical product development to support labeling claims. *Federal Register* 74 (235): 65132–65133.

McLeod, L.D., Cappelleri, J.C., and Hays, R.D. (2016). Best (but of forgotten) practices: expressing and interpreting meaning and effect sizes in clinical outcome assessments. *American Journal of Clinical Nutrition* 103: 685–693. (Erratum: https://doi.org/10.3945/ajcn.116.148593).

Mohs, R.C., Rosen, W.G., and Davis, K.L. (1983). The Alzheimer's disease assessment scale: an instrument for assessing treatment efficacy. *Psychopharmacology Bulletin* 19: 448–450.

Mokkink, L.B., Terwee, C.B., Patrick, D.L. et al. (2010). International consensus on taxonomy, terminology, and definitions of measurement properties for health-related patient-reported outcomes: results of the COSMIN study. *Journal of Clinical Epidemiology* 63: 737–745.

Nunnally, J.C. and Bernstein, I.H. (1994). *Psychometric Theory*, 3e. New York: McGraw-Hill.

Powers, J.H., Patrick, D.L., Walton, M.K. et al. (2017). Clinician-reported outcome assessments of treatment benefit: report of the ISPOR clinical outcome assessment emerging good practices task force. *Value in Health* 20: 2–14.

Reeve, B.B., Wyrwich, K.W., Wu, A.W. et al. (2013). ISOQOL recommends minimum standards for patient-reported outcome measures used in patient-centered outcomes and comparative effectiveness research. *Quality of Life Research* 22: 1889–1905.

Roland, M.O. and Morris, R.W. (1983). A study of the natural history of back pain. Part 1: development of a reliable and sensitive measure of disability in low back pain. *Spine* 8: 141–144.

Schroeder, K.W., Tremaine, W.J., and Ilstrup, D.M. (1987). Coated oral 5-aminosalicylic acid therapy for mildly to moderately active ulcerative colitis. A randomized study. *New England Journal of Medicine* 317: 1625–1629.

Squires, J.E., Estabrooks, C.A., Newburn-Cool, C.V., and Gierl, M. (2011). Validation of the conceptual research utilization scale: an application of the standards for educational and psychological testing in healthcare. *BMC Health Services Research* 11: 107.

Streiner, D.L. (2003). Being inconsistent about consistency: when coefficient does and doesn't matter. *Journal of Personality Assessment* 80: 217–222.

Streiner, D.L., Norman, G.R., and Cairney, J. (2015). *Health Measurement Scales*, 5e. New York: Oxford University Press.

5

Construct Validity and Criterion Validity

Construct validity can be defined as "the degree to which the scores of a measurement instrument are consistent with hypotheses (for instance, with regard to internal relationships, relationship with scores of other instruments or difference between relevant groups)" (Mokkink et al. 2010a). As such, this major type of validity involves constructing and evaluating postulated relationships on a scale purported to measure a particular concept or construct of interest, the phenomenon or characteristic of measurement (the "thing" intended to be measured). Construct validity of a target PRO scale is determined by evidence that its relationships among items, domains, and concepts conform to a priori hypotheses concerning logical relationships that should exist with other measures or characteristics of patients and patient groups (FDA 2009). If these hypotheses are confirmed, there is evidence that supports the construct validity of a PRO scale in measuring its intended construct. If not all of these hypotheses are confirmed, then the mismatch could be attributed to the scale being good but the theory being wrong, the theory being correct but the scale being invalid, or both the theory and the scale are void or misplaced. Assessments of construct validity are quantified through descriptive statistics, correlations, and regression analyses.

In situations when a gold standard is lacking, construct validation relies on structural validity, an aspect of construct validity, which is defined as "the degree to which scores of a measurement instrument are an adequate reflection of the dimensionality of the construct to be measured" (Mokkink et al. 2010b). Structural validity can be assessed with factor analysis. Section 5.1 covers exploratory factor analysis where there are no clear ideas about the number and types of dimensions or domains. Section 5.2 addresses confirmatory factor analysis where a priori hypotheses about the construct are available based on theory or previous research.

A Practical Approach to Quantitative Validation of Patient-Reported Outcomes: A Simulation-Based Guide Using SAS, First Edition. Andrew G. Bushmakin and Joseph C. Cappelleri.
© 2023 John Wiley & Sons, Inc. Published 2023 by John Wiley & Sons, Inc.

Another aspect of construct validity is conceptual hypothesis testing. In addition to addressing structural validity, confirmatory factor analysis is such an example of conceptual hypothesis testing in the sense of whether and how well the observed data conform to the hypothesized factor structure. Hypothesis testing, in the context of construct validation, involves formulating relationships of scores on the target PRO instrument with scores on other instruments measuring the characteristics of being similar or dissimilar. When these other instruments are similar, then convergent validity is being assessed; when dissimilar, discriminant (or divergent) validity is being examined. Convergent validity addresses the relationships of the target PRO scale to other variables or measures to which it is expected to be appreciably or substantially related, according to the theory postulated. Discriminant validity, on the other hand, addresses the relationships of the target PRO scale to other variables or measures to which it is expected to be weakly or insignificantly related (according to the theory postulated). Section 5.3 centers on convergent validity and discriminant validity.

Known-groups validity is another empirical vehicle central to hypothesis testing as ingrained within construct validity. Here, hypotheses are formulated about differences in scores on the PRO instrument under study with respect to subgroups of patients known to differ on a salient characteristic (e.g., severity of illness), which is expected to be meaningfully related to the concept being measured by the PRO instrument. Known-groups validity is based on the principle that the measurement scale of interest should be sensitive to differences between specific groups of subjects known to differ in a relevant way. A scale that cannot clearly distinguish between such distinct groups is hardly likely to be of much value. Section 5.5 centers on known-groups validity.

Another facet of construct validity is cross-cultural validity, "the degree to which the performance on a translated or culturally adapted PRO instrument are an adequate reflection of the performance of items in the original version of the instrument" (Mokkink et al. 2010b). Methods to assess cross-cultural validity include structural equation modeling (such as confirmatory factor analysis), logistic regression, and item response theory. Although not covered directly in this chapter, details on cross-cultural validity are found elsewhere (de Vet et al. 2011; Fayers and Machin 2016; Streiner et al. 2015).

Although criterion validity is often intermingled with construct validity, criterion validity deserves its own classification (DeVellis 2017). Criterion validity has been defined by the COSMIN panel as the "degree to which the scores of a measurement instrument are an adequate reflection of a gold standard" (Mokkink et al. 2010b). This definition indicates that criterion validity of a target PRO measure involves a comparison of it with a gold standard, or a proxy gold standard, which serves as a criterion variable. Section 5.6 concentrates on criterion validity.

5.1 Exploratory Factor Analyses

5.1.1 Modeling Assumptions

Let's consider a scale with n items (observed variables $v_1, v_2, \ldots, v_n$). Every item represents a patient-reported measurement for a particular aspect of the measured concept. The framework that follows also applies generally to clinician-reported and observer-reported measurements. Since the goal of factor analysis is to model the interrelationships among items, we focus primarily on the variance and covariance rather than the mean. Factor analysis assumes that variance can be partitioned into two types of variance, common and unique. Common variance is the amount of variance that is shared among a set of items. Items that are highly correlated will share a lot of variance. Unique variance of an item is any portion of variance that's distinctive and not common to the item.

Let's also assume that the measurement model for this scale is represented by k domains ($k < n$). Exploratory factor analysis assumes that the variable v_i is represented as a mixture of $k + 1$ components: the k components are the common factors $F_1, F_2, \ldots, F_k$ and the $k + 1$ component represents the unique contribution not related to any factor (represented by U_i). All those components are not observed and hence referred to as latent variables, but they sum up to yield v_i.

This relationship can generally be represented by the following equation:

$$v_i = lf_1 v_i F_1 + lf_2 v_i F_2 + \ldots + lf_k v_i F_k + lu_i v_i U_i \tag{5.1}$$

The coefficients, often referenced as loadings, $lf_j v_i$ ($j = 1, 2, \ldots, k; i = 1, 2, \ldots, n$) represent the impacts of the factor F_j onto variable v_i. The coefficients $lu_i v_i$ represent impacts of unique factors U_i. A portion of the full causal model related only to variable v_i is graphically represented by Figure 5.1. For illustrative purposes, Figure 5.1 limits the relationship between only one variable v_i, all common factors, and the unique factor specific to this particular variable. The full model, which can be viewed as a system of the n equations based on the general Eq. (5.1) and Figure 5.1, encompasses all variables $v_1, v_2, \ldots, v_n$ and all their unique corresponding factors $U_1, U_2, \ldots, U_n$. It is assumed here that unique factors $U_1, U_2, \ldots, U_n$ are independent and therefore that $cov(U_i, U_j) = 0$ for any i and j ($i \neq j$). Moreover, the unique factors are independent of the common factor and hence $cov(U_i, F_j) = 0$ for any i and j ($j = 1, 2, \ldots, k; i = 1, 2, \ldots, n$).

Consider an example of a scale with just two domains (factors) F_1 and F_2 that are operationalized or represented by six items (variables $v_1, v_2, \ldots, v_6$).

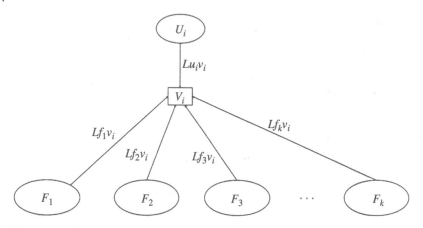

Figure 5.1 Exploratory factor analysis model for the item v_i.

The relationships between the observed variables $v_1, v_2, \ldots, v_6$ and the latent factors can be represented by the following six equations:

$$\begin{cases} v_1 = lf_1v_1F_1 + lf_2v_1F_2 + lu_1v_1U_1 \\ v_2 = lf_1v_2F_1 + lf_2v_2F_2 + lu_2v_2U_2 \\ v_3 = lf_1v_3F_1 + lf_2v_3F_2 + lu_3v_3U_3 \\ v_4 = lf_1v_4F_1 + lf_2v_4F_2 + lu_4v_4U_4 \\ v_5 = lf_1v_5F_1 + lf_2v_5F_2 + lu_5v_5U_5 \\ v_6 = lf_1v_6F_1 + lf_2v_6F_2 + lu_6v_6U_6 \end{cases} \qquad (5.2)$$

The above system of equations is graphically represented by Figure 5.2. Note that this figure represents a link among all variables (both observed and latent) in the exploratory factor analysis.

By constructing every variable v_i as a linear combination of two factors, F_1 and F_2, and unique factor U_i (as shown by Eq. (5.1)) leads to important consequences regarding the relationships between those observed variables. Let's estimate correlations between variables v_1 and v_2 based on Eq. (5.2). For simplicity, the first two equations can be rewritten as follows:

$$v_1 = a_1F_1 + b_1F_2 + c_1U_1$$

$$v_2 = a_2F_1 + b_2F_2 + c_2U_2$$

where the a's and b's are factor loadings or path coefficients. Then the correlation between variables v_1 and v_2 is

$$corr(v_1, v_2) = cov(v_1, v_2) / \sqrt{Var(v_1)Var(v_2)}. \qquad (5.3)$$

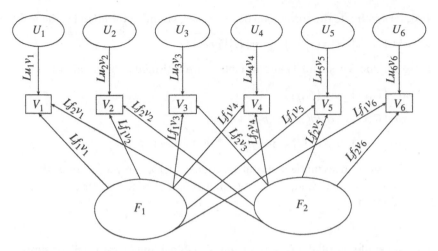

Figure 5.2 Exploratory factor analysis model for six items and two domains.

Without loss of generality, let's assume that $Var(v_1) = Var(v_2) = Var(F_1) = Var(F_2) = 1$ and, additionally, $cov(F_1, F_2) = 0$. Then Eq. (5.3) can be revised as follows:

$$corr\left(v_1, v_2\right) = cov\left(v_1, v_2\right)$$

$$corr\left(v_1, v_2\right) = cov\left(a_1 F_1 + b_1 F_2 + c_1 U_1, a_2 F_1 + b_2 F_2 + c_2 U_2\right)$$

$$corr\left(v_1, v_2\right) = a_1 a_2 \, cov\left(F_1, F_1\right) + a_1 b_2 \, \boldsymbol{cov}\left(\boldsymbol{F_1, F_2}\right) + a_1 c_2 \, \boldsymbol{cov}\left(\boldsymbol{F_1, U_2}\right)$$
$$+ b_1 a_2 \, \boldsymbol{cov}\left(\boldsymbol{F_2, F_1}\right) + b_1 b_2 \, cov\left(F_2, F_2\right) + b_1 c_2 \, \boldsymbol{cov}\left(\boldsymbol{F_2, U_2}\right)$$
$$+ c_1 a_2 \, \boldsymbol{cov}\left(\boldsymbol{U_1, F_1}\right) + c_1 b_2 \, \boldsymbol{cov}\left(\boldsymbol{U_1, F_2}\right) + c_1 c_2 \, \boldsymbol{cov}\left(\boldsymbol{U_1, U_2}\right). \tag{5.4}$$

In Eq. (5.4), the covariances marked in bold are equal to zero, as it was assumed that all factors (common and unique) are independent. Note also that $cov(F_1, F_1) = cov(F_2, F_2) = 1$. As a result, Eq. (5.4) will be reduced to

$$corr\left(v_1, v_2\right) = a_1 a_2 + b_1 b_2. \tag{5.5}$$

If we assume that only one latent factor (F_1) is present, then Eq. (5.5) would be simplified to

$$corr\left(v_1, v_2\right) = a_1 a_2. \tag{5.6}$$

More generally, for any two variables v_i and v_j ($i \neq j$) represented by Eq. (5.1), the correlation will be represented by following equation

$$corr\left(v_i, v_j\right) = lf_1 v_i lf_1 v_j + lf_2 v_i lf_2 v_j + \ldots + lf_k v_i lf_k v_j. \tag{5.7}$$

Next, let's estimate the correlation between, say, latent factor F_1 and variable v_2:

$$corr\left(F_1, v_2\right) = \text{cov}\left(F_1, v_2\right) \Big/ \sqrt{Var\left(F_1\right)Var\left(v_2\right)}. \tag{5.8}$$

Because variances of factor F_1 and variable v_2 are assumed to be equal to 1, then

$$corr\left(F_1, v_2\right) = \text{cov}\left(F_1, v_2\right)$$

$$corr\left(F_1, v_2\right) = \text{cov}\left(F_1, a_2F_1 + b_2F_2 + c_2U_2\right)$$

$$corr\left(F_1, v_2\right) = a_2 \text{cov}\left(F_1, F_1\right) + b_2 \, \boldsymbol{cov}\left(\boldsymbol{F_1, F_2}\right) + c_2 \, \boldsymbol{cov}\left(\boldsymbol{F_1, U_2}\right). \tag{5.9}$$

Here the covariances marked in bold are equal to zero, as it was assumed that all factors are independent and, by definition, $cov(F_1, F_1) = 1$. As a result, Eq. (5.9) will be reduced to

$$corr\left(F_1, v_2\right) = a_2. \tag{5.10}$$

More generally, correlations between any variable v_i and factor F_j will be simply equal to the loading (or path coefficient) for the path from this factor F_j to observed variable v_i:

$$corr\left(v_i, F_j\right) = lf_j v_i. \tag{5.11}$$

To simulate data to illustrate the aforementioned set of relationships and to further highlight assumptions of the exploratory factor analysis, we will continue with the example represented by Figure 5.2. The first step in this process is to simulate latent factors (Figure 5.3). When generating the latent factors, we assume, as noted previously, that factor F_1 and factor F_2 are not correlated (later, we will relax this assertion). As before, it is also assumed that unique factors $U_1, U_2, \ldots, U_6$ are

```
data _corr_(type=corr);
input
_TYPE_ $    _NAME_ $   F1      F2      U1      U2      U3      U4      U5      U6;
datalines;
  CORR      F1         1       0       0       0       0       0       0       0
  CORR      F2         0       1       0       0       0       0       0       0
  CORR      U1         0       0       1       0       0       0       0       0
  CORR      U2         0       0       0       1       0       0       0       0
  CORR      U3         0       0       0       0       1       0       0       0
  CORR      U4         0       0       0       0       0       1       0       0
  CORR      U5         0       0       0       0       0       0       1       0
  CORR      U6         0       0       0       0       0       0       0       1
  MEAN      .          0       0       0       0       0       0       0       0
  STD       .          1       1       1       1       1       1       1       1
  N         .          500     500     500     500     500     500     500     500
;
run;
proc simnormal data=_corr_ out=_sim_ds numreal=500 seed=12345;
var F1 F2 U1 U2 U3 U4 U5 U6;
run;
proc corr data=_sim_ds ;
Var F1 F2 U1 U2 U3 U4 U5 U6;
Run;
```

Figure 5.3 Generating latent factors F_1 and factor F_2 and unique factors $U_1, U_2, \ldots, U_6$.

independent, meaning that the correlation between U_i and U_j ($i \neq j$) is equal to zero and correlation between U_i ($i = 1, \ldots, 6$) and F_j ($j = 1, 2$) is also equal to zero.

First, we create a dataset (data _corr_(type=corr);...) representing postulated relationships between latent factors and unique factors – all pairwise correlations are zeroes. Then we use the SIMNORMAL procedure to generate 500 observations based on predefined correlations. The last procedure in Figure 5.3 estimates correlations between simulated factors (see Figure 5.4 for partial output – as expected, all pairwise correlations are very close to zero).

Figure 5.5 demonstrates how items of a scale can be simulated. Let's start with the third part of the data step (code under "/* Step 3:...."). The SAS code lines

$$v1 = Lf1v1*F1 + Lf2v1*F2 + Lu1v1*U1;$$
$$v2 = Lf1v2*F1 + Lf2v2*F2 + Lu2v2*U2;$$
$$v3 = Lf1v3*F1 + Lf2v3*F2 + Lu3v3*U3;$$

	F1	F2	U1	U2	U3	U4	U5	U6
	Pearson Correlation Coefficients, N = 500							
	Prob > |r| under H0: Rho=0							
F1	1.00000	-0.02490	0.04613	-0.02732	-0.04577	0.03016	0.01606	0.02289
		0.5785	0.3033	0.5422	0.3071	0.5011	0.7201	0.6096
F2	-0.02490	1.00000	0.02413	-0.03352	0.01316	0.00563	0.01575	0.04302
	0.5785		0.5904	0.4546	0.7692	0.9001	0.7253	0.3370
U1	0.04613	0.02413	1.00000	0.00162	0.05191	0.01695	-0.04573	-0.01982
	0.3033	0.5904		0.9712	0.2466	0.7054	0.3075	0.6584
U2	-0.02732	-0.03352	0.00162	1.00000	-0.03273	-0.02015	0.00533	0.04306
	0.5422	0.4546	0.9712		0.4652	0.6530	0.9054	0.3366
U3	-0.04577	0.01316	0.05191	-0.03273	1.00000	0.02581	0.02699	0.05638
	0.3071	0.7692	0.2466	0.4652		0.5648	0.5471	0.2082
U4	0.03016	0.00563	0.01695	-0.02015	0.02581	1.00000	-0.00010	-0.04288
	0.5011	0.9001	0.7054	0.6530	0.5648		0.9982	0.3386
U5	0.01606	0.01575	-0.04573	0.00533	0.02699	-0.00010	1.00000	-0.02363
	0.7201	0.7253	0.3075	0.9054	0.5471	0.9982		0.5981
U6	0.02289	0.04302	-0.01982	0.04306	0.05638	-0.04288	-0.02363	1.00000
	0.6096	0.3370	0.6584	0.3366	0.2082	0.3386	0.5981	

Figure 5.4 Simulated correlations for latent factors F_1, F_2 and unique factors $U_1, U_2, \ldots, U_6$.

```
Data _efa_;
Set   _sim_ds;
/* Step 1: Setting values of loadings for latent factors*/
Lf1v1 = 0.9; Lf2v1 = 0.2; Lf1v2 = 0.9; Lf2v2 = 0.2; Lf1v3 = 0.9; Lf2v3 = 0.2;
Lf1v4 = 0.2; Lf2v4 = 0.9; Lf1v5 = 0.2; Lf2v5 = 0.9; Lf1v6 = 0.2; Lf2v6 = 0.9;
/* Step 2: Estimating loadings for unique factors (Lu1v1, Lu2v2....)*/
Lu1v1 =sqrt(1-Lf1v1**2-Lf2v1**2); Lu2v2 =sqrt(1-Lf1v2**2-Lf2v2**2);
Lu3v3 =sqrt(1-Lf1v3**2-Lf2v3**2);
Lu4v4 =sqrt(1-Lf1v4**2-Lf2v4**2); Lu5v5 =sqrt(1-Lf1v5**2-Lf2v5**2);
Lu6v6 =sqrt(1-Lf1v6**2-Lf2v6**2);
/* Step 3: Creating variable v1, v2,..v6 */
v1 = Lf1v1*F1 + Lf2v1*F2 + Lu1v1*U1; v2 = Lf1v2*F1 + Lf2v2*F2 + Lu2v2*U2;
v3 = Lf1v3*F1 + Lf2v3*F2 + Lu3v3*U3;
v4 = Lf1v4*F1 + Lf2v4*F2 + Lu4v4*U4; v5 = Lf1v5*F1 + Lf2v5*F2 + Lu5v5*U5;
v6 = Lf1v6*F1 + Lf2v6*F2 + Lu6v6*U6;
Run;
proc corr data=_efa_ ; Var F1 F2 v1-v6; Run;
```

Figure 5.5 Simulating items $v_1, v_2, \ldots, v_6$.

v4 = Lf1v4*F1 + Lf2v4*F2 + Lu4v4*U4;
v5 = Lf1v5*F1 + Lf2v5*F2 + Lu5v5*U5;
v6 = Lf1v6*F1 + Lf2v6*F2 + Lu6v6*U6;

are exact replica of the system of Eq. (5.2), but simulation of the loadings needs further explanation. First, (see code under "/* Step 1:") we assign value of 0.9 and 0.2 for loading from latent factor F_1 and F_2 to variables v_1, v_2, and v_3 (and for variables v_4, v_5, and v_6 we simply reverse those loadings). Therefore, the latent factor F_1 is more likely to be related to variables v_1, v_2, and v_3 and latent factor F_2 is more likely to be related to variables v_4, v_5, and v_6.

In Figures 5.1 and 5.2 and the system of Eq. (5.2), we did not make any assumptions about relationships between loadings from latent factors and loadings from unique factors to an item. The second part (see code under "/* Step 2:") reveals the main assumption (basically the essence) of the exploratory factor analysis. It shows that loadings for the unique factors (U_1, U_2, . . ., U_6) are not independent from loadings for latent factors (F_1, F_2) – they are linked via an explicit formula, which in our example will be

$$lu_i v_i = \sqrt{1 - \left(\left(lf_1 v_i\right)^2 + \left(lf_2 v_i\right)^2\right)} \tag{5.12}$$

for any i ($i = 1, 2, . . ., 6$).

To explain Eq. (5.12), we need to introduce the general communality formula as

$$Communality\ for\ item\ v_i = \sum_{j=1}^{k} \left(lf_j v_i\right)^2 \tag{5.13}$$

where k is the number of latent factors F_1, F_2, . . ., F_k. A communality for an observed variable (item) refers to the amount of variance in the item that is accounted for by the latent factors. With two latent factors the

$$Communality\ for\ item\ v_i = \left(lf_1 v_i\right)^2 + \left(lf_2 v_i\right)^2 \tag{5.14}$$

which in our simulated example will be the same $(0.9)^2 + (0.2)^2 = 0.85$ for every item v_i. This means that 85% of the variance for item v_i ($i = 1, . . ., 6$) is accounted for by the two latent factors. It also means that 15% of the variance of v_i is accounted for by the unique factor U_i. In this particular simulated example, the communality for each item is the same, but, in practice, it is expected that different items will have different communality estimates. Note that defining loadings for unique factors as shown by Eq. (5.12) will also assure that variances of the simulated items v_i will be equal to 1.

Figure 5.6 represents a correlation matrix for dataset "_efa_," which was generated by SAS code from Figure 5.5. As expected, correlations between latent factors

```
                        Pearson Correlation Coefficients, N = 500
                               Prob > |r| under H0: Rho=0

             F1          F2          v1          v2          v3          v4          v5          v6

F1        1.00000    -0.02490     0.89329     0.89767     0.89158     0.18691     0.18023     0.18109
                       0.5785      <.0001      <.0001      <.0001      <.0001      <.0001      <.0001

F2       -0.02490     1.00000     0.18664     0.17053     0.18938     0.90554     0.90065     0.90235
           0.5785                  <.0001      0.0001      <.0001      <.0001      <.0001      <.0001

v1        0.89329     0.18664     1.00000     0.84278     0.84924     0.35947     0.34301     0.34798
           <.0001      <.0001                  <.0001      <.0001      <.0001      <.0001      <.0001

v2        0.89767     0.17053     0.84278     1.00000     0.83584     0.34066     0.33745     0.34440
           <.0001      0.0001      <.0001                  <.0001      <.0001      <.0001      <.0001

v3        0.89158     0.18938     0.84924     0.83584     1.00000     0.36336     0.35657     0.36213
           <.0001      <.0001      <.0001      <.0001                  <.0001      <.0001      <.0001

v4        0.18691     0.90554     0.35947     0.34066     0.36336     1.00000     0.85796     0.85362
           <.0001      <.0001      <.0001      <.0001      <.0001                  <.0001      <.0001

v5        0.18023     0.90065     0.34301     0.33745     0.35657     0.85796     1.00000     0.85037
           <.0001      <.0001      <.0001      <.0001      <.0001      <.0001                  <.0001

v6        0.18109     0.90235     0.34798     0.34440     0.36213     0.85362     0.85037     1.00000
           <.0001      <.0001      <.0001      <.0001      <.0001      <.0001      <.0001
```

Figure 5.6 Simulated correlations between latent factors and variables.

and observed items are very close to the loadings we used to generate simulated data. For example, the correlation between latent factor F_1 and variable v_1 is 0.89329 and between latent factor F_1 and variable v_4 is 0.18691 (which were defined, respectively, 0.9 and 0.2 in the simulation). Now let's look at the correlation between variables v_1 and v_2. Earlier (see Eq. (5.5)), we showed that the theoretical value for this correlation can be calculated as

$$corr\left(v_1, v_2\right) = a_1 a_2 + b_1 b_2$$
$$corr\left(v_1, v_2\right) = 0.9 \times 0.9 + 0.2 \times 0.2 = 0.85.$$

From Figure 5.6 the simulated value for $corr(v_1, v_2)$ is 0.84278. The theoretical correlation between variables v_1 and v_4 can be estimated as

$$corr\left(v_1, v_4\right) = a_1 a_4 + b_1 b_4$$
$$corr\left(v_1, v_4\right) = 0.9 \times 0.2 + 0.2 \times 0.9 = 0.36.$$

And the simulated value for $corr(v_1, v_4)$ is practically the same 0.35947.

5.1.2 Exploratory Factor Analysis Implementation

Figure 5.7 represents the implementation of the exploratory factor analysis using the FACTOR procedure in SAS. There are several parameters which are needed to be defined. First is the number of factors – we simulated data based on two factors (`nfactors=2`) and hence pretend to know the truth. But, in real life, we will not know how many latent factors should be defined.

```
Proc Factor data=_efa_ method=prin priors=SMC scree rotate=VARIMAX nfactors=2;
Var v1-v6;
Run;
```

Figure 5.7 Exploratory factor analysis implementation.

Second is the method to extract factors. In our example, we use principal factor analysis (method=prin). Note that this parameter "prin" will define different methods depending on the option priors, which is defined as priors=SMC. It means that, first, we need to define the initial communality for every variable. We know that the simulated value for communalities in our example, which happens to be same for every variable, and equals 0.85. Then those initial communalities will replace values of 1 (i.e., diagonal elements) in the correlation matrix (see Figure 5.6). Next, the principal component analysis will be performed using this *reduced* correlation matrix, which generally will lead to the presence of negative eigenvalues. Because we defined the number of factors to be two, two first principal components will be selected and loadings for these two components will be used to represent the relationship between latent factors and observed variables.

The last important option to define is the rotation of the initial extracted latent factors to optimize and simplify the interpretation of the latent factors. In the simulation, we defined the latent factors to be independent and, knowing this, we use rotate=VARIMAX as the best option. This VARIMAX rotation, while keeping latent factors orthogonal, will also attempt to maximize loadings for the smallest possible number of factors. The best outcome from a rotation is if every variable will have a large loading for just one factor, with relatively small loadings for other factors.

SAS code from Figure 5.7 will produce several sets of results, which should be examined jointly. The first set of results is titled as "Initial Factor Solution" (see Figures 5.8 and 5.13 for partial output). As mentioned earlier, the important first step is to approximate initial communalities (Prior Communality Estimates). Those initial communalities are simply the r-squared values when a variable is regressed on all other variables. For a given item as the outcome

```
Initial Factor Method: Principal Factors
                     Prior Communality Estimates: SMC
         v1             v2             v3             v4             v5             v6
0.78146452     0.76284538     0.77359120     0.79369334     0.78808055     0.78286847

Eigenvalues of the Reduced Correlation Matrix: Total = 4.68254346  Average = 0.78042391
         Eigenvalue    Difference    Proportion    Cumulative
    1     3.52906501    2.10369955      0.7537        0.7537
    2     1.42536546    1.48524271      0.3044        1.0581
    3     -.05987725    0.00544369     -0.0128        1.0453
    4     -.06532094    0.00321088     -0.0139        1.0313
    5     -.06853183    0.00962517     -0.0146        1.0167
    6     -.07815699                   -0.0167        1.0000
2 factors will be retained by the NFACTOR criterion.
```

Figure 5.8 Initial factor solution.

```
Proc Reg data=_efa_;
Communality_v1: Model v1= v2 v3 v4 v5 v6;
Communality_v2: Model v2= v1 v3 v4 v5 v6;
Communality_v3: Model v3= v1 v2 v4 v5 v6;
Communality_v4: Model v4= v1 v2 v3 v5 v6;
Communality_v5: Model v5= v1 v2 v3 v4 v6;
Communality_v6: Model v6= v1 v2 v3 v4 v5;
Run;Quit;
```

Figure 5.9 Estimation of the initial communalities.

(dependent variable) in multiple linear regression, the r-square can be interpreted as the percentage of variance in that item that can be explained by the remaining variables as predictors (independent variables).

As an illustration, Figure 5.9 shows how REG procedure can be used to produce initial communalities (Table 5.1 gives r-squared for six regression models estimated by REG procedure). For example, the FACTOR procedure estimated the initial communality for the variable v1 as 0.78146452 (see Figure 5.8) and Table 5.1; as such, the r-squared for the first model Communality_v1 is also the same value of 0.7815.

The next segment in the output is the Eigenvalues of the Reduced Correlation Matrix. To illustrate this part of the analysis, let's create a reduced correlation matrix and estimate eigenvalues for this matrix. Based on Figure 5.6, the reduced correlation matrix between variables is represented by Figure 5.10. Note that we deleted correlations with latent factors and replaced

Table 5.1 Estimated r-squared.

Model	Dependent variable	R-square
Communality_v1	v1	0.7815
Communality_v2	v2	0.7628
Communality_v3	v3	0.7736
Communality_v4	V4	0.7937
Communality_v5	V5	0.7881
Communality_v6	V6	0.7829

	v1	v2	v3	v4	v5	v6
v1	**0.7815**	0.84278	0.84924	0.35947	0.34301	0.34798
v2	0.84278	**0.7628**	0.83584	0.34066	0.33745	0.34440
v3	0.84924	0.83584	**0.7736**	0.36336	0.35657	0.36213
v4	0.35947	0.34066	0.36336	**0.7937**	0.85796	0.85362
v5	0.34301	0.33745	0.35657	0.85796	**0.7881**	0.85037
v6	0.34798	0.34440	0.36213	0.85362	0.85037	**0.7829**

Figure 5.10 Reduced correlation matrix (with prior or initial communalities on the diagonal).

diagonal elements with r-squared values (bold numbers in Figure 5.10) from Table 5.1. Figure 5.11 demonstrates the estimation of the eigenvalues (see Figure 5.12 for resultant output). As we can see, those values match the values produced by FACTOR procedure (see Figure 5.8).

Figure 5.13 represents the last set of results under "Initial Factor Solution." First is the "Factor Pattern" presenting initial loadings, which, usually, is difficult to interpret and, generally, those loadings are considered simply as transitional results. Next is the "Variance Explained by Each Factor." Recall that every variable $v_1, v_2, \ldots, v_6$ in our simulation has a variance of 1 (see Eqs. (5.12)–(5.14)), which means that the overall variance will be equal to the number of variables used in the simulation, which is six.

```
Proc IML;
corr_reduced = {
0.7815      0.84278     0.84924     0.35947     0.34301     0.34798,
0.84278     0.7628      0.83584     0.34066     0.33745     0.34440,
0.84924     0.83584     0.7736      0.36336     0.35657     0.36213,
0.35947     0.34066     0.36336     0.7937      0.85796     0.85362,
0.34301     0.33745     0.35657     0.85796     0.7881      0.85037,
0.34798     0.34440     0.36213     0.85362     0.85037     0.7829};
Eigenvalue=eigval(corr_reduced);
print Eigenvalue;
Quit;
```

Figure 5.11 Estimation of eigenvalues.

```
Eigenvalue
  3.529072
  1.4253726
 -0.059869
 -0.065297
 -0.068538
 -0.078141
```

Figure 5.12 Estimated eigenvalues (based on IML procedure).

```
Initial Factor Method: Principal Factors
          Factor Pattern
          Factor1          Factor2
v1        0.76292          0.49733
v2        0.75013          0.49585
v3        0.76658          0.48226
v4        0.77834         -0.48192
v5        0.77083         -0.48780
v6        0.77246         -0.47894

Variance Explained by Each Factor
   Factor1          Factor2
  3.5290650        1.4253655

                    Final Communality Estimates: Total = 4.954430
          v1               v2               v3               v4               v5               v6
  0.82938545       0.80856078       0.82022080       0.83806396       0.83212218       0.82607730
```

Figure 5.13 Initial factor pattern and estimated communalities.

Variance explained by Factor 1 and by Factor 2 is 3.5290650 and 1.4253655, respectively. Note that those variances are numerically equal to the first two eigenvalues in Figure 5.8. The sum of those two values is 4.954430, meaning that these two factors explain about 83% ($4.954430/6$) of total variance. Note also that the value of 4.954430 is exactly the same as the total final communality (see Figure 5.13). And, obviously, sum of final communalities will also be equal to 4.954430. The final communalities are in range from 0.81 (0.80856078) to 0.84 (0.83806396), which are slightly smaller than the theoretical simulated communality of 0.85.

The second set of results is labeled "Rotated Factor Solution" (see Figure 5.14), with the VARIMAX rotation applied. In this simulation, the VARIMAX rotation with two factors attempts to maximize the loading for one factor while keeping factors orthogonal. Figure 5.14 shows that loadings are close to what we used to generate variables (Figure 5.5). For example, the loading from Factor 1 to variable v_1 is 0.19522, and the loading from Factor 2 is 0.88954 – both values are close to the simulated values of 0.2 and 0.9 (note also that factors switched positions relative to the simulation – see Figure 5.5).

Now both factors explain almost the same amount of variance (2.4947529 and 2.4596775), as they should. This result also highlights the important property of the rotation. It does not change the overall amount of explained variance and keeps the communalities for every variable the same. For example, for variable v_1 the initial loadings (Figure 5.13) are 0.76292 and 0.49733 and, after VARIMAX rotation, those loadings (Figure 5.14) become 0.19522 and 0.88954, then

$$\text{Communality for item } v_1 = (0.76292)^2 + (0.49733)^2$$
$$= (0.19522)^2 + (0.88954)^2 = 0.8294.$$

The results from the Figure 5.14 indicate that exploratory factor analysis is capable of extracting the underlying structure of the data, but, unfortunately, it is not that simple. In the simulation we knew the number of factors and that they

```
Rotation Method: Varimax
      Rotated Factor Pattern
            Factor1          Factor2
v1          0.19522          0.88954
v2          0.18714          0.87951
v3          0.20840          0.88136
v4          0.89286          0.20217
v5          0.89162          0.19270
v6          0.88657          0.20017

Variance Explained by Each Factor
    Factor1          Factor2
  2.4947529        2.4596775

                    Final Communality Estimates: Total = 4.954430
        v1              v2              v3              v4              v5              v6
  0.82938545      0.80856078      0.82022080      0.83806396      0.83212218      0.82607730
```

Figure 5.14 Rotated factor solution.

were orthogonal, instructing the FACTOR procedure to extract two orthogonal factors. But, in real life, we do not know how many factors exist and the relationship between factors. Are those factors orthogonal or correlated? If a dataset is a result of a clinical or observation study, then the number of factors is needed to be determined (see the next Section 5.1.3 for more details). For the relationship between factors, usually the most conservative approach is assumed, namely, that factors are rather correlated than orthogonal.

Let's investigate how results of the analyses will be changed if we assume that factors are not independent and hence correlated. In order to do that the option in Figure 5.7

```
rotate= VARIMAX
```

is replaced by

```
rotate=PROMAX.
```

This option represents oblique rotation; therefore, it does not assume that factors are independent. As with the VARIMAX rotation in this simulation, the PROMAX rotation with two factors is attempting to maximize the loading for one factor, but now the factors can be correlated. After running code from Figure 5.7 with "rotate=PROMAX" option the first set of results ("Initial Factor Solution") will be exactly the same as previously in Figure 5.13. The second set of results will have the new title "Prerotated Factor Solution," but, in fact, those results are the same as those were titled previously as "Rotated Factor Solution" in Figure 5.14. And now we have a new third set of results titled as "Rotated Factor Solution" with subtitle "Rotation Method: Promax (power = 3)" (see Figure 5.15 for key fragments of the output).

Several observations are noteworthy. First, we see that this rotation leads to a solution with factors that are clearly correlated: the correlation between Factor 1 and Factor 2 is 0.40622. Knowing that the original factors in the simulation

```
             Inter-Factor Correlations
                   Factor1        Factor2
Factor1           1.00000        0.40622
Factor2           0.40622        1.00000

Rotated Factor Pattern (Standardized Regression Coefficients)
                  Factor1        Factor2
v1               0.00693        0.90787
v2               0.00055        0.89898
v3               0.02289        0.89612
v4               0.90990        0.01347
v5               0.91073        0.00362
v6               0.90363        0.01276

                     Final Communality Estimates: Total = 4.954430
          v1            v2            v3            v4            v5            v6
0.82938545     0.80856078     0.82022080     0.83806396     0.83212218     0.82607730
```

Figure 5.15 Promax rotation method.

were orthogonal, we find this result somewhat disappointing. It shows that when the oblique rotation method is applied, the underlying relationship between factors may not be assessed correctly.

The next part represents the loadings. It is clear that with this Promax rotation, the loadings are even more different between factors while still keeping the same communality for every variable (compare communalities in Figures 5.13–5.15). It should be stressed that it does not mean that oblique rotation is not a good option for exploratory factor analysis. In fact, we think that it is, generally, the most appropriate (conservative) approach to explore data. The most important point is that the results of the exploratory factor analysis should be treated as hypothesis-generated results about the underlying structure of the data. The exploratory factor analysis suggested structure should always be tested with confirmatory factor analysis (see Section 5.2).

5.1.3   Evaluating the Number of Factors and Factor Loadings

5.1.3.1   Scree Plot

When investigating the measurement structure of data with exploratory factor analysis the first, and most important, step is to identify the number of latent factors. Previously we discussed the very first portion of results titled "Initial Factor Solution" (Figure 5.8). The most relevant part needed to decide on how many latent factors should be is the set of Eigenvalues of the Reduced Correlation Matrix. Figure 5.16 represents a scree plot based on eigenvalues from Figure 5.8.

One rule of thumb is to try to draw a straight line (a dashed line in Figure 5.16) starting with last eigenvalue in a way that it will approximately go through as many eigenvalues as possible. In our example eigenvalues 3, 4, 5, and 6 are remarkably close to be approximated by a straight line. This realization means that the rest of eigenvalues, which are not close to this straight line, represent latent factors – the first and second eigenvalues in our simulation represent dimensionality or number of latent factors. This implies that the first two eigenvalues are associated with the two common factors, and the rest of the eigenvalues are associated with unique factors.

As powerful and simple to use as a scree test is, it is not always obvious when working with real-life data to identify "the break" (or discontinuity) on the scree plot, which can be somewhat subjective. However, another method, the parallel analysis, was shown to be an effective approach to assess the number of latent factors (even though it is important to understand the particular implementation). A parallel analysis, as a part of the FACTOR procedure, simulates random correlation matrices (of the same size as the initial correlation matrix) based on a multivariate standard normal distribution. Eigenvalues for every simulated random correlation matrix are estimated and recorded. Then, say, the 95th percentile is estimated for every eigenvalue. If an observed eigenvalue for a factor is larger

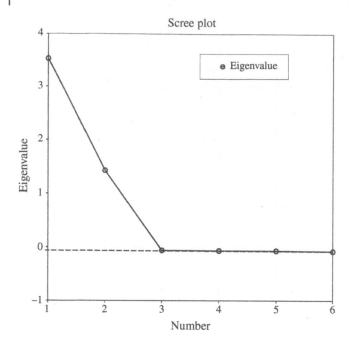

Figure 5.16 Scree plot.

than that estimated 95th percentiles, then this factor is assumed to be one of the vital latent factors.

To invoke this feature, we simply need to redefine NFACTORS option (see Figure 5.17; note that we continue to use the same dataset "_efa_" created earlier): 1000 simulations are requested and 95th percentile for every eigenvalue will be estimated and plotted.

The first portion of the output titled "Initial Factor Solution" (after running code from Figure 5.17) has a new section Parallel Analysis (see Figure 5.18) and corresponding plot (see Figure 5.19). It shows that two dimensions should be retained (as anticipated for this simulated "_efa_" dataset). We would like to highlight important and somewhat unexpected characteristic of this implementation. As we can see, the observed eigenvalues are different from eigenvalues we found earlier in Figure 5.8. The difference is that in Figure 5.8, the reduced

```
proc factor data=_efa_ method=prin PRIORS=SMC scree rotate=PROMAX
NFACTORS=PARALLEL(ALPHA=.05 NSIMS=1000 SEED=123) PLOTS=PARALLEL;
Var v1-v6;
Run;
```

Figure 5.17 Procedure FACTOR with parallel analysis.

```
Initial Factor Method: Principal Factors
        Parallel Analysis:
        NSims=1000 Seed=123

            Observed      Simulated
            Eigenvalue    Crit Val
    1        3.7485        1.2114*
    2        1.6451        1.1168*
    3        0.1660        1.0553
    4        0.1541        1.0039
    5        0.1492        0.9560
    6        0.1372        0.9061
* Retained Dimension (Obs > Crit, alpha=0.05)
```

Figure 5.18   Observed and simulated eigenvalues.

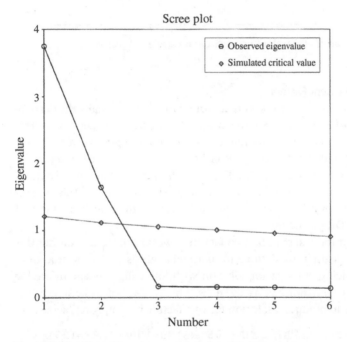

Figure 5.19   Plot of the observed and simulated eigenvalues.

correlation matrix was used (with the initial communality estimates on the diagonal), but in Figure 5.18, the original correlation matrix is used (with 1's on the diagonal). To demonstrate this, we can simply run the code from Figure 5.11 but replace the initial communalities on the diagonal of the correlation matrix by values of 1. See Figure 5.20 for SAS code and for its output; note that the observed eigenvalues from Figure 5.18 are virtually same as in Figure 5.20, allowing for simulation error.

```
Proc IML;
corr = {
1           0.84278     0.84924     0.35947     0.34301     0.34798,
0.84278     1           0.83584     0.34066     0.33745     0.34440,
0.84924     0.83584     1           0.36336     0.35657     0.36213,
0.35947     0.34066     0.36336     1           0.85796     0.85362,
0.34301     0.33745     0.35657     0.85796     1           0.85037,
0.34798     0.34440     0.36213     0.85362     0.85037     1};
Eigenvalue=eigval(corr);
print Eigenvalue;
Quit;

Estimated eigenvalue of the original correction matrix (output from above IML,procedure)
Eigenvalue
 3.7484661
 1.6450704
 0.1659752
 0.1540981
 0.1492013
 0.1371889
```

Figure 5.20   Estimation of eigenvalues using original correlation matrix.

5.1.3.2   Correlated Latent Factors

In previous simulations, the factors were assumed to be orthogonal – the correlations between two factors was initially postulated to be zero. Let's relax this assumption and generate a new simulated, dataset assuming that latent factors are not orthogonal and that the correlation between those latent factors is 0.5. Figure 5.21 contains the simulation, and Figures 5.22 and 5.23 contain the output. First, we see in Figure 5.22 that the parallel analysis implied that this dataset could be summarized by just one latent factor, which is also depicted by Figure 5.23 generated by FACTOR procedure.

But we know that there should be two factors – we simulated the dataset this way. Because of the settings we defined for parallel analysis, FACTOR procedure stopped after producing initial factor solution with following message in the log file "NOTE: Rotation not possible with 1 factor." Let's force the FACTOR procedure to produce a solution for two factors by simply replacing

```
NFACTORS=PARALLEL(ALPHA=.05 NSIMS=1000 SEED=123)
PLOTS=PARALLEL;
```

with

```
NFACTORS=2;.
```

Figure 5.24 represents the results of the analysis: eigenvalues for the reduced correlation matrix and the final structure of the two requested factors after PROMAX rotation. As we learned previously, we should not expect that loadings [see results under Rotated Factor Pattern (Standardized Regression Coefficients)] will correspond to the loadings used to

```
data _corr_(type=corr);
input
_TYPE_ $    _NAME_ $   F1       F2      U1      U2      U3      U4      U5      U6;
datalines;
  CORR       F1        1        .5      0       0       0       0       0       0
  CORR       F2        .5       1       0       0       0       0       0       0
  CORR       U1        0        0       1       0       0       0       0       0
  CORR       U2        0        0       0       1       0       0       0       0
  CORR       U3        0        0       0       0       1       0       0       0
  CORR       U4        0        0       0       0       0       1       0       0
  CORR       U5        0        0       0       0       0       0       1       0
  CORR       U6        0        0       0       0       0       0       0       1
  MEAN       .         0        0       0       0       0       0       0       0
  STD        .         1        1       1       1       1       1       1       1
  N          .         500      500     500     500     500     500     500     500
;
run;
proc simnormal data=_corr_ out=_sim_ds numreal=500 seed=12345;
var F1 F2 U1 U2 U3 U4 U5 U6;
run;
Data _efa_1;
Set  _sim_ds;
/* Step 1: Setting values of loading for latent factors */
Lf1v1 = 0.8; Lf2v1 = 0.2; Lf1v2 = 0.8; Lf2v2 = 0.2; Lf1v3 = 0.8; Lf2v3 = 0.2;
Lf1v4 = 0.2; Lf2v4 = 0.8; Lf1v5 = 0.2; Lf2v5 = 0.8; Lf1v6 = 0.2; Lf2v6 = 0.8;
/* Step 2: Estimating loadings for unique factors (Lu1v1, Lu2v2....)*/
Lu1v1 =sqrt(1-Lf1v1**2-Lf2v1**2); Lu2v2 =sqrt(1-Lf1v2**2-Lf2v2**2);
Lu3v3 =sqrt(1-Lf1v3**2-Lf2v3**2);
Lu4v4 =sqrt(1-Lf1v4**2-Lf2v4**2); Lu5v5 =sqrt(1-Lf1v5**2-Lf2v5**2);
Lu6v6 =sqrt(1-Lf1v6**2-Lf2v6**2);
/* Step 3: Creating variable v1, v2,..v6 */
v1 = Lf1v1*F1 + Lf2v1*F2 + Lu1v1*U1; v2 = Lf1v2*F1 + Lf2v2*F2 + Lu2v2*U2;
v3 = Lf1v3*F1 + Lf2v3*F2 + Lu3v3*U3;
v4 = Lf1v4*F1 + Lf2v4*F2 + Lu4v4*U4; v5 = Lf1v5*F1 + Lf2v5*F2 + Lu5v5*U5;
v6 = Lf1v6*F1 + Lf2v6*F2 + Lu6v6*U6;
Run;
proc factor data=_efa_1 method=prin PRIORS=SMC scree rotate=PROMAX
NFACTORS=PARALLEL(ALPHA=.05 NSIMS=1000 SEED=123) PLOTS=PARALLEL;
Var v1-v6;
Run;
```

Figure 5.21 Exploratory factor analysis with using parallel analysis and correlated factors.

```
        Parallel Analysis:
      NSims=1000 Seed=123

            Observed      Simulated
            Eigenvalue    Crit Val
     1      4.1296        1.2114*
     2      0.7511        1.1168
     3      0.3055        1.0553
     4      0.2835        1.0039
     5      0.2760        0.9560
     6      0.2542        0.9061
 * Retained Dimension (Obs > Crit, alpha=0.05)
```

Figure 5.22 Parallel analysis results (based on initial correlation matrix).

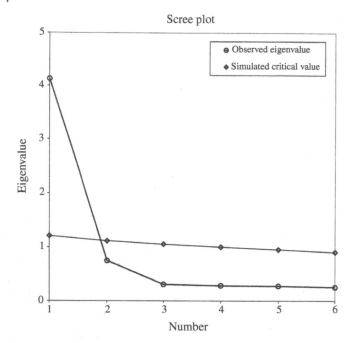

Figure 5.23 Scree plot and critical values from parallel analysis (based on initial correlation matrix).

```
Initial Factor Solution
Eigenvalues of the Reduced Correlation Matrix: Total = 3.73729872 Average = 0.62288312
           Eigenvalue    Difference    Proportion    Cumulative
      1    3.75274781    3.37886627      1.0041        1.0041
      2    0.37388154    0.45659483      0.1000        1.1042
      3    -.08271329    0.00932933     -0.0221        1.0820
      4    -.09204262    0.00484766     -0.0246        1.0574
      5    -.09689028    0.02079414     -0.0259        1.0315
      6    -.11768443                   -0.0315        1.0000
2 factors will be retained by the NFACTOR criterion.

Rotated Factor Solution
        Inter-Factor Correlations
                 Factor1         Factor2
Factor1         1.00000         0.70100
Factor2         0.70100         1.00000

Rotated Factor Pattern (Standardized Regression Coefficients)
           Factor1         Factor2
v1         0.08685         0.77100
v2         0.10425         0.73607
v3         0.13074         0.73002
v4         0.75604         0.11475
v5         0.76856         0.08765
v6         0.74585         0.11320
```

Figure 5.24 Eigenvalues for initial factor solution and rotated factor pattern.

simulate data, but we clearly see that we have a robust two-factor structure of the scale with large loadings on one factor and small loadings for another. Note that FACTOR procedure also attempts to estimate the correlation between latent factors but performs poorly – the simulated correlation between latent factors was defined as 0.5, but in Figure 5.24, the estimated correlation is 0.70100.

There is another important property of the parallel analysis: The critical values have no relationship with the data itself; the only important number is the number of items (variables) in a scale and, to some degree, the number of observations. If we would run the analysis using the code from Figure 5.21 and change the correlation between latent factors and also change the loadings, but keep the same number of observations, the critical values from parallel analysis will not change. There can be small changes when a different SEED is used, but with a sufficient number of simulations even this difference disappears.

5.1.3.3 Parallel Analysis with Reduced Correlation Matrix
In the previous section, the parallel analysis, as implemented in FACTOR procedure, is based on the initial (full) correlation matrix. It is as if we would do exploratory factor analysis specifying that communalities should be equal to 1 (this option is implemented by PRIORS=ONE). But we are not interested in explaining or understanding all variance represented by the data; instead, we are interested in the understanding of the common variance. To investigate the possible measurement structure of a scale based on the common variance, we use the reduced correlation matrix with diagonal elements equal to communalities for every variable.

If we want to do parallel analysis base on a reduced correlation matrix, then the simulations should be programed from the ground up. To perform this analysis, we consider the following five-step algorithm.

First step: to simulate the random dataset based only on the number of variables, number of observations, and possible range distribution of those variables;
Second step: to create a reduced correlation matrix corresponding to the hypothesized common variance;
Third step: to estimate the eigenvalues of this reduced correlation matrix and keep them to analyze later;
Fourth step: to repeat the above steps a sufficient number of times (say, 1000 or more times);
Fifth step: to estimate critical values as the 95th percentile for every eigenvalue.

Figure 5.25 represents the implementation of the above-described algorithm. To simplify and highlight some additional elements of the LUA language, the parallel analysis was implemented via three functions. The first function is the CreateSimDataset and corresponds to the first step of the creating random dataset. In our simulation (datasets "_efa_1"; see Figure 5.21) the variable

```
Proc Lua restart;
submit;
-- Beginning of the CreateSimDataset function
function CreateSimDataset(seed,n)
sas.submit
[[
Data _tmp_1;
Do id=1 to @n@;call streaminit(@seed@);
v1 = RAND('NORMAL',  0, 1);
v2 = RAND('NORMAL',  0, 1);
v3 = RAND('NORMAL',  0, 1);
v4 = RAND('NORMAL',  0, 1);
v5 = RAND('NORMAL',  0, 1);
v6 = RAND('NORMAL',  0, 1);
output;
End;
Drop ID;
Run;
]]
end
-- End of the CreateSimDataset function

-- Beginning of the SimEigenvalues function
function SimEigenvalues()
sas.submit
[[
Proc Factor data=_tmp_1
method=prin
PRIORS=SMC;
ODS Output Eigenvalues=Eigenvalues ;
Var v1-v6;
Run;

PROC APPEND BASE=EIGENVAL DATA=Eigenvalues; Run;
]]
end
-- End of the SimEigenvalues function

-- Beginning of the Eigenvalues95pct function
function Eigenvalues95pct()
sas.submit
[[
Proc Sort Data=EIGENVAL; By Number; Run;
Proc Univariate data=EIGENVAL;
Var Eigenvalue ;
Output out=Percentiles pctlpre=P_ pctlpts=95;
By Number;
Run;

Proc Print Data=Percentiles NOOBS; Run;
]]
end
-- End of the Eigenvalues95pct function

endsubmit;
run;
/*----------------------------------------*/
Proc Lua ;
submit;
for i=1,1000
do
 CreateSimDataset(i,500)
 SimEigenvalues()
end
Eigenvalues95pct()
endsubmit;
run;
```

Figure 5.25 Parallel analysis implementation based on reduced correlation matrix.

values are normally distributed and, as such, the random values for parallel analysis for every variable will also be taken from normal distribution. For example, for the first variable v_1, Figure 5.25 includes the following line of code

```
v1 = RAND('NORMAL', 0, 1);.
```

With real data, those lines should be replaced based on the definition of the responses for a scale under investigation. Suppose, for instance, that a scale has responses for every item ranging from 1 to 5, then the following code can be used (example for variable v_1):

```
v1 = RAND('UNIFORM', 1, 5);.
```

The SimEigenvalues function (Figure 5.25) corresponds to steps two and three. This function estimates eigenvalues for the reduced correlation matrix by simply running FACTOR procedure with option PRIORS=SMC. The APPEND procedure is then used to add estimated eigenvalues to a dataset.

The last function Eigenvalues95pct calculates 95th percentiles for every eigenvalue by using UNIVARIATE procedure.

In Figure 5.26, critical value (95th percentile) is presented for every eigenvector (after running code from Figure 5.25). Figure 5.27 shows the original eigenvalues (from Figure 5.24) overlaid with those critical values. It is clear that parallel analysis based on a reduced correlation matrix predicted correctly that the number of factors is two.

Let's also demonstrate that code from the Figure 5.25 can be used to mimic the implementation of the parallel analysis by the FACTOR procedure. To do so we just need to replace

```
PRIORS=SMC
```

by

```
PRIORS=ONE
```

in the SimEigenvalues function (inside the FACTOR procedure). Figure 5.28 represents results for the estimation of critical eigenvalues after 1000

```
Number       P_95
   1       0.22875
   2       0.13560
   3       0.06906
   4       0.01100
   5      -0.03528
   6      -0.09056
```

Figure 5.26 95th percentiles for eigenvalues based on 1000 randomly simulated datasets using reduced correlation matrix (critical values with PRIOR = SMC using code from 5.25).

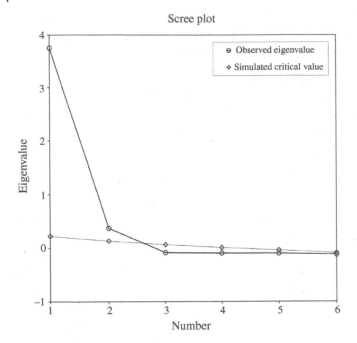

Figure 5.27 95th percentiles for eigenvalues from parallel analysis overlaid over scree plot with original eigenvalues.

Number	P_95
1	1.20951
2	1.12027
3	1.05730
4	1.00475
5	0.95972
6	0.90164

Figure 5.28 95th percentiles for eigenvalues based on 1000 randomly simulated datasets using full correlation matrix (critical values with PRIOR = ONE using code from 5.25).

simulations – comparing those values with the simulated critical values from Figure 5.22, we can see that they are practically the same.

Given the previous illustration, a logical question to ask is which approach is most appropriate to be used. The answer is that we recommend exploring all of them, if possible. It should be somewhat clear after this section that exploratory factor analysis is just, well, "exploratory." We should not rely just on the results of parallel analysis to define the number of factors. Ideally, a suggested factor structure should be evaluated through a logical connection between items. Do items suggested by exploratory factor analysis as belonging to a given factor represent a plausible latent factor? Can those items be considered as representing facets of the same underlying factor? We recommended, therefore, to confirm the factor structure by using confirmatory factor analysis.

5.1.3.4 Factor Loadings

In the simulations we presented previously in this section, the factors loadings were simple to interpret. For example, in Figure 5.24, variables v_1, v_2, and v_3 have large loadings for factor 2 (with observed loadings values of 0.77100, 0.73607, and 0.73002) and notably smaller loadings for factor 1 (and opposite pattern for variables v_4, v_5, and v_6). If, as a result of the exploratory factor analysis, a suggested factor structure for a scale has three or more domains, then the same type of pattern should be applied, namely, for a variable to be representative of a factor it should have a large loading for one and only factor, with noticeably smaller loadings for other factors.

Now consider a hypothetical example presented by Figure 5.29 with three known factors. It is clear that variables v_1, v_2, and v_3 represent factor 3 and variables v_6, v_7, and v_8 represent factor 1. But variables v_4 and v_5 have large loadings for two domains and, as such, can be generally considered flawed items, which can be deleted, as they measure or represent two concepts (factors) simultaneously. Variable v_9 represents the opposite situation in that this item does not load on any factor and, again, the general suggestion is simply to remove this item from the scale. Those are the general recommendations but, with real scales, the situation could be somewhat more complicated and not as straightforward.

The one possible situation, for example, is that the variable v_9 is the single variable that also represents a new and distinct concept, different from factors 1 and 3 (note that the loadings were low for all three factors). Variables v_4 and v_5 could be representative also of a distinct, but related to factors 1, 2, and 3, concept (note high loadings for factors 1, 2, and 3). The point is that if the items were generated as a result of well-conducted qualitative work, all those items are important for subjects and cannot be simply dismissed outright.

Rotated Factor Pattern (Standardized Regression Coefficients)			
	Factor1	Factor2	Factor3
v1	0.08685	0.04501	**0.77100**
v2	0.10425	0.23200	**0.73607**
v3	0.13074	0.09789	**0.73002**
v4	**0.75604**	**0.66475**	0.11475
v5	**0.76856**	0.17651	**0.88765**
v6	**0.74585**	0.11320	0.11320
v7	**0.63445**	0.11320	0.11320
v8	**0.89701**	0.11320	0.11320
v9	0.20456	0.11320	0.11320

Figure 5.29 Hypothetical rotated factor pattern.

For example, on the nine-item Minnesota Nicotine Withdrawal Scale, scree plots and rotated factor patterns from the exploratory factor analyses revealed two multi-item domains – Negative Affect with four items and Insomnia with two items – and three individual items (Craving, Restlessness, Increased Appetite) (Cappelleri et al. 2005). Specifically, the four items on Negative Affect had large loadings on factor 1 and a low loading on factor 2. Similarly, the two items on Insomnia had large loadings on factor 2 and a low loading on factor 1. While the remaining three items were judged to be retained for their clinical relevance (based on prior research and specialty knowledge), the Increased Appetite item loaded tenuously, Restlessness item loaded ambiguously, and Craving item loaded inconsistently across assessments. These three items lacked the cohesiveness and stability desired across states of withdrawal, suggesting that each of the three items represented a singular aspect of withdrawal rather than one belonging to a multi-item domain. The two domains (negative affect and insomnia) and the three individual items (increased restlessness, and especially craving) are each relevant in evaluating and understanding comprehensively the effect that smoking cessation treatment has on distinctive aspects of withdrawal symptoms (Gonzales et al. 2006; Jorenby et al. 2006).

How large must a factor loading be to be considered "large" and thus "substantial"? We suggest that a loading equal to or greater than 0.40 be treated as meaningful and that loadings under 0.40 generally be ignored (O'Rourke and Hatcher 2013; Stevens 2009).

Consider the following simulation presented by Figure 5.30. The simulated scale has three orthogonal factors (their pairwise correlations are zero), seven items, and the last factor is represented by just one variable v_7. This type of variable commonly referenced as a *manifest* or a directly observable variable, is distinct from a latent variable representing a hypothetical construct. For the first run of this simulation, three factors are requested to be extracted. Figure 5.31 shows the scree plot based on reduced correlation matrix, which indicates that three factors can be considered – the straight dashed line goes through eigenvalues 7, 6, 5, and 4, but below eigenvalues 3 (by a small margin), 2, and 1.

Knowing that original factors are orthogonal, let's first look at the orthogonal Rotated Factor Pattern (in output section titled "Prerotated Factor Solution"). Figure 5.32 indicates that the first six variables correctly attributed to the two factors (as simulated), but the last variable v_7 has small loadings for all three factors. As stated previously, in a vast majority of cases we should not assume that latent factors are orthogonal; an oblique solution should be examined (see the "Rotated Factor Solution" in Figure 5.33).

The oblique solution correctly identified the association between first six variables and factors 1 and 2. But loadings for variable v_7 have been drastically changed. Now we have large (in absolute values) loadings (0.78555

```
data _corr_(type=corr);
input
_TYPE_ $   _NAME_ $   F1     F2     F3     U1     U2     U3     U4     U5     U6     U7;
datalines;
 CORR       F1         1      0      0      0      0      0      0      0      0      0
 CORR       F2         0      1      0      0      0      0      0      0      0      0
 CORR       F3         0      0      1      0      0      0      0      0      0      0
 CORR       U1         0      0      0      1      0      0      0      0      0      0
 CORR       U2         0      0      0      0      1      0      0      0      0      0
 CORR       U3         0      0      0      0      0      1      0      0      0      0
 CORR       U4         0      0      0      0      0      0      1      0      0      0
 CORR       U5         0      0      0      0      0      0      0      1      0      0
 CORR       U6         0      0      0      0      0      0      0      0      1      0
 CORR       U7         0      0      0      0      0      0      0      0      0      1
 MEAN       .          0      0      0      0      0      0      0      0      0      0
 STD        .          1      1      1      1      1      1      1      1      1      1
 N          .          500    500    500    500    500    500    500    500    500    500
;
run;

proc simnormal data=_corr_ out=_sim_ds numreal=500 seed=12345;
var F1 F2 F3 U1 U2 U3 U4 U5 U6 U7;
run;

Data _efa_2;
Set _sim_ds;
/* Step 1: Setting values of loading for latent factors */
Lf1v1 = 0.8; Lf2v1 = 0.2;  Lf3v1 = 0.2;
Lf1v2 = 0.8; Lf2v2 = 0.2;  Lf3v2 = 0.2;
Lf1v3 = 0.8; Lf2v3 = 0.2;  Lf3v3 = 0.2;
Lf1v4 = 0.2; Lf2v4 = 0.8;  Lf3v4 = 0.1;
Lf1v5 = 0.2; Lf2v5 = 0.8;  Lf3v5 = 0.1;
Lf1v6 = 0.2; Lf2v6 = 0.8;  Lf3v6 = 0.1;
Lf1v7 = 0. ; Lf2v7 = 0. ;  Lf3v7 = 0.7;
/* Step 2: Estimating loadings for unique factors (Lu1v1, Lu2v2....)*/
Lu1v1 =sqrt(1-Lf1v1**2-Lf2v1**2-Lf3v1**2);
Lu2v2 =sqrt(1-Lf1v2**2-Lf2v2**2-Lf3v2**2);
Lu3v3 =sqrt(1-Lf1v3**2-Lf2v3**2-Lf3v3**2);
Lu4v4 =sqrt(1-Lf1v4**2-Lf2v4**2-Lf3v4**2);
Lu5v5 =sqrt(1-Lf1v5**2-Lf2v5**2-Lf3v5**2);
Lu6v6 =sqrt(1-Lf1v6**2-Lf2v6**2-Lf3v6**2);
Lu7v7 =sqrt(1-Lf1v7**2-Lf2v7**2-Lf3v7**2);
/* Step 3: Creating variable v1, v2,..v6, and v7 */
v1 = Lf1v1*F1 + Lf2v1*F2 + Lf3v1*F3 + Lu1v1*U1;
v2 = Lf1v2*F1 + Lf2v2*F2 + Lf3v2*F3 + Lu2v2*U2;
v3 = Lf1v3*F1 + Lf2v3*F2 + Lf3v3*F3 + Lu3v3*U3;
v4 = Lf1v4*F1 + Lf2v4*F2 + Lf3v4*F3 + Lu4v4*U4;
v5 = Lf1v5*F1 + Lf2v5*F2 + Lf3v5*F3 + Lu5v5*U5;
v6 = Lf1v6*F1 + Lf2v6*F2 + Lf3v6*F3 + Lu6v6*U6;
v7 = Lf1v7*F1 + Lf2v7*F2 + Lf3v7*F3 + Lu7v7*U7;
Run;
proc factor data=_efa_2 method=prin PRIORS=SMC rotate=PROMAX NFACTORS=3;
Var v1-v7;
Run;
```

Figure 5.30 Exploratory factor analysis with manifest variables.

and -0.60602) for factors 2 and 3 and a small loading for factor 1. Note also that two large loadings observed from the output have different signs, meaning that an assumed positive change in factors 2 and 3 will affect variable seven in two different directions. While negative loadings can be tolerated when small (assuming that all items are scored in the same direction in reflecting the concept of interest), but to have a large negative loading means that something is not right (recall discussion on negative Cronbach's coefficient alpha in Section 4.2.1).

Applying the parallel analysis (as implemented by FACTOR procedure or based on the approach from Figure 5.25) suggested that only two factors are needed to

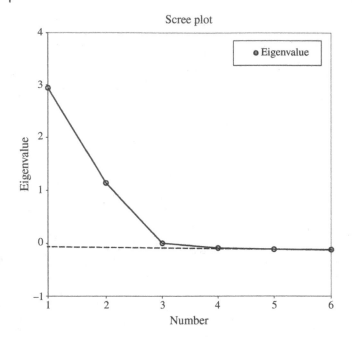

Figure 5.31   Scree plot based on reduced correlation matrix (for simulation from Figure 5.30).

```
              Rotated Factor Pattern
              Factor1          Factor2          Factor3
v1            0.23018          0.79683          0.06172
v2            0.27703          0.76753          0.05559
v3            0.19689          0.80855          0.07468
v4            0.80928          0.13134          0.02280
v5            0.79027          0.15680          0.01054
v6            0.80511          0.13991          0.01695
v7           -0.01589          0.19348         -0.04378
```

Figure 5.32   Prerotated factor solution (orthogonal solution; results of the simulation based on Figure 5.30).

```
Rotated Factor Pattern (Standardized Regression Coefficients)
              Factor1          Factor2          Factor3
v1            0.01929          0.82656         -0.00314
v2            0.08169          0.82741         -0.04710
v3           -0.03179          0.72489          0.12469
v4            0.81649         -0.07987          0.07508
v5            0.80315          0.08931         -0.07102
v6            0.81612         -0.00630          0.00785
v7           -0.01323          0.78555         -0.60602
```

Figure 5.33   Rotated factor pattern (oblique solution; results of the simulation based on Figure 5.30).

```
Rotated Factor Pattern (Standardized Regression Coefficients)
            Factor1        Factor2
v1          0.02241        0.82168
v2          0.08108        0.77927
v3         -0.01679        0.84258
v4          0.83267       -0.02966
v5          0.80518        0.00118
v6          0.82583       -0.01989
v7         -0.07116        0.21050
```

Figure 5.34 Rotated factor pattern (oblique solution; results of the simulation from Figure 5.30 with "NFACTORS=2").

describe simulated dataset "_efa_2" (note that the SAS code is not included, and readers are encouraged to run those analysis by altering SAS code in Figures 5.25 and 5.30 accordingly). It indicates that even parallel analysis has trouble to identify the correct number of factors. Figure 5.34 represents the Rotated Factor Pattern if only two factors are requested to be extracted. The corresponding result for variable seven is likely to be erroneously interpreted for deletion, as it does not have substantial or even logical loadings in both analyses (with three factors or two factors extracted). But we know that variable seven is a manifest variable – it was simulated as such. This lesson shows the importance of a rigorous examination of not only the suggested structure of the scale but also the variables themselves, which may be mistaken initially as being unnecessary or redundant. Manifest single-item variables can be crucial in the measurement the underlying conditions and effect of the treatment, as illustrated previously with the Minnesota Nicotine Withdrawal Scale.

In conclusion, historically the exploratory factor analysis has been applied to identify sets of factors for a measurement scale. The implication is that we are, basically, saying we are not sure how many latent factors (sub-concepts) this scale has and what factor-specific items in this scale are measuring (i.e., measurement model is completely undetermined). In the modern approach, we should have very good appraisal for the number of factors and items measuring those factors – that is, we should have a predefined *conceptual framework based on qualitative work*. This means that we do not need to determine the number of factors or items measuring those factors – we only (best case scenario) need to confirm the measurement structure of a scale using confirmatory factor analysis.

5.2 Confirmatory Factor Analyses

5.2.1 Confirmatory Factor Analysis Model

Let's again start with a hypothetical scale with n items (variables $v_1, v_2, \ldots, v_n$). Every item, as in the exploratory factor analysis, represents a patient-reported (or clinician or observer-) reported measurement for a particular aspect of the measured concept. And, let's also assume that the measurement model for this scale is represented by k domains ($k < n$). Confirmatory factor analysis assumes that the variable v_i is represented as a mixture of just two components: (i) a factor this variable is associated with and (ii) the error term (Brown 2015; Cappelleri et al. 2013; Kline 2011; O'Rourke and Hatcher 2013). Both components are not observed (latent), but they sum up to yield v_i. This relationship can generally be represented by the following equation (assuming that variable v_i is associated with latent factor F_k):

$$v_i = lf_k v_i F_k + e_i \tag{5.15}$$

The coefficient $lf_k v_i$ (also referenced as a factor loading) represents the impact of the factor F_k on variable v_i. The error term e_i is assumed to be from a normal distribution with mean 0 and a variance σ_e^2 [$e_i \sim N(0, \sigma_e^2)$]. Both of those parameters ($lf_k v_i$ and σ_e^2) are need to be estimated. Note that this Eq. (5.15) (and graphical depiction of this equation by Figure 5.35) represents only a fragment of the larger full confirmatory factor analysis model, but this fragment matches almost exactly the initial measurement error model, which served as the basis for the test–retest analyses and was discussed in Chapter 4 (specifically in Section 4.1.1 – compare Figures 5.35 and 4.1). It shows that at its elemental level the confirmatory factor analysis model for relationships between a latent factor and an observed variable is also deeply rooted in classical measurement theory.

Figure 5.36 depicts a typical confirmatory factor analysis model. This figure represents relationships among latent factors, observed variables and error terms for a hypothetical scale. The scale includes nine items, which are representative of three domains. The first three items represent factor 1, next three items represent factor 2, and last three items represent factor 3.

The most important part, which serves as a basic building block of the full model, is the part represented by Figure 5.37 (example for the variable v_4). This figure illustrates the fundamental relationship between a latent factor and an

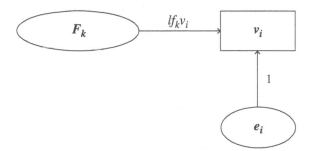

Figure 5.35 Confirmatory factor analysis: a fragment depicting the relationship between item v_i, corresponding latent factor, and the error.

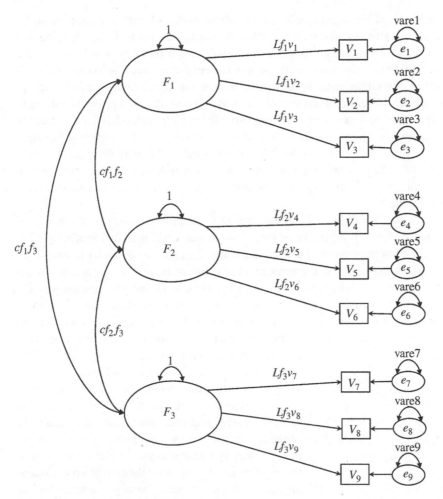

Figure 5.36 Confirmatory factor analysis model for a scale with nine items and three domains.

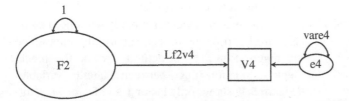

Figure 5.37 The segment of the *measurement* part of the model: a fundamental element of the confirmatory factor analysis model.

observed variable – changes in the latent (unobserved) factors are the cause for the changes in the observed variables. It should be noted that in this chapter, unless stated otherwise, almost all examples and discussions are based on the assumption that the relationship between latent factors and observed variables is consistent with the reflective model (formative models with casual indicators will be discussed later in this chapter). Unknown loading Lf2v4 represents a strength of the effect of factor 2 on observed variable V4 (it is, essentially, a slope in the regression Eq. (5.15)). Variable V4 is also affected by another unobserved component represented by the oval with letters e4 inside – this is an error term. Note a curved two-headed arrow connected to the oval with letters vare4 above, which symbolizes the variance of the error term for variable (or item) 4; it also needs to be estimated.

The next important detail in Figure 5.37 is the curved two-headed arrow connected to the oval representing factor 2 – in this case, it is also symbolizes the variance but here the variance of the latent factor is set equal to 1. This is an important distinction in the assessment of the confirmatory factor analysis models vs. causal models. When causal models are considered, the variances of the latent factors are usually set to be free parameters, but, as a result, one of the loadings from a latent factor to a variable is needed to be set to the value of 1. By doing so, we create measurement units for this factor (i.e., the factor can now be considered as if measured using the same units as that of the corresponding variable). In confirmatory factor analysis, on the other hand, the loadings for every variable are one of the central parameters needed to be estimated and then evaluated. As a result, we generally keep latent factors as unitless components in confirmatory factor analysis modeling and postulate or predefine variance for them to be equal, generally, to 1 (in fact, it could be any number) for the model to be estimable. Figure 5.37 also corresponds to the *measurement* part of the model, the part which outlines the relationships between latent factors and corresponding observed variables.

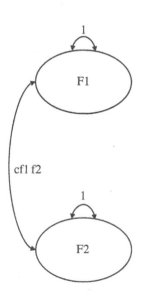

Figure 5.38 Example of the *structural* part of the confirmatory factor analysis model.

Another essential block, generally referenced as the *structural* part of the model, is partially represented by Figure 5.38. The structural part of the model depicts relationships between latent variables (Figure 5.38 shows only factor 1 and factor 2). A different kind of curved two-headed arrow is present: It is connected to both ovals representing factor 1 and factor 2 with letters cf1f2 attached to it – representing the covariance between factor 1 and factor 2, which also needs to be estimated. This type of the curved two-headed arrow implies that we assume that latent factors are less likely to be independent and, as such, they will covary. In a full model (Figure 5.36), we assume that all three latent factors can covary and variables `cf1f2`, `cf1f3`, and `cf2f3` represent those covariances (which need to be estimated). Figure 5.38 (and in part 5.36) represents the simplest relationship between latent factors. In fact, we can even predefine a relationship between any two latent factors. For example, we can define that `cf1f2` to be equal to 0, which would mean that factor 1 and factor 2 are postulated as orthogonal or independent, although this assumption is generally not recommended; it is better for a model to estimate those parameters based on the empirical data.

5.2.2 Confirmatory Factor Analysis Model Implementation

Consider the same hypothetical scale presented by Figure 5.36 with nine observed items (variables) and three domains (factors). Figure 5.39 represents the generations of the simulated dataset. The first data step creates a correlation type dataset

```
data _corr_(type=corr);
input
_TYPE_ $ _NAME_ $  F1    F2    F3    e1   e2   e3   e4   e5   e6   e7   e8   e9;
datalines;
CORR        F1     1     0.4   0.5   0    0    0    0    0    0    0    0    0
CORR        F2     0.4   1     0.6   0    0    0    0    0    0    0    0    0
CORR        F3     0.5   0.6   1     0    0    0    0    0    0    0    0    0
CORR        e1     0     0     0     1    0    0    0    0    0    0    0    0
CORR        e2     0     0     0     0    1    0    0    0    0    0    0    0
CORR        e3     0     0     0     0    0    1    0    0    0    0    0    0
CORR        e4     0     0     0     0    0    0    1    0    0    0    0    0
CORR        e5     0     0     0     0    0    0    0    1    0    0    0    0
CORR        e6     0     0     0     0    0    0    0    0    1    0    0    0
CORR        e7     0     0     0     0    0    0    0    0    0    1    0    0
CORR        e8     0     0     0     0    0    0    0    0    0    0    1    0
CORR        e9     0     0     0     0    0    0    0    0    0    0    0    1
MEAN        .      0     0     0     0    0    0    0    0    0    0    0    0
STD         .      1     1     1     1    1    1    1    1    1    1    1    1
N           .      500   500   500   500  500  500  500  500  500  500  500 500
;
run;
proc simnormal data=_corr_ out=_sim_ds numreal=500 seed=345;
var F1 F2 F3 e1 e2 e3 e4 e5 e6 e7 e8 e9;
run;
Data _cfa_1;
Set  _sim_ds;
/* Step 1: Setting values of loadings for latent factors*/
Lf1v1 = 1.2; Lf1v2 = 1.4; Lf1v3 = 1.3;
Lf2v4 = 2.1; Lf2v5 = 1.9; Lf2v6 = 1.7;
Lf3v7 = 0.9; Lf3v8 = 1.0; Lf3v9 = 1.4;
/* Step 2: Setting values of variances for error terms */
vare1 = sqrt(2.5); vare2 = sqrt(1.5); vare3 = sqrt(2.0);
vare4 = sqrt(2.6); vare5 = sqrt(3.7); vare6 = sqrt(3.1);
vare7 = sqrt(2.2); vare8 = sqrt(2.7); vare9 = sqrt(1.8);
/* Step 3: Creating variable v1, v2,...v8, and v9 */
v1 = Lf1v1*F1 + vare1*e1; v2 = Lf1v2*F1 + vare2*e2; v3 = Lf1v3*F1 + vare3*e3;
v4 = Lf2v4*F2 + vare4*e4; v5 = Lf2v5*F2 + vare5*e5; v6 = Lf2v6*F2 + vare6*e6;
v7 = Lf3v7*F3 + vare7*e7; v8 = Lf3v8*F3 + vare8*e8; v9 = Lf3v9*F3 + vare9*e9;
Keep v1 v2 v3 v4 v5 v6 v7 v8 v9;
Run;
```

Figure 5.39 Generation of the simulated dataset for confirmatory factor analysis.

representing relationships between latent variables in the model (note that error terms are also considered as latent components in the model). This data step ("data _corr_ ..") should be pretty familiar by now. We define three correlated factors: correlation between factors 1 and 2 is postulated to be 0.4, the correlation between factors 1 and 3 is 0.5, and between factors 2 and 3 is 0.6. The error terms (e1 e2 ... e9) are considered to be independent of each other and also not related (independent) to factors 1, 2, and 3. As pointed out in Figure 5.38, the variance of the latent factors is postulated to be equal to 1. We also define here variances (and standard deviations) of the error terms to be 1, as we will define actual variances of error terms later.

The SIMNORMAL procedure is generating 500 observations with random values representing latent factors and errors. The next data step ("Data _cfa_1;...") creates simulated observed variables (v1 v2 ... v9). To simulate every variable, we only need to define a loading for this variable and the variance of the error term. Note this principal dissimilarity between exploratory factor analysis and confirmatory factor analysis: there is no any relationship between factor loadings and variances of the error terms, and an observed variable is affected by only one latent factor (compare SAS code from Figure 5.5 with current code from Figure 5.39).

Figure 5.40 represents the implementation of the confirmatory factor analysis model using the CALIS procedure. It is the same CALIS procedure introduced in Chapter 4 and was used to show how test–retest analysis works. This introductory example has three essential segments working together to describe the model titled as LINEQS, VARIANCE, and COV. It should be noted that there are several different approaches implemented as a part of the CALIS procedure to define a model, which is markedly different. While we find that the approach described below is most intuitive, other researchers could find other modeling "languages" more suitable.

Under the section titled LINEQS (Figure 5.40), the causal relationships among observed variables, latent factors, and error terms are described in terms of what is affecting what. Note that every line under LINEQS, for example

```
v1 = lf1v1 f1 + e1,
```

is almost an exact replica of Eq. (5.15).

```
Proc Calis COV data=_cfa_1 G4=200 GCONV=1E-10 Method=ML ALL;
LINEQS
  v1    = lf1v1 f1 + e1,   v2   = lf1v2 f1 + e2,   v3   = lf1v3 f1 + e3,
  v4    = lf2v4 f2 + e4,   v5   = lf2v5 f2 + e5,   v6   = lf2v6 f2 + e6,
  v7    = lf3v7 f3 + e7,   v8   = lf3v8 f3 + e8,   v9   = lf3v9 f3 + e9;
VARIANCE
f1=1,f2=1,f3=1,
e1 = vare1, e2 = vare2, e3 = vare3, e4 = vare4, e5 = vare5, e6 = vare6, e7 = vare7,
e8 = vare8, e9 = vare9;
COV
f1 f2 = cf1f2, f1 f3 = cf1f3, f2 f3 = cf2f3;
Run;
```

Figure 5.40 Confirmatory factor analysis model implementation.

The next integral part in the description of the model is the section VARIANCE. In this section, we define which latent variables variances will be predefined or should be estimated. In this example, variances for latent factors 1, 2, and 3 are postulated to be equal to 1 (see Figure 5.36 and discussion of Figure 5.38). But the variances for the error terms are needed to be estimated. We instruct to do this by assigning a parameter to be estimated to the error term. For example, the following statement

```
e1 = vare1
```

directs CALIS procedure to estimate the variance for the error term e1 and assign it to variable vare1. Compare this with the implementation from Figure 4.3, where an opposite tactic was implemented – the variance of the latent factor was a free parameter, but the variance of the error term was postulated. Note that for this particular type, generally called first-order confirmatory factor analysis, the variances of the latent factors should be postulated, and the variances of the error terms should be estimated.

The last section titled COV defines not causal relationships between variables in the model (causal relationships defined under LINEQS). The first-order confirmatory factor analysis (CFA) corresponds to the measurement model of a scale with two or more domains (latent factors), which scored separately and a scale, generally, will not have any aggregated/total score. In this case, it is generally assumed that domains are not independent, which means that they co-vary. And to express this under the COV section, we instruct the CALIS procedure to estimate covariances between latent factors.

The CALIS procedure generates a lot of information. Here the most relevant output parts will be discussed. First is the "Modeling specifications" (see Figure 5.41) - the information on how many observations available for analysis (500) and model type (LINEQS) is showed. As mentioned previously, model type here represents the specific SAS "language" to describe relationships between observed and latent variables; it does not represent anything else. The next subsection specifies the variables in the model in terms of the Endogenous, Exogenous, Manifest, Latent, and Error. *Manifest* variables are simply observed variables – variables in the dataset representing responses of subjects to the items of a scale. *Latent* variables are not observed factors (domains) in the model, and it is important to emphasize that the input dataset should not have any variable named as f1, f2, or f3. *Error* obviously represents errors (again the input dataset should not have any variables named as e1, e2, . . .e9). *Endogenous* is referred to variables that are affected by other variables in the model. If a single-headed arrow is pointing to a variable, then this variable is endogenous. *Exogenous* variables, in contrast, are the variables that are not affected by any variable in the model and, as such, there should be no single-headed arrow pointing to this variable. Note that observed (manifest) and latent variables can be

```
         Modeling Information
      Maximum Likelihood Estimation

      Data Set                WORK._CFA_1
      N Records Read          500
      N Records Used          500
      N Obs                   500
      Model Type              LINEQS
      Analysis                Covariances

                    Variables in the Model
      Endogenous    Manifest      v1  v2  v3  v4  v5  v6  v7  v8  v9
                    Latent
      Exogenous     Manifest
                    Latent        f1  f2  f3
                    Error         e1  e2  e3  e4  e5  e6  e7  e8  e9

                 Number of Endogenous Variables = 9
                 Number of Exogenous Variables  = 12

      Initial Estimates for Linear Equations
      v1 =    1f1v1(.) f1  +  1 e1
      v2 =    1f1v2(.) f1  +  1 e2
      v3 =    1f1v3(.) f1  +  1 e3
      v4 =    1f2v4(.) f2  +  1 e4
      v5 =    1f2v5(.) f2  +  1 e5
      v6 =    1f2v6(.) f2  +  1 e6
      v7 =    1f3v7(.) f3  +  1 e7
      v8 =    1f3v8(.) f3  +  1 e8
      v9 =    1f3v9(.) f3  +  1 e9

      Initial Estimates for Variances of Exogenous Variables
      Variable
      Type               Variable     Parameter       Estimate
      Latent             f1                            1.00000
                         f2                            1.00000
                         f3                            1.00000
      Error              e1           vare1               .
                         e2           vare2               .
                         e3           vare3               .
                         e4           vare4               .
                         e5           vare5               .
                         e6           vare6               .
                         e7           vare7               .
                         e8           vare8               .
                         e9           vare9               .

      Initial Estimates for Covariances Among Exogenous Variables
      Var1     Var2     Parameter        Estimate
      f1       f2       cf1f2               .
      f1       f3       cf1f3               .
      f2       f3       cf2f3               .
```

Figure 5.41 Modeling specifications.

endogenous or exogeneous as a part of a CFA model, but error variables will always be exogeneous.

The sections Initial Estimates for Linear Equations, Initial Estimates for Variances of Exogenous Variables, and Initial Estimates for Covariances Among Exogenous Variables simply repeat the description of the model highlighting which parameters are postulated and which parameters need to be estimated, with the dot (.) symbolizing an unknown parameter.

```
Covariance Structure Analysis: Maximum Likelihood Estimation

                         Fit Summary
Modeling Info      Number of Observations                500
                   Number of Variables                    9
                   Number of Moments                     45
                   Number of Parameters                  21
                   Number of Active Constraints           0
                   Baseline Model Function Value     2.0861
                   Baseline Model Chi-Square      1040.9440
                   Baseline Model Chi-Square DF          36
                   Pr > Baseline Model Chi-Square    <.0001
Absolute Index     Fit Function                      0.0582
                   Chi-Square                       29.0473
                   Chi-Square DF                         24
                   Pr > Chi-Square                   0.2184
                   Elliptic Corrected Chi-Square    29.1717
                   Pr > Elliptic Corr. Chi-Square    0.2137
                   Z-Test of Wilson & Hilferty       0.7789
                   Hoelter Critical N                   626
                   Root Mean Square Residual (RMR)   0.1044
                   Standardized RMR (SRMR)           0.0234
                   Goodness of Fit Index (GFI)       0.9872
Parsimony Index    Adjusted GFI (AGFI)               0.9760
                   Parsimonious GFI                  0.6581
                   RMSEA Estimate                    0.0205
                   RMSEA Lower 90% Confidence Limit  0.0000
                   RMSEA Upper 90% Confidence Limit  0.0437
                   Probability of Close Fit          0.9861
                   ECVI Estimate                     0.1441
                   ECVI Lower 90% Confidence Limit   0.1350
                   ECVI Upper 90% Confidence Limit   0.1800
                   Akaike Information Criterion      71.0473
                   Bozdogan CAIC                    180.5541
                   Schwarz Bayesian Criterion      159.5541
                   McDonald Centrality               0.9950
Incremental Index  Bentler Comparative Fit Index     0.9950
                   Bentler-Bonett NFI                0.9721
                   Bentler-Bonett Non-normed Index   0.9925
                   Bollen Normed Index Rho1          0.9581
                   Bollen Non-normed Index Delta2    0.9950
                   James et al. Parsimonious NFI     0.6481
```

Figure 5.42 Fit statistics.

Figure 5.42 represents the next important section of the output, namely, the fit statistics. Modeling Info portion provides additional information for the initial specification of the model. There are two important values: Number of Parameters and Number of Moments. The Number of Parameters is simply the number of loadings, variances, and covariances needed to be estimated – which in this example is 21. It is generally suggested (Jackson 2003; Kyriazos 2018) that it should be from 5 to 20 observations available for every parameter to estimate – although note that it is just a rule of thumb. With 21 parameters we would need at least 105 observations (we simulated 500).

Another very important value is Number of Moments that is simply the number of distinct covariances between pairs of observed variables and variances of those variables. Basically, it is the number of diagonal elements (representing variances) and number of elements in upper-triangular (covariances) of the variance–covariance matrix. The Number of Parameters should always be less (or equal) but never larger than `Number of Moments`. It is important to stress that the variance–covariance matrix is *the input data* for the CALIS procedure, not the dataset with observations. In fact, we can simply use the variance–covariance matrix (or correlation matrix as will be shown later) as the input dataset for CALIS procedure. It does not mean, however, that the number of observations does not matter, as more observations will provide a more accurate variance–covariance matrix, which in turn can lead to more precise estimations of the parameters of the model.

Figure 5.42 also gives us the variety of the fit indexes. In our experience, all of them usually move more or less together but favoring some distinct aspect of the fit. To gauge the fit of the CFA model, we suggest to use Bentler's Comparative Fit Index (CFI). In our experience with many datasets from clinical studies, values of 0.9 (a cut-off value) or more are associated with good or acceptable fit (Bentler and Bonnett 1990). While a CFI threshold of 0.95 is often cited for adequate fit, it has been demonstrated as unduly conservative in rejecting acceptable models (Brown 2015; Fan and Sivo 2005; Marsh et al. 2004; Yuan 2005).

We focus on Bentler's CFI for goodness of model fit. While it has demonstrated strong performance (power and robustness) as a fit index (Bentler and Bonnett 1990), other fit indices are available but their statistical properties have documented shortcomings and are not expected to be on par with CFI, including the chi-square test statistic (West et al. 2012), goodness-of-fit statistic (Hooper et al. 2008), standardized root mean square residual (Canjur and Ercan 2015), and root mean square error of approximation (RMSEA) (Chen et al. 2008; Cook et al. 2009). Nonetheless, other researchers (for whatever reason) may favor a different fit index as evidence that the model fits the data. The general approach is that the one single fit index (including a cut-off value) should be preselected and used throughout all CFA analyses (for example, at different time points in the study).

As in case with Cronbach's alpha and exploratory factor analysis, we stress again that applying the CFA model to baseline data could lead to the small Bentler's CFI (less than 0.9) due to the restricted range in the data. The post-baseline observations are good candidates to investigate measurement model of a scale.

There are another two important sets of the results, which are also essential in the assessment of the model fit. Figure 5.43 presents the results of the estimations of the unstandardized loadings, which represent simply the effect of the latent factor on an item in the original units for this item. If a measurement model fits the data, it is anticipated that all loadings should be significant (p-value <0.05); in this example, all p-values are less than 0.0001.

The comparison of the estimated loadings with values preset in simulation (see Figure 5.44) shows that, with 500 simulated observations (based on the simulated dataset from Figure 5.39), loadings are somewhat close to the values defined in simulation. For example, loading from factor 2 to item 4 was predefined as 2.1

```
Covariance Structure Analysis: Maximum Likelihood Estimation

            Linear Equations
v1 =     0.9790(**) f1  +   1.0000 e1
v2 =     1.4125(**) f1  +   1.0000 e2
v3 =     1.3618(**) f1  +   1.0000 e3
v4 =     2.0664(**) f2  +   1.0000 e4
v5 =     1.8020(**) f2  +   1.0000 e5
v6 =     1.5674(**) f2  +   1.0000 e6
v7 =     1.0102(**) f3  +   1.0000 e7
v8 =     1.0499(**) f3  +   1.0000 e8
v9 =     1.3774(**) f3  +   1.0000 e9


                          Effects in Linear Equations
                                                  Standard
Variable     Predictor     Parameter     Estimate    Error     t Value    Pr > |t|
v1           f1            lf1v1         0.97903    0.09393    10.4224     <.0001
v2           f1            lf1v2         1.41249    0.09314    15.1660     <.0001
v3           f1            lf1v3         1.36181    0.09113    14.9441     <.0001
v4           f2            lf2v4         2.06641    0.11901    17.3627     <.0001
v5           f2            lf2v5         1.80198    0.11698    15.4048     <.0001
v6           f2            lf2v6         1.56744    0.10573    14.8257     <.0001
v7           f3            lf3v7         1.01024    0.09131    11.0638     <.0001
v8           f3            lf3v8         1.04990    0.09147    11.4779     <.0001
v9           f3            lf3v9         1.37741    0.09800    14.0553     <.0001
```

Figure 5.43   Unstandardized loadings.

Loadings in the simulation (from figure 5.39)		Estimated loadings (500 observations)		Estimated loadings (5000 observations)	
Lf1v1 = **1.2**;		lf1v1	0.97903	lf1v1	1.16704
Lf1v2 = **1.4**;		lf1v2	1.41249	lf1v2	1.35581
Lf1v3 = **1.3**;		lf1v3	1.36181	lf1v3	1.32278
Lf2v4 = **2.1**;		lf2v4	2.06641	lf2v4	2.10783
Lf2v5 = **1.9**;		lf2v5	1.80198	lf2v5	1.94278
Lf2v6 = **1.7**;		lf2v6	1.56744	lf2v6	1.70238
Lf3v7 = **0.9** ;		lf3v7	1.01024	lf3v7	0.89825
Lf3v8 = **1.0** ;		lf3v8	1.04990	lf3v8	1.00007
Lf3v9 = **1.4** ;		lf3v9	1.37741	lf3v9	1.37612

Figure 5.44   Predefined vs. estimated loadings.

(Lf2v4 = 2.1) and the estimated value for this loading was 2.06641 (lf2v4 2.06641). Loading from factor 1 to item 1 was predefined as 1.2 (Lf1v1 = 1.2), but its estimated value is 0.97903 (lf1v1 0.97903).

Generally, CFA requires a large number of observations to have stable estimations of the parameters of the model. The third column in Figure 5.44 shows that, if we run analyses with 5000 simulated observations, the estimated loadings for all items are now very close to the values predefined in the simulation (to run this analysis we only need to replace parameter numreal in the SIMNORMAL procedure [numreal = 5000] in Figure 5.39).

Confirmatory factor analysis can be viewed as a subclass of structural equation modeling or causal analysis. Estimated unstandardized loadings discussed above play an important role in CFA. But, for CFA, we need to have a standardized approach, which would allow us to interpret the strength of the relationship between a latent factor and items representing it. This approach also should be general and can be applied to any scale and is not dependent on the range of responses for every item in a scale. Standardized loadings provide this uniform and consistent solution in this context. Figure 5.45 represents standardized loadings.

It is important to note how standardized loadings are estimated: (i) the input dataset is recalculated so that every variable has a mean of zero and standard deviation of 1, and (ii) parameters of the model are then estimated using this newly created dataset. To illustrate this, we can simply apply the STANDARD procedure to dataset "_cfa_1" and then run the CALIS procedure (see Figure 5.46). In this calculation, unstandardized loadings and standardized loadings will be the same and equal to their respective loadings represented by Figure 5.45. This is somewhat analogous to the Cronbach's coefficient alpha calculations with

```
Standardized Results for Linear Equations
v1 =      0.5075(**) f1  +   1.0000 e1
v2 =      0.7476(**) f1  +   1.0000 e2
v3 =      0.7352(**) f1  +   1.0000 e3
v4 =      0.7743(**) f2  +   1.0000 e4
v5 =      0.6947(**) f2  +   1.0000 e5
v6 =      0.6714(**) f2  +   1.0000 e6
v7 =      0.5505(**) f3  +   1.0000 e7
v8 =      0.5697(**) f3  +   1.0000 e8
v9 =      0.6973(**) f3  +   1.0000 e9
```

			Standardized Effects in Linear Equations			
				Standard		
Variable	Predictor	Parameter	Estimate	Error	t Value	Pr > |t|
v1	f1	1f1v1	0.50749	0.04159	12.2024	<.0001
v2	f1	1f1v2	0.74758	0.03709	20.1550	<.0001
v3	f1	1f1v3	0.73523	0.03716	19.7834	<.0001
v4	f2	1f2v4	0.77429	0.03011	25.7123	<.0001
v5	f2	1f2v5	0.69475	0.03240	21.4412	<.0001
v6	f2	1f2v6	0.67140	0.03321	20.2157	<.0001
v7	f3	1f3v7	0.55052	0.04182	13.1638	<.0001
v8	f3	1f3v8	0.56969	0.04122	13.8211	<.0001
v9	f3	1f3v9	0.69731	0.03839	18.1656	<.0001

Figure 5.45 Standardized loadings.

```
Proc Standard DATA=_cfa_1 Mean=0 Std=1 Out=_cfa_2;
  Var v1 v2 v3 v4 v5 v6 v7 v8 v9 ;
RUN;

Proc Calis COV data=_cfa_2 G4=200 GCONV=1E-10 Method=ML  ALL;
LINEQS
  v1    = 1f1v1 f1 + e1,   v2    = 1f1v2 f1 + e2,   v3    = 1f1v3 f1 + e3,
  v4    = 1f2v4 f2 + e4,   v5    = 1f2v5 f2 + e5,   v6    = 1f2v6 f2 + e6,
  v7    = 1f3v7 f3 + e7,   v8    = 1f3v8 f3 + e8,   v9    = 1f3v9 f3 + e9;
VARIANCE
f1=1,  f2=1,  f3=1,
e1 =vare1, e2 =vare2, e3 =vare3, e4 =vare4, e5 =vare5, e6 =vare6, e7 =vare7,
e8 =vare8, e9 =vare9;
Cov
f1 f2 =cf1f2, f1 f3 =cf1f3, f2 f3 =cf2f3;
Run;
```

Figure 5.46 Performing CFA with standardized variables.

standardized variables. Although in CFA the results using standardized variables play a fundamental role (which is completely opposite to the recommendation given in Section 4.2.1 on the use of the Cronbach's coefficient alpha results using standardized variables).

For the effect of a latent factor on an item to be considered as meaningful, we recommend that a standardized loading should be at least 0.4 (Cappelleri et al. 2013; Brown 2015; O'Rourke and Hatcher 2013; Stevens 2009) and significant (p-value<0.05). Figure 5.45 shows that all standardized loadings are greater than 0.4 and significant (p-values<0.0001). As discussed previously, baseline data are not optimal for the assessment of the fit of the measurement model of a scale (the same was noted for Cronbach's coefficient alpha in Chapter 4). Baseline values for loadings are also likely be less than a cut-off of 0.4 or not significant or both. Using baseline data should not be considered as the only option to test the measurement model of a scale.

The joint evaluation of the above-described results finalizes the assessment of the measurement model fit. In summary, for the measurement model to fit the data, the Bentler CFI should be at least 0.9, unstandardized and standardized loadings should be significant (p-value<0.05) and, in addition, all standardized loadings should be at least 0.4.

While for the assessment of model fit, we highlighted the need to evaluate three sets of results (fit index, unstandardized and standardized loadings) at the different time points, there are two other sets of results that are important for understanding how well CFA can estimate other parameters defined in the simulation. Recall that in the simulation, we also predefined the variances of error terms and correlations between latent factors. Figures 5.47 and 5.48 show estimations of those parameters in comparison with simulated values. Most estimations of the variances and correlations using the dataset with 500 simulated observations were close to predefined values. For example, the correlation between latent factor 1 and latent factor 2 was predefined to be equal to 0.4 and the estimated value was 0.33909. But when the same analysis was performed using simulated dataset

Variances in the simulation (from Figure 5.39)	Estimated variances (500 observations)		Estimated variances (5000 observations)	
vare1 = sqrt(2.5);	vare1	2.76308	vare1	2.56851
vare2 = sqrt(1.5);	vare2	1.57478	vare2	1.54137
vare3 = sqrt(2.0);	vare3	1.57622	vare3	1.87236
vare4 = sqrt(2.6);	vare4	2.85239	vare4	2.70073
vare5 = sqrt(3.7);	vare5	3.48025	vare5	3.60792
vare6 = sqrt(3.1);	vare6	2.99344	vare6	3.02779
vare7 = sqrt(2.2);	vare7	2.34685	vare7	2.16698
vare8 = sqrt(2.7);	vare8	2.29405	vare8	2.60657
vare9 = sqrt(1.8);	vare9	2.00461	vare9	1.83067

Figure 5.47 Predefined vs. estimated variances.

Correlations in the simulation (from Figure 5.39)			Estimated correlations (500 observations)				Estimated correlations (5000 observations)			
	F1	F2	F3	Var1	Var2	Parameter	Estimate	Var1	Var2	Parameter	Estimate
F1	1	0.4	0.5	f1	f2	cf1f2	0.33909	f1	f2	cf1f2	0.40077
F2	0.4	1	0.6	f1	f3	cf1f3	0.50375	f1	f3	cf1f3	0.49332
F3	0.5	0.6	1	f2	f3	cf2f3	0.64134	f2	f3	cf2f3	0.60110

Figure 5.48 Predefined vs. estimated correlations.

with 5000 observations, the estimations of the corresponding variances and correlations were much closer to the predefined values. For example, estimated correlations between latent factors were practically the same as defined in the simulation. This indicates that if a measurement model is defined correctly, then CFA will be able to extract asymptotically correct estimations of the parameters of the model, given a sufficient number of observations.

It is also important to note that the algorithm implemented in the CALIS procedure can produce zero or even negative (!) estimations of the variances. Fortunately, it almost always is linked to the incorrect specification of the measurement model and, as such, can be fixed by providing the correct specifications. But sometimes, even if everything is correct in the programmatic definition of the measurement model, the CALIS procedure during the convergence process can generate negative variances. In this case, we can force the CALIS procedure to make the positive estimation of the variance parameters. To constrain the variances to be positive, we add the following as a part of the CALIS procedure:

```
Bounds
vare1-vare9 > 1.0e-8;
```

Note that the `Bounds` statement can be invoked not only to escape issues with negative variances but also to constrain any parameter in the model.

5.2.3 Confirmatory Factor Analysis with Domains Represented by a Single Item

Earlier in the chapter, the example of the scale which included multi-item domains alongside with single items representing unique aspects of nicotine withdrawal was described (see Section 5.1.3.4). The distinct property of this type of scales is the present of at least one domain represented by only one item – a manifest variable. Consider a scale with three multi-item latent domains $F1$, $F2$, $F3$ measured by nine items (variables v_1, v_2, ... v_9) and two single-item domains $F4$ and $F5$ with domain $F4$ represented by single manifest variable v_{10} and domain $F5$ represented by single manifest variable v_{11} (see Figure 5.49 representing the CFA model for this scale).

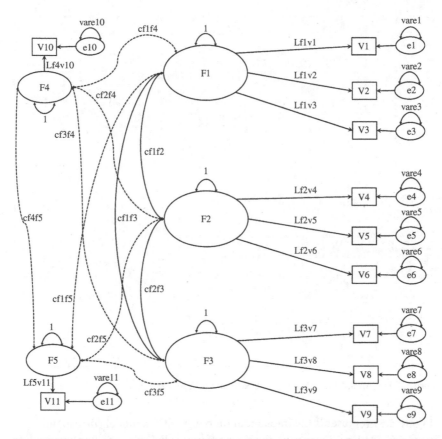

Figure 5.49 CFA model with single variables v_{10} and v_{11} (representing domains $F4$ and $F5$).

A comparison of Figure 5.49 with Figure 5.36 shows that two additional single item domains $F4$ and $F5$ follow the same pattern as that found for multi-item domains. For instance, manifest variable v_{10} is affected by latent factor $F4$ and error e_{10} (as generally any observed variables will be as a part of the CFA). To highlight the new parts of the model (relative to Figure 5.36) the covariances between factors $F4$ and $F5$ and between these factors with factors $F1$, $F2$, and $F3$ are represented by curved two-headed dashed arrows.

Figure 5.50 represents the simulation of the dataset. The simulation of this dataset was detailed earlier in the previous section (see Figure 5.39), but here we only add information on two new latent domains and two error terms as a part of the data step "data _corr_(type=corr);..." to produce a correlation matrix and an updated data step "Data _cfa_3;..." in order to simulate two additional variables v_{10} and v_{11}.

```
data _corr_(type=corr);
input
_TYPE_ $    _NAME_ $   F1     F2     F3     F4     F5     e1    e2    e3    e4    e5    e6    e7    e8    e9    e10   e11;
datalines;
 CORR        F1         1      0.4    0.5    0.5    0.4    0     0     0     0     0     0     0     0     0     0     0
 CORR        F2         0.4    1      0.6    0.3    0.5    0     0     0     0     0     0     0     0     0     0     0
 CORR        F3         0.5    0.6    1      0.2    0.3    0     0     0     0     0     0     0     0     0     0     0
 CORR        F4         0.5    0.3    0.2    1      0.4    0     0     0     0     0     0     0     0     0     0     0
 CORR        F5         0.4    0.5    0.3    0.4    1      0     0     0     0     0     0     0     0     0     0     0
 CORR        e1         0      0      0      0      0      1     0     0     0     0     0     0     0     0     0     0
 CORR        e2         0      0      0      0      0      0     1     0     0     0     0     0     0     0     0     0
 CORR        e3         0      0      0      0      0      0     0     1     0     0     0     0     0     0     0     0
 CORR        e4         0      0      0      0      0      0     0     0     1     0     0     0     0     0     0     0
 CORR        e5         0      0      0      0      0      0     0     0     0     1     0     0     0     0     0     0
 CORR        e6         0      0      0      0      0      0     0     0     0     0     1     0     0     0     0     0
 CORR        e7         0      0      0      0      0      0     0     0     0     0     0     1     0     0     0     0
 CORR        e8         0      0      0      0      0      0     0     0     0     0     0     0     1     0     0     0
 CORR        e9         0      0      0      0      0      0     0     0     0     0     0     0     0     1     0     0
 CORR        e10        0      0      0      0      0      0     0     0     0     0     0     0     0     0     1     0
 CORR        e11        0      0      0      0      0      0     0     0     0     0     0     0     0     0     0     1
 MEAN        .          0      0      0      0      0      0     0     0     0     0     0     0     0     0     0     0
 STD         .          1      1      1      1      1      1     1     1     1     1     1     1     1     1     1     1
 N           .          500    500    500    500    500    500   500   500   500   500   500   500   500   500   500   500
;
run;


proc simnormal data=_corr_ out=_sim_ds numreal=500 seed=345;
var F1 F2 F3 F4 F5 e1 e2 e3 e4 e5 e6 e7 e8 e9 e10 e11;
run;

Data _cfa_3;
Set _sim_ds;
/* Step 1: Setting values of loadings for latent factors */
Lf1v1 = 1.2; Lf1v2 = 1.4; Lf1v3 = 1.3;
Lf2v4 = 2.1; Lf2v5 = 1.9; Lf2v6 = 1.7;
Lf3v7 = 0.9; Lf3v8 = 1.0; Lf3v9 = 1.4;
Lf4v10 = 1.0 ;
Lf5v11 = 1.0 ;
/* Step 2: Setting values of variances for error terms */
vare1 = sqrt(2.5); vare2 = sqrt(1.5); vare3 = sqrt(2.0);
vare4 = sqrt(2.6); vare5 = sqrt(3.7); vare6 = sqrt(3.1);
vare7 = sqrt(2.2); vare8 = sqrt(2.7); vare9 = sqrt(1.8);
vare10 = sqrt(0.2); vare11 = sqrt(0.5);
/* Step 3: Creating variable v1, v2,..v10, and v11 */
v1 = Lf1v1*F1 + vare1*e1; v2 = Lf1v2*F1 + vare2*e2; v3 = Lf1v3*F1 + vare3*e3;
v4 = Lf2v4*F2 + vare4*e4; v5 = Lf2v5*F2 + vare5*e5; v6 = Lf2v6*F2 + vare6*e6;
v7 = Lf3v7*F3 + vare7*e7; v8 = Lf3v8*F3 + vare8*e8; v9 = Lf3v9*F3 + vare9*e9;
v10 = Lf4v10*F4 + vare10*e10;
v11 = Lf5v11*F5 + vare11*e11;

Keep v1 v2 v3 v4 v5 v6 v7 v8 v9 v10 v11;
Run;
```

Figure 5.50 Simulation of the dataset with single item domains.

Figure 5.51 represents the implementation of the CFA model corresponding to Figure 5.49. At first, there is no tangible difference between the implementation of this model compared with the model implementation in Figure 5.40. The "LINEQS" statement is similar – only two additional equations describing relationships between single item factors and variables representing them are added. The "VARIANCE" statement also looks conventional. Variances of additional latent factors are added and defined to be equal to 1, and error terms for variables v_{10} and v_{11} are also added. The "Cov" statement now has all pairwise covariances between all latent variables in the model. In addition, a new part of the model "Bounds" is added, which was introduced in the previous section.

Let's "extract" a part of the model (from Figure 5.49) related to the relationship between variable v_{10}, corresponding latent factor $F4$, and error e_{10} (see Figure 5.52). Figure 5.52 is exactly the same as the general Figure 5.35 in Section 5.2.1, yet it also very close to Figure 4.1. As discussed in Chapter 4, there is not enough information to split a single measurement (represented by, for example, variable v_{10}) into two components: a latent factor $F4$ and error term. As a result, we constrain loading "lf4v10" to value of 1 (as was done in Section 4.1.1, although without

```
Proc Calis COV data=_cfa_3 G4=200 GCONV=1E-10 Method=ML ALL;
LINEQS
  v1   = 1f1v1 f1 + e1,   v2   = 1f1v2 f1 + e2,   v3   = 1f1v3 f1 + e3,
  v4   = 1f2v4 f2 + e4,   v5   = 1f2v5 f2 + e5,   v6   = 1f2v6 f2 + e6,
  v7   = 1f3v7 f3 + e7,   v8   = 1f3v8 f3 + e8,   v9   = 1f3v9 f3 + e9,
  v10 = 1f4v10 f4 + e10,
  v11 = 1f5v11 f5 + e11;
VARIANCE
f1=1, f2=1, f3=1, f4=1, f5=1,
e1=vare1, e2=vare2, e3=vare3, e4=vare4, e5=vare5, e6=vare6, e7=vare7, e8=vare8,
e9=vare9, e10=vare10, e11=vare11;
Cov
f1 f2 =cf1f2, f1 f3 =cf1f3, f2 f3 =cf2f3,
f4 f1 =cf1f4, f4 f2 =cf2f4, f4 f3 =cf3f4,
f5 f1 =cf1f5, f5 f2 =cf2f5, f5 f3 =cf3f5,
f4 f5 =cvf4f5;
Bounds
1f4v10=1, 1f5v11=1;
Run;
```

Figure 5.51   CFA implementation with single item domains.

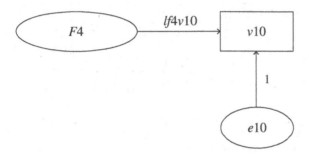

Figure 5.52   Confirmatory factor analysis: a fragment depicting the relationship between variable v_{10}, corresponding latent factor $F4$, and error e_{10}.

introduction a variable representing a loading). Conceptually, in this case, the "Bounds" statement can be viewed as directing the CALIS procedure that loadings "1f4v10" and "1f5v11" should not be estimated and during the minimization process should be kept being equal to 1. Figure 5.53 represents a partial output for the key parameters: fit index, loadings, variances, and covariances.

This approach to model single-item domains (see Figure 5.49 as an example) is based on the same blueprint used for the multi-item domains, but it can lead to unusual results in some situations. To illustrate this, let's first introduce the alternative approach to modeling single-item domains. In this alternative approach (which the authors actually recommend), a single item representing a latent domain is treated as an exogenous variable (note that generally items are considered to be endogenous variables) that measures the corresponding domain without any error (see Figure 5.54 for a depiction of the CFA model using this approach). In this model for variables v_{10} and v_{11}, the only parameters that need to

```
                              Fit Summary
Modeling Info          Number of Observations                500
                       Number of Variables                   11
                       Number of Moments                     66
                       Number of Parameters                  32
Parsimony Index        RMSEA Estimate                        0.0347
                       RMSEA Lower 90% Confidence Limit       0.0163
                       RMSEA Upper 90% Confidence Limit       0.0508
Incremental Index      Bentler Comparative Fit Index          0.9839


             Linear Equations
v1  =    1.1609(**) f1  +  1.0000 e1
v2  =    1.4182(**) f1  +  1.0000 e2
v3  =    1.3704(**) f1  +  1.0000 e3
v4  =    2.2633(**) f2  +  1.0000 e4
v5  =    1.8194(**) f2  +  1.0000 e5
v6  =    1.6099(**) f2  +  1.0000 e6
v7  =    0.8890(**) f3  +  1.0000 e7
v8  =    0.8421(**) f3  +  1.0000 e8
v9  =    1.5239(**) f3  +  1.0000 e9
v10 =    1.0000     f4  +  1.0000 e10
v11 =    1.0000     f5  +  1.0000 e11
```

```
                 Estimates for Variances of Exogenous Variables
Variable                                          Standard
Type                 Variable    Parameter    Estimate    Error      t Value    Pr > |t|
Latent               f1                        1.00000
                     f2                        1.00000
                     f3                        1.00000
                     f4                        1.00000
                     f5                        1.00000
Error                e1          vare1         2.69120    0.19861    13.5499    <.0001
                     e2          vare2         1.45944    0.15439     9.4529    <.0001
                     e3          vare3         2.02815    0.17635    11.5008    <.0001
                     e4          vare4         2.38697    0.30321     7.8723    <.0001
                     e5          vare5         3.55087    0.29075    12.2126    <.0001
                     e6          vare6         2.94238    0.23666    12.4328    <.0001
                     e7          vare7         2.17846    0.15775    13.8099    <.0001
                     e8          vare8         2.54335    0.17782    14.3026    <.0001
                     e9          vare9         1.35846    0.20885     6.5045    <.0001
                     e10         vare10        0.25074    0.07918     3.1666    0.0015
                     e11         vare11        0.55514    0.09845     5.6386    <.0001
```

```
                 Covariances Among Exogenous Variables
                                              Standard
Var1    Var2    Parameter    Estimate         Error      t Value    Pr > |t|
f1      f2      cf1f2        0.39359          0.05195     7.5770     <.0001
f1      f3      cf1f3        0.58099          0.05042    11.5222     <.0001
f2      f3      cf2f3        0.62077          0.04626    13.4205     <.0001
f4      f1      cf1f4        0.55647          0.05420    10.2671     <.0001
f4      f2      cf2f4        0.26373          0.05517     4.7801     <.0001
f4      f3      cf3f4        0.15047          0.05956     2.5265     0.0115
f5      f1      cf1f5        0.45938          0.06255     7.3443     <.0001
f5      f2      cf2f5        0.48823          0.05980     8.1644     <.0001
f5      f3      cf3f5        0.27603          0.06600     4.1822     <.0001
f4      f5      cf4f5        0.46871          0.06587     7.1162     <.0001
```

Figure 5.53 Partial output of the CFA modeling (based on the dataset from Figure 5.50 and the CALIS procedure from Figure 5.51).

be estimated are their variances (represented by variables varv10 and varv11) and pairwise covariances among variables v_{10} and v_{11} and other latent factors $F1$, $F2$, and $F3$ (cf_1v_{10}, cf_2v_{10}, cf_3v_{10}, . . .).

Doing so simplifies this model and, more importantly, does not change the overall results of the modeling for key parameters, such as fit index, loadings, variances and covariances. To demonstrate this, we need to change SAS code from Figure 5.51 to be representative of the model from Figure 5.54. This alternative implementation is represented by Figure 5.55. There are three notable changes. First, under

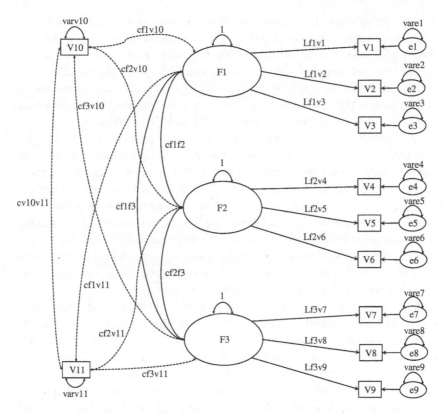

Figure 5.54 CFA model with single variables v_{10} and v_{11} as exogenous variables.

```
Proc Calis COV data=_cfa_3 G4=200 GCONV=1E-10 Method=ML  ALL;
LINEQS
  v1  = lf1v1 f1 + e1,  v2  = lf1v2 f1 + e2,  v3  = lf1v3 f1 + e3,
  v4  = lf2v4 f2 + e4,  v5  = lf2v5 f2 + e5,  v6  = lf2v6 f2 + e6,
  v7  = lf3v7 f3 + e7,  v8  = lf3v8 f3 + e8,  v9  = lf3v9 f3 + e9;
VARIANCE
f1=1, f2=1, f3=1,
v10=varv10, v11=varv11,
e1=vare1, e2=vare2, e3=vare3, e4=vare4, e5=vare5, e6=vare6, e7=vare7, e8=vare8,
e9=vare9;
Cov
f1 f2 =cf1f2,   f1 f3 =cf1f3,   f2 f3 =cf2f3,
v10 f1 =cf1v10, v10 f2 =cf2v10, v10 f3 =cf3v10,
v11 f1 =cf1v11, v11 f2 =cf2v11, v11 f3 =cf3v11,
v10 v11 =cv10v11;
Run;
```

Figure 5.55 CFA implementation with single items v_{10} and v_{11} as exogenous variables.

"LINEQS" we only describe relationships between multi-item latent domains and variables measuring or representing them – this part is the same as in Figure 5.40. Second, under "VARIANCE" we also have the same code as in Figure 5.40 but with two extra lines defining that variances of the variables v_{10} and v_{11} should be estimated (in addition to variances of the error terms). And third, under "Cov" (compare with code in Figure 5.40) the covariances to be estimated among variables v_{10} and v_{11} themselves and with latent factors $F1$, $F2$, and $F3$ are added.

After application of this implementation to the same dataset "_cfa_3", Figure 5.56 represents partial output for key parameters. Let's compare results from Figure 5.53 with results from Figure 5.56. Under "Fit Summary" this latest analysis shows that the only difference is the number of parameters to be estimated. In the latest analysis, we only need to estimate 30 parameters – the variances of the variables v_{10} and v_{11} still needed to be estimated, but in the implementation using latent factors (from Figure 5.53), the loadings from the factor to the variable and the variance of the error term were needed to be estimated (even though loadings were constrained to be 1, CALIS procedure still counted them as parameters). Note, again, that fit indexes are exactly the same in both analyses.

Under "Linear Equations" the same estimations of the loadings from factors $F1$, $F2$, and $F3$ are generated by both models, showing that both approaches (used to add single-item domains in the CFA) do not affect loadings for the multi-item domains.

The presentation of the results under "Estimates for Variances of Exogenous Variables" is slightly different, however. In Figure 5.53, we only have variances for "Latent" variables and for "Error" terms, whereas in Figure 5.56, we also have variances for "Observed" variables. The estimated variances for the errors e1, e2, . . ., e9 are the same in both analyses, but we need to reconcile results for the estimations of the variances for errors e10 and e11 (from Figure 5.53) with variances for "Observed" variables v10 and v11 (from Figure 5.56). Recall (see, for example, Figure 5.52) that variable v10 was modeled as the sum of the factor f4 and error term e10. Because loading lf4v10 in Figure 5.52 is constrained to be equal to 1 and the variance of the factor f4 is also constrained to 1, then (based on results for variances from Figure 5.53)

$$Var(v10) = Var(f4) + Var(e10)$$
$$Var(v10) = 1 + 0.25074$$
$$Var(v10) = 1.25074.$$

Therefore, in Figure 5.56, we find that the variance for "Observed" variables v10 is also 1.25074 (and the same pattern can be observed for variable v11). It shows the agreement between both models in their estimation of the variances.

The last part is "Covariances Among Exogenous Variables." Comparing Figures 5.53 and 5.56, we can see that estimated covariances between variables v_{10}

```
                            Fit Summary
Modeling Info          Number of Observations                500
                       Number of Variables                   11
                       Number of Moments                     66
                       Number of Parameters                  30
Parsimony Index        RMSEA Estimate                      0.0347
                       RMSEA Lower 90% Confidence Limit    0.0163
                       RMSEA Upper 90% Confidence Limit    0.0508
Incremental Index      Bentler Comparative Fit Index       0.9839


            Linear Equations
v1 =    1.1609(**) f1  +   1.0000 e1
v2 =    1.4182(**) f1  +   1.0000 e2
v3 =    1.3704(**) f1  +   1.0000 e3
v4 =    2.2633(**) f2  +   1.0000 e4
v5 =    1.8194(**) f2  +   1.0000 e5
v6 =    1.6099(**) f2  +   1.0000 e6
v7 =    0.8890(**) f3  +   1.0000 e7
v8 =    0.8421(**) f3  +   1.0000 e8
v9 =    1.5239(**) f3  +   1.0000 e9


                 Estimates for Variances of Exogenous Variables
Variable                                            Standard
Type            Variable   Parameter    Estimate      Error    t Value    Pr > |t|
Latent          f1                       1.00000
                f2                        1.00000
                f3                        1.00000
Observed        v10        varv10        1.25074     0.07918   15.7956    <.0001
                v11        varv11        1.55514     0.09845   15.7956    <.0001
Error           e1         vare1         2.69119     0.19861   13.5498    <.0001
                e2         vare2         1.45945     0.15439    9.4530    <.0001
                e3         vare3         2.02815     0.17635   11.5007    <.0001
                e4         vare4         2.38698     0.30321    7.8723    <.0001
                e5         vare5         3.55087     0.29075   12.2126    <.0001
                e6         vare6         2.94238     0.23666   12.4328    <.0001
                e7         vare7         2.17846     0.15775   13.8099    <.0001
                e8         vare8         2.54334     0.17782   14.3026    <.0001
                e9         vare9         1.35846     0.20885    6.5045    <.0001

                 Covariances Among Exogenous Variables
                                              Standard
Var1    Var2    Parameter    Estimate          Error      t Value    Pr > |t|
f1      f2      cf1f2         0.39359          0.05195     7.5769     <.0001
f1      f3      cf1f3         0.58099          0.05042    11.5222     <.0001
f2      f3      cf2f3         0.62078          0.04626    13.4206     <.0001
v10     f1      cf1v10        0.55647          0.05420    10.2671     <.0001
v10     f2      cf2v10        0.26373          0.05517     4.7801     <.0001
v10     f3      cf3v10        0.15047          0.05956     2.5265     0.0115
v11     f1      cf1v11        0.45938          0.06255     7.3443     <.0001
v11     f2      cf2v11        0.48823          0.05980     8.1644     <.0001
v11     f3      cf3v11        0.27603          0.06600     4.1822     <.0001
v10     v11     cv10v11       0.46871          0.06587     7.1162     <.0001
```

Figure 5.56 Partial output of the CFA modeling (based on dataset from Figure 5.50 and the CALIS procedure from Figure 5.55).

and v_{11} and latent factors $F1$, $F2$, and $F3$ in Figure 5.56 are exactly the same as covariances between latent factors $F4$ and $F5$ and latent factors $F1$, $F2$, and $F3$. For example, the covariance between variable v_{10} and factor $F1$ (Figure 5.56) is given as

```
                                    Standard
Var1    Var2    Parameter    Estimate     Error    t Value    Pr > |t|
v10     f1      cv10f1        0.55647    0.05420   10.2671     <.0001
```

and the covariance between variable $F4$ and factor $F1$ (Figure 5.53) is

				Standard		
Var1	Var2	Parameter	Estimate	Error	t Value	Pr > |t|
f4	f1	cvf1f4	0.55647	0.05420	10.2671	<.0001.

To reiterate, the difference between two implementations is the way the observed single item representing a latent factor is included in the CFA model. In the implementation represented by Figure 5.51, the single item is treated as an endogenous variable with a latent factor affecting it, whereas in Figure 5.55, a more simple model is implemented by treating the single item as an exogenous variable. The results indicate that both implementations of the CFA (Figures 5.51 and 5.55) are identical in terms of the estimation of the parameters for this simulated dataset.

Let's now manufacture the situation when those two implementations will produce different results. Note that initial simulation (Figure 5.50) in this section is based on the CFA model represented by Figure 5.49. But to be consistent with the CFA model represented by Figure 5.54, the simulation of the data should be changed. We do not need to simulate latent factors and error terms first for single-item domains and then to create observed variables v_{10} and v_{11}; instead, we can simulate data for variables v_{10} and v_{11} directly. Figure 5.57 represents the

```
data _corr_ (type=corr);
input
_TYPE_ $  _NAME_ $  F1   F2   F3   e1  e2  e3  e4  e5  e6  e7  e8  e9  v10  v11;
datalines;
  CORR      F1       1    0.4  0.5  0   0   0   0   0   0   0   0   0   0.5  0.4
  CORR      F2       0.4  1    0.6  0   0   0   0   0   0   0   0   0   0.3  0.5
  CORR      F3       0.5  0.6  1    0   0   0   0   0   0   0   0   0   0.2  0.3
  CORR      e1       0    0    0    1   0   0   0   0   0   0   0   0   0    0
  CORR      e2       0    0    0    0   1   0   0   0   0   0   0   0   0    0
  CORR      e3       0    0    0    0   0   1   0   0   0   0   0   0   0    0
  CORR      e4       0    0    0    0   0   0   1   0   0   0   0   0   0    0
  CORR      e5       0    0    0    0   0   0   0   1   0   0   0   0   0    0
  CORR      e6       0    0    0    0   0   0   0   0   1   0   0   0   0    0
  CORR      e7       0    0    0    0   0   0   0   0   0   1   0   0   0    0
  CORR      e8       0    0    0    0   0   0   0   0   0   0   1   0   0    0
  CORR      e9       0    0    0    0   0   0   0   0   0   0   0   1   0    0
  CORR      v10      0.5  0.3  0.2  0   0   0   0   0   0   0   0   0   1    0.4
  CORR      v11      0.4  0.5  0.3  0   0   0   0   0   0   0   0   0   0.4  1
  MEAN      .        0    0    0    0   0   0   0   0   0   0   0   0   0    0
  STD       .        1    1    1    1   1   1   1   1   1   1   1   1   0.5  0.6
  N         .        500  500  500  500 500 500 500 500 500 500 500 500 500 500
;
run;
proc simnormal data=_corr_ out=_sim_ds numreal=500 seed=678;
var F1 F2 F3 e1 e2 e3 e4 e5 e6 e7 e8 e9 v10 v11;
run;
Proc Corr Data=_sim_ds; Run;
Data _cfa_4; Set _sim_ds;
/* Step 1: Setting values of loadings for latent factors */
Lf1v1 = 1.2; Lf1v2 = 1.4; Lf1v3 = 1.3;
Lf2v4 = 2.1; Lf2v5 = 1.9; Lf2v6 = 1.7;
Lf3v7 = .9; Lf3v8 = 1.0; Lf3v9 = 1.4 ;
/* Step 2: Setting values of variances for error terms */
vare1 = sqrt(2.5); vare2 = sqrt(1.5); vare3 = sqrt(2.0);
vare4 = sqrt(2.6); vare5 = sqrt(3.7); vare6 = sqrt(3.1);
vare7 = sqrt(2.2); vare8 = sqrt(2.7); vare9 = sqrt(1.8);
/* Step 3: Creating variable v1, v2,..v8, and v9 */
v1 = Lf1v1*F1 + vare1*e1; v2 = Lf1v2*F1 + vare2*e2; v3 = Lf1v3*F1 + vare3*e3;
v4 = Lf2v4*F2 + vare4*e4; v5 = Lf2v5*F2 + vare5*e5; v6 = Lf2v6*F2 + vare6*e6;
v7 = Lf3v7*F3 + vare7*e7; v8 = Lf3v8*F3 + vare8*e8; v9 = Lf3v9*F3 + vare9*e9;
Keep v1 v2 v3 v4 v5 v6 v7 v8 v9 v10 v11;
Run;
```

Figure 5.57 Dataset simulation with additional correlations for variables v_{10} and v_{11}.

simulation of the new dataset "_cfa_4" based on the interrelationship among variables (observed, latent, errors) represented by Figure 5.54. Note that the following is now added as a part of the initial definition of the correlations matrix ("data _corr_(type=corr);...") : (i) correlations between variables v_{10} and v_{11} and latent factors, (ii) correlation between variables v_{10} and v_{11}, and (iii) standard deviations for v_{10} and v_{11} (those are also the parameters in the CFA related to the variables v_{10} and v_{11}).

Now we can use this newly generated dataset "_cfa_4" as a source for the CFA analysis. There is no need to change SAS implementation represented by Figures 5.51 and 5.55 (except changing the input dataset; instead of "Proc Calis COV data=_cfa_3..." it should be "Proc Calis COV data=_ cfa_4"). Figures 5.58 and 5.59 represent partial output using both CFA implementations. We can see that almost all estimated parameters are the same (fit indexes, loadings for factors $F1$, $F2$, and $F3$, variances for the variables $v_1, v_2, \ldots,$ v_8, v_9). The only peculiar result is the estimation of the variances for factors $F4$ and $F5$ based on the model implementation from Figure 5.51. The variances of the error terms are paradoxically negative ("e10 vare10 -0.74125 ..." and "e11 vare11 -0.62124...").

As discussed earlier, the variance for variable v_{10} can be represented as

$$Var(v10) = Var(f4) + Var(e10).$$

If we replace $Var(f4)$ with a value of 1 and $Var(e10)$ with an obviously logically and methodically incorrect estimation of the -0.74125 (variance cannot be negative), then

$$Var(v10) = 1 - 0.74125$$

$$Var(v10) = 0.25875.$$

But the value of 0.25875 is exactly the value of the variance in Figure 5.59 ("Observed v10 varv10 0.25875...").

There are two important lessons from this simulation. The first lesson is that the algorithm to perform CFA can produce illogical results, such as negative variances. It should be noted that it is not some kind of oversight in SAS implementation; it is in the nature of the algorithm itself. The second lesson is that parametrization of the measurement model matters. By deliberately setting variances of the factors $F4$ and $F5$ to a value of 1 and also constraining loadings to a value of 1, we caused this result. Although the CALIS procedure produced those negative estimations of the variances, it also produced the following warning message in the SAS log:

```
WARNING: The estimated variance of error variable e10 is
negative.
```

WARNING: The estimated variance of error variable e11 is negative.
WARNING: Although all predicted variances for the observed variables and latent factors are positive, the corresponding predicted covariance matrix is not positive definite. It has 2 negative eigenvalues.

	Fit Summary		
Modeling Info	Number of Observations		500
	Number of Variables		11
	Number of Moments		66
	Number of Parameters		32
Parsimony Index	RMSEA Estimate		0.0000
	RMSEA Lower 90% Confidence Limit		0.0000
	RMSEA Upper 90% Confidence Limit		0.0278
Incremental Index	Bentler Comparative Fit Index		1.0000

Linear Equations

v1	=	1.2476(**) f1	+	1.0000 e1
v2	=	1.3866(**) f1	+	1.0000 e2
v3	=	1.2574(**) f1	+	1.0000 e3
v4	=	2.1999(**) f2	+	1.0000 e4
v5	=	1.9092(**) f2	+	1.0000 e5
v6	=	1.6600(**) f2	+	1.0000 e6
v7	=	0.9245(**) f3	+	1.0000 e7
v8	=	1.0446(**) f3	+	1.0000 e8
v9	=	1.3852(**) f3	+	1.0000 e9
v10	=	1.0000 f4	+	1.0000 e10
v11	=	1.0000 f5	+	1.0000 e11

Estimates for Variances of Exogenous Variables

Variable Type	Variable	Parameter	Estimate	Standard Error	t Value	Pr > |t|
Latent	f1		1.00000			
	f2		1.00000			
	f3		1.00000			
	f4		1.00000			
	f5		1.00000			
Error	e1	vare1	2.14197	0.17363	12.3362	<.0001
	e2	vare2	1.41764	0.15179	9.3393	<.0001
	e3	vare3	1.90185	0.16115	11.8015	<.0001
	e4	vare4	2.20919	0.26643	8.2920	<.0001
	e5	vare5	3.79918	0.30559	12.4323	<.0001
	e6	vare6	2.91455	0.23343	12.4856	<.0001
	e7	vare7	2.09345	0.16110	12.9949	<.0001
	e8	vare8	2.60282	0.20154	12.9147	<.0001
	e9	vare9	1.89683	0.21517	8.8155	<.0001
	e10	vare10	-0.74125	0.01638	-45.2499	<.0001
	e11	vare11	-0.62124	0.02398	-25.9080	<.0001

Covariances Among Exogenous Variables

Var1	Var2	Parameter	Estimate	Standard Error	t Value	Pr > |t|
f1	f2	cf1f2	0.43194	0.05010	8.6211	<.0001
f1	f3	cf1f3	0.52298	0.05419	9.6502	<.0001
f2	f3	cf2f3	0.57817	0.04940	11.7030	<.0001
f4	f1	cvf1f4	0.24064	0.02470	9.7429	<.0001
f4	f2	cvf2f4	0.17508	0.02456	7.1295	<.0001
f4	f3	cvf3f4	0.07761	0.02813	2.7586	0.0058
f5	f1	cvf1f5	0.21661	0.03081	7.0298	<.0001
f5	f2	cvf2f5	0.33990	0.02803	12.1258	<.0001
f5	f3	cvf3f5	0.19366	0.03340	5.7989	<.0001
f4	f5	cvf4f5	0.12663	0.01512	8.3763	<.0001

Figure 5.58 Partial output of the CFA modeling (based on the dataset from Figure 5.57 and CFA implementation based on Figure 5.51).

```
                          Fit Summary
Modeling Info        Number of Observations              500
                     Number of Variables                 11
                     Number of Moments                   66
                     Number of Parameters                30
Parsimony Index      RMSEA Estimate                  0.0000
                     RMSEA Lower 90% Confidence Limit 0.0000
                     RMSEA Upper 90% Confidence Limit 0.0278
Incremental Index    Bentler Comparative Fit Index   1.0000


         Linear Equations
v1 =     1.2476(**) f1  +   1.0000 e1
v2 =     1.3866(**) f1  +   1.0000 e2
v3 =     1.2574(**) f1  +   1.0000 e3
v4 =     2.1999(**) f2  +   1.0000 e4
v5 =     1.9092(**) f2  +   1.0000 e5
v6 =     1.6600(**) f2  +   1.0000 e6
v7 =     0.9245(**) f3  +   1.0000 e7
v8 =     1.0447(**) f3  +   1.0000 e8
v9 =     1.3852(**) f3  +   1.0000 e9
```

```
                Estimates for Variances of Exogenous Variables
Variable                                      Standard
Type          Variable  Parameter   Estimate     Error   t Value   Pr > |t|
Latent        f1                    1.00000
              f2                    1.00000
              f3                    1.00000
Observed      v10       varv10      0.25875    0.01638   15.7956    <.0001
              v11       varv11      0.37876    0.02398   15.7956    <.0001
Error         e1        vare1       2.14197    0.17363   12.3362    <.0001
              e2        vare2       1.41765    0.15179    9.3393    <.0001
              e3        vare3       1.90185    0.16115   11.8015    <.0001
              e4        vare4       2.20919    0.26643    8.2919    <.0001
              e5        vare5       3.79918    0.30559   12.4322    <.0001
              e6        vare6       2.91455    0.23343   12.4856    <.0001
              e7        vare7       2.09345    0.16110   12.9949    <.0001
              e8        vare8       2.60281    0.20154   12.9146    <.0001
              e9        vare9       1.89687    0.21517    8.8157    <.0001
```

```
                Covariances Among Exogenous Variables
                                          Standard
Var1   Var2    Parameter    Estimate        Error    t Value   Pr > |t|
f1     f2      cf1f2        0.43194       0.05010     8.6211    <.0001
f1     f3      cf1f3        0.52298       0.05419     9.6503    <.0001
f2     f3      cf2f3        0.57817       0.04940    11.7029    <.0001
v10    f1      cv10f1       0.24064       0.02470     9.7429    <.0001
v10    f2      cv10f2       0.17508       0.02456     7.1295    <.0001
v10    f3      cv10f3       0.07760       0.02813     2.7586    0.0058
v11    f1      cv11f1       0.21661       0.03081     7.0298    <.0001
v11    f2      cv11f2       0.33990       0.02803    12.1258    <.0001
v11    f3      cv11f3       0.19366       0.03340     5.7989    <.0001
v10    v11     cv10v11      0.12663       0.01512     8.3763    <.0001
```

Figure 5.59 Partial output of the CFA modeling (based on the dataset from Figure 5.57 and CFA implementation based on Figure 5.55).

It is just a reminder to always check the log for warning or error messages when performing analyses of this type.

Earlier, we introduced the "Bounds" statement as a part of the CALIS procedure with a suggestion that if negative variances are estimated, then we can simply constrain them to be positive. The above example shows that the use of the "Bounds" statement for this purpose is not a blank check and thus should be used very carefully. For example, in this simulation (when using CFA implementation based on Figure 5.51) it will not solve the issue and only will lead to even more methodologically confusing results.

5.2.4 Second-Order Confirmatory Factor Analysis

5.2.4.1 Implementation of the Model with at Least Three First-Order Latent Domains

In the previous sections, the implementation of the most simple cases of CFA models was described. If a scale has an aggregated or a global domain – high-level (second-order) factor encompassing or enveloping low-level (first-order) factors – then the assessment of the fit of a measurement model became more complicated. Consider a scale with three latent domains (factors $F1$, $F2$, and $F3$) measured by nine items and one aggregated domain (factor $F4$), which generally is calculated as a mean (or a sum) of the three-domain scores (see Figure 5.60 representing the CFA model for this scale).

Comparing this Figure 5.60 with Figure 5.36, we note that the measurement part of the model stays the same, but the structural part representing the relationships among latent factors is different. In this model, we have an additional second-order latent factor, which causes changes in the first-order latent factors. To determine the order of the factor (first-order or second-order), the relationship between a factor and other elements of the measurement model should be examined. If a latent factor only affects observed items, this factor is the first-order factor. If a latent exogenous factor affects at least one other first-order latent factor, then this factor is a second-order factor.

The aggregated factor should be considered for scales for which first-order factors can be considered as related. This assessment can be made by calculating correlations between factors (domain) scores. If correlations are sizeable (say more than 0.4), then a second-order CFA can be contemplated. If correlations between domain scores are relatively low or close to zero, then an aggregated factor is not likely. After all, if factors are independent (close to being orthogonal with correlations close to zero), then the aggregated factor will be inappropriate as first-order factors in this case have nothing in common.

It can then be conceptualized (Figure 5.60) as if factors $F1$, $F2$, and $F3$ play the same role in the measurement of the aggregated factor as the observed items v_1, v_2, . . ., v_9 play in the measurement of the latent factors $F1$, $F2$, and $F3$. For example, we assume that variables v_1, v_2, and v_3 are measuring the same latent concept represented by factor $F1$ and, as such, those variables v_1, v_2, and v_3 should be related (generally should be substantially correlated). Similarly, and subsequently, factors $F1$, $F2$, and $F3$ that are measuring the same latent (underlying) concept represented by factor $F4$ should also be substantially correlated.

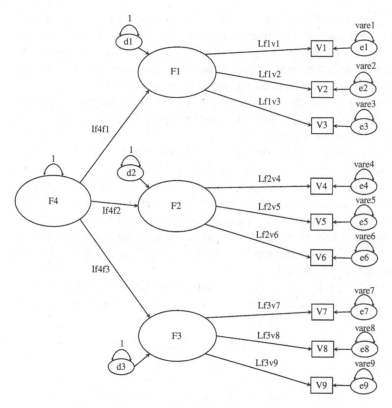

Figure 5.60 Depiction of the second-order CFA measurement model.

In the CFA model with only first-order factors, the structural part of the model is represented merely by covariances between those latent factors – there is no causal relationship between latent factors. If the CFA model has a second-order factor, however, then its structural part is markedly different. The relationships between second-order factors and the first-order factors now become causal. For example, in Figure 5.60, factor $F4$ causes changes in factor $F1$ then, in turn, factor $F1$ causes changes in observed variable v_1. If we look at Figure 5.60 as a representation of the causal model, factor $F4$ can be viewed as the ultimate source of the changes in observed variables $v_1, v_2, \ldots, v_8, v_9$. Note that in Figure 5.60, only factor $F4$ is the exogenous latent factor (alongside with error terms, which are always exogenous latent elements in CFA).

If an element of the model (be it a latent factor or an observed variable) is affected by another element of the same model, the error term should be associated with the affected variable. For the measurement part of the model, they are regarded as *errors* (latent variables $e_1, e_2, \ldots, e_9$). To distinguish error terms associated with latent factors, they are generally referenced as *disturbances* (latent variables $d1$, $d2$, and $d3$ in Figure 5.60). The variances of the error terms are the parameters in the CFA, and they are needed to be estimated (parameters $vare_1$, $vare_2$, ..., $vare_9$ in Figure 5.60), but variances of the disturbances for the identification purposes, as well as the variance of the second-order latent factor $F4$, are set to be equal to value of one.

Figure 5.61 represents the implementation of the second-order CFA corresponding to the hypothetical scale represented by Figure 5.60. Compared with the implementation discussed earlier (see Figure 5.40) under "LINEQS" section, we now have three additional lines representing relationships between latent factor $F4$ and latent factors $F1$, $F2$, and $F3$. As a part of the "VARIANCE" section, instead of defining variances for factors $F1$, $F2$, and $F3$, the variances for the aggregated factor $F4$ and the disturbances associated with first-order factors are set to 1. Note that there is no "COV" section. The "Bounds" part of the model description is also included, but the estimated variances should be carefully investigated to be sure that zero variances are not the result of the wrong implementation of the CFA model or some errors in the data.

To run this second-order model the same simulated dataset "_cfa_1" produced by the code from Figure 5.39 is used. Figure 5.62 represents the

```
Proc Calis COV data=_cfa_1 G4=200 GCONV=1E-10 Method=ML  ALL;
LINEQS
   v1   = lf1v1 f1 + e1,   v2   = lf1v2 f1 + e2,   v3   = lf1v3 f1 + e3,
   v4   = lf2v4 f2 + e4,   v5   = lf2v5 f2 + e5,   v6   = lf2v6 f2 + e6,
   v7   = lf3v7 f3 + e7,   v8   = lf3v8 f3 + e8,   v9   = lf3v9 f3 + e9,
   f1   = lf4f1 f4 + d1,   f2   - lf4f2 f4 + d2,   f3   = lf4f3 f4 + d3;
VARIANCE
f4=1,
d1=1, d2=1, d3=1,
e1=vare1, e2=vare2, e3=vare3, e4=vare4, e5=vare5, e6=vare6, e7=vare7, e8=vare8,
e9=vare9;
Bounds
vare1-vare9 > 1.0e-8;
Run;
```

Figure 5.61 Implementation of the second-order CFA corresponding to the hypothetical scale represented by Figure 5.60.

```
          Linear Equations
v1 =    0.8386(**) f1  +   1.0000 e1
v2 =    1.2099(**) f1  +   1.0000 e2
v3 =    1.1664(**) f1  +   1.0000 e3
v4 =    1.5578(**) f2  +   1.0000 e4
v5 =    1.3584(**) f2  +   1.0000 e5
v6 =    1.1816(**) f2  +   1.0000 e6
v7 =    0.2196(ns) f3  +   1.0000 e7
v8 =    0.2282(ns) f3  +   1.0000 e8
v9 =    0.2994(ns) f3  +   1.0000 e9
f1 =    0.6025(**) f4  +   1.0000 d1
f2 =    0.8716(**) f4  +   1.0000 d2
f3 =    4.4912(ns) f4  +   1.0000 d3
```

Figure 5.62 Unstandardized loadings for the second-order CFA model.

```
Standardized Results for Linear Equations
v1 =       0.5075(**) f1  +   1.0000 e1
v2 =       0.7476(**) f1  +   1.0000 e2
v3 =       0.7352(**) f1  +   1.0000 e3
v4 =       0.7743(**) f2  +   1.0000 e4
v5 =       0.6947(**) f2  +   1.0000 e5
v6 =       0.6714(**) f2  +   1.0000 e6
v7 =       0.5505(**) f3  +   1.0000 e7
v8 =       0.5697(**) f3  +   1.0000 e8
v9 =       0.6973(**) f3  +   1.0000 e9
f1 =       0.5161(**) f4  +   1.0000 d1
f2 =       0.6570(**) f4  +   1.0000 d2
f3 =       0.9761(**) f4  +   1.0000 d3
```

Figure 5.63 Standardized loadings for second-order CFA model.

estimated unstandardized loadings, and Figure 5.63 represents the estimated standardized loadings. The interesting detail about this model is that the fit indexes are precisely the same as in Figure 5.42 (and, as a result, we do not show them here).

The results for unstandardized loadings show that path coefficients from factor $F3$ to variables v_7, v_8, and v_9 are not significant, nor is the path coefficient from second-order factor $F4$ to factor $F3$. As such, we cannot confirm that this second-order model fits the data (yet Bentler's CFI is large with value of 0.9950, indicating the possibility of a good fit). Note that we do not anticipate that the estimated unstandardized loadings will be close to the values used in the simulation, as the dataset was simulated to represent a first-order CFA model. But this second-order model reveals another surprising result – the standardized loadings (all significant; Figure 5.63) for the measurement part of the model are identical to the standardized loadings from Figure 5.45.

5.2.4.2 Implementation of the Model with Two First-Order Latent Domains

Figure 5.64 represents an example of the second-order model of two first-order latent domains. Note that, compared with Figure 5.60, in Figure 5.64 we simply delete all elements of the model related to the factor $F3$. Following the same approach, we can take the implementation from Figure 5.61 and also simply delete all code related to factor $F3$ (see Figure 5.65). In the previous section, we used dataset "_cfa_1" as the input for analyses, which will be employed here also, but only variables v_1, v_2, . . ., v_5, v_6 will be used in analyses.

After running the SAS code from Figure 5.65, we first notice the following message in the log:

NOTE: Convergence criterion (ABSGCONV=0.00001) satisfied.
NOTE: The Moore-Penrose inverse is used in computing the covariance matrix for parameter estimates.

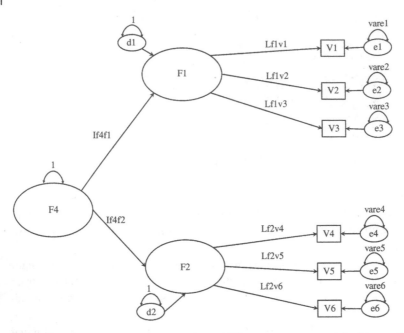

Figure 5.64 Depiction of the second-order CFA measurement model with two first-order latent factors.

```
Proc Calis COV data=_cfa_1 G4=200 GCONV=1E-10 Method=ML   ALL;
LINEQS
  v1    = lf1v1 f1 + e1,   v2    = lf1v2 f1 + e2,   v3    = lf1v3 f1 + e3,
  v4    = lf2v4 f2 + e4,   v5    = lf2v5 f2 + e5,   v6    = lf2v6 f2 + e6,
  f1    = lf4f1 f4 + d1,   f2    = lf4f2 f4 + d2;
VARIANCE
f4=1,
d1=1, d2=1,
e1=vare1, e2=vare2, e3=vare3, e4=vare4, e5=vare5, e6=vare6;
Bounds
vare1-vare6 > 1.0e-8;
Run;
```

Figure 5.65 Implementation of the second-order CFA corresponding to the hypothetical scale represented by Figure 5.64.

WARNING: Standard errors and t values might not be accurate with the use of the Moore-Penrose inverse.
NOTE: The stability coefficient is 0, which is less than one. The condition for converged total and indirect effects is satisfied.
WARNING: Lagrange multiplier statistics and Wald statistics might not be accurate with the use of the Moore-Penrose inverse in computing the covariance matrix for parameter estimates.

Although a WARNING message can be legitimate in some cases (and, at times even can be ignored if we are absolutely sure that we have a valid and correctly structured dataset and the implementation of the model is appropriate), it is important to investigate why we have this kind of message. The first place to examine is the output part titled as "Covariance Structure Analysis: Optimization." Convergence status is the part of the optimization output and presented below:

```
Convergence criterion (ABSGCONV=0.00001) satisfied.
NOTE: The Moore-Penrose inverse is used in computing the
covariance matrix for parameter estimates.
WARNING: Standard errors and t values might not be
accurate with the use of the Moore-Penrose inverse.
NOTE: Covariance matrix for the estimates is not
full rank.
NOTE: The variance of some parameter estimates is zero
or some parameter estimates are linearly related to other
parameter estimates as shown in the following equations:
lf2v4 = -0.418842 + 0.037311 *lf1v1 + 0.055457 *lf1v2
+ 0.052099 *lf1v3 - 0.572519*lf2v5 - 0.507225*lf2v6 -
0.115675*lf4f1 + 1.396251*lf4f2
```

The most important information in the above is that the CALIS procedure found that a loading from factor $F2$ to variable v_4 (represented by parameter lf2v4) is a linear combination of the all other loadings in the model and, because of this, the Covariance matrix for the estimates is not full rank. What does it mean in terms of the results? The simple answer is that results will not be unique. Therefore, if we or someone else will use the same data and identical implementation of the CFA model, but using a different software package, then a different set of estimations could be obtained.

This situation is related to the non-identification problem, which could arise even in simple cases. Recall, for example, the discussion on test–retest analyses with only one observation per subject (Chapter 4). To illustrate the above issue, let's consider a simplest situation – a scale with just two items (v_1 and v_2) representing one factor $F1$ (see Figure 5.66 for graphical depiction and 5.67 for SAS implementation). After running the SAS code from Figure 5.67, we will get almost the same message in the log file and also under "Covariance Structure Analysis: Optimization" the linear dependency between parameters in the model will be highlighted as follows:

```
NOTE: The variance of some parameter estimates is zero
or some parameter estimates are linearly related to
```

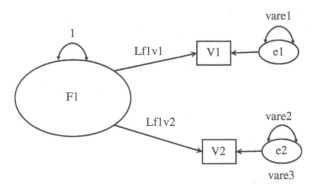

Figure 5.66 Depiction of the CFA measurement model with only two items and one latent factor.

```
Proc Calis COV data=_cfa_1 G4=200 GCONV=1E-10 Method=ML   ALL;
LINEQS
  v1   = lf1v1 f1 + e1,
  v2   = lf1v2 f1 + e2;
VARIANCE
f1=1,
e1 = vare1, e2 = vare2;
Bounds
vare1-vare2 > 1.0e-8;
Run;
```

Figure 5.67 Implementation of the CFA model for a scale with only two items and one latent factor (represented by Figure 5.66).

other parameter estimates as shown in the following equations:
vare1 = −17.705888 + 4.053012*lf1v1 − 3.647299*lf1v2 + 8.172245*vare2

As discussed previously, the "true" input for the analysis is the variance–covariance matrix of the observed variables. For this simple example, this matrix will have only three unique elements: variance of the variable v_1, variance of the variable v_2, and covariance between v_1 and v_2 (in the output under "Fit Summary" this information represented by "Number of Moments" and equals 3 in this example). But the number of parameters needed to estimate this model is four: two loadings (lf1v1 and lf1v2) and two variances (vare1 and vare2). In the "Fit Summary" this information is represented by "Number of Parameters" and equals 4. For the estimated parameters to be unique, the number of parameters should be less or equal to the number of unique elements.

To escape this identification problem, we add yet another element in the description of the CFA model. Generally, every model description element in CALIS procedure starts with the keyword, such as, for example, "LINEQS," and finishes with semicolon (";"), with sub-elements divided by commas (","). There is an additional element that does not start with any keyword: It is a program statement. Although a program statement can be put anywhere between model description elements, we recommend to put it at the very end of the CALIS procedure, after the last semicolon and just before the "Run;" statement. In Figure 5.67, the following program statement

```
lf1v1=lf1v2;
```

should be added as the very last code line in the description of the model. After rerunning code from Figure 5.67, with the additional code line forcing the loadings to be equal, the identification issue that previously manifested itself via linear dependency between estimated parameters in the model is eliminated.

Now let's go back to the previously discussed second-order model. The identification problem we had for relationships between the second-order factor and the first-order factor is the same as just discussed and explained above for the simple example with two items and one latent factor. To overcome this identification problem in the current context, we need to follow the same analytic strategy but this time for the loadings between the second-order factor $F4$ and the first-order factors $F1$ and $F2$. Thus, in Figure 5.65 the following program statement

```
lf4f1 = lf4f2;
```

should also be added as the very last code line in the description of the model (just before the "Run;" statement). Figures 5.68 and 5.69 represent estimation results for the unstandardized and standardized parameters with original code from Figure 5.65 without any changes. Figures 5.70 and 5.71 represent the results of the estimations using code from Figure 5.65 with the addition of program statement "lf4f1 = lf4f2;".

```
            Linear Equations
v1 =     0.8866(**) f1  +    1.0000 e1
v2 =     1.3177(**) f1  +    1.0000 e2
v3 =     1.2380(**) f1  +    1.0000 e3
v4 =     1.0650(**) f2  +    1.0000 e4
v5 =     0.9261(**) f2  +    1.0000 e5
v6 =     0.8205(**) f2  +    1.0000 e6
f1 =     0.4316(**) f4  +    1.0000 d1
f2 =     1.6541(**) f4  +    1.0000 d2

             Estimates for Variances of Exogenous Variables
Variable                                      Standard
Type          Variable   Parameter   Estimate   Error     t Value   Pr > |t|
Latent        f4                      1.00000
Disturbance   d1                      1.00000
              d2                      1.00000
Error         e1         vare1        2.78919   0.20073   13.8951   <.0001
              e2         vare2        1.50999   0.21548    7.0077   <.0001
              e3         vare3        1.61272   0.19909    8.1004   <.0001
              e4         vare4        2.88477   0.35351    8.1603   <.0001
              e5         vare5        3.52280   0.32187   10.9446   <.0001
              e6         vare6        2.93500   0.26057   11.2638   <.0001
```

Figure 5.68 Unstandardized loadings for the second-order CFA model (not unique solution).

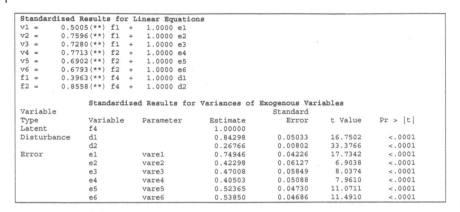

```
Standardized Results for Linear Equations
v1 =      0.5005(**) f1  +    1.0000 e1
v2 =      0.7596(**) f1  +    1.0000 e2
v3 =      0.7280(**) f1  +    1.0000 e3
v4 =      0.7713(**) f2  +    1.0000 e4
v5 =      0.6902(**) f2  +    1.0000 e5
v6 =      0.6793(**) f2  +    1.0000 e6
f1 =      0.3963(**) f4  +    1.0000 d1
f2 =      0.8558(**) f4  +    1.0000 d2

            Standardized Results for Variances of Exogenous Variables
Variable                                            Standard
Type          Variable   Parameter   Estimate       Error      t Value    Pr > |t|
Latent        f4                      1.00000
Disturbance   d1                      0.84298        0.05033    16.7502    <.0001
              d2                      0.26766        0.00802    33.3766    <.0001
Error         e1         vare1        0.74946        0.04226    17.7342    <.0001
              e2         vare2        0.42298        0.06127     6.9038    <.0001
              e3         vare3        0.47008        0.05849     8.0374    <.0001
              e4         vare4        0.40503        0.05088     7.9610    <.0001
              e5         vare5        0.52365        0.04730    11.0711    <.0001
              e6         vare6        0.53850        0.04686    11.4910    <.0001
```

Figure 5.69 Standardized loadings for the second-order CFA model (not unique solution).

```
            Linear Equations
v1 =      0.7850(**) f1  +    1.0000 e1
v2 =      1.1668(**) f1  +    1.0000 e2
v3 =      1.0961(**) f1  +    1.0000 e3
v4 =      1.6735(**) f2  +    1.0000 e4
v5 =      1.4553(**) f2  +    1.0000 e5
v6 =      1.2893(**) f2  +    1.0000 e6
f1 =      0.7163(**) f4  +    1.0000 d1
f2 =      0.7163(**) f4  +    1.0000 d2

            Estimates for Variances of Exogenous Variables
Variable                                            Standard
Type          Variable   Parameter   Estimate       Error      t Value    Pr > |t|
Latent        f4                      1.00000
Disturbance   d1                      1.00000
              d2                      1.00000
Error         e1         vare1        2.78918        0.20073    13.8951    <.0001
              e2         vare2        1.51001        0.21547     7.0079    <.0001
              e3         vare3        1.61271        0.19909     8.1004    <.0001
              e4         vare4        2.88489        0.35351     8.1607    <.0001
              e5         vare5        3.52280        0.32188    10.9446    <.0001
              e6         vare6        2.93495        0.26057    11.2635    <.0001
```

Figure 5.70 Unstandardized loadings for the second-order CFA model (unique solution).

```
Standardized Results for Linear Equations
v1 =      0.5005(**) f1  +    1.0000 e1
v2 =      0.7596(**) f1  +    1.0000 e2
v3 =      0.7280(**) f1  +    1.0000 e3
v4 =      0.7713(**) f2  +    1.0000 e4
v5 =      0.6902(**) f2  +    1.0000 e5
v6 =      0.6793(**) f2  +    1.0000 e6
f1 =      0.5823(**) f4  +    1.0000 d1
f2 =      0.5823(**) f4  +    1.0000 d2

            Standardized Results for Variances of Exogenous Variables
Variable                                            Standard
Type          Variable   Parameter   Estimate       Error      t Value    Pr > |t|
Latent        f4                      1.00000
Disturbance   d1                      0.66088        0.05486    12.0458    <.0001
              d2                      0.66088        0.05486    12.0458    <.0001
Error         e1         vare1        0.74946        0.04226    17.7341    <.0001
              e2         vare2        0.42298        0.06127     6.9040    <.0001
              e3         vare3        0.47008        0.05849     8.0374    <.0001
              e4         vare4        0.40504        0.05088     7.9614    <.0001
              e5         vare5        0.52365        0.04730    11.0711    <.0001
              e6         vare6        0.53849        0.04686    11.4907    <.0001
```

Figure 5.71 Standardized loadings for the second-order CFA model (unique solution).

Figures 5.69 and 5.71 show that the estimated parameters of the measurement part of the model (loadings from factors $F1$ and $F2$ to variables $v_1, v_2, \ldots, v_5, v_6$ and variances for variables $v_1, v_2, \ldots, v_5, v_6$) are the same for unique vs. not unique solutions.

5.2.5 Formative vs. Reflective Model

It was noted earlier that the vast majority of multi-item patient-reported outcomes are classified as reflective models. The main assumption for this type of model is that a latent factor affects items that can be observed and measured. The formative model represents the opposite way of thinking about the relationship between items and the domain they represent. An example of the relationships between items and a domain for a formative model can be depicted as shown in Figure 5.72.

In a formative scale, items affect the latent variable and, importantly, items representing a formative domain are not expected to correlate. This relationship can be regarded as if items form a domain; thus, the name of this model is "formative." The relationship corresponding to Figure 5.72 can be written as (compare Eq. (5.16) with Eq. (5.15))

$$F = v_1 + v_2 + v_3. \tag{5.16}$$

Although Eq. (5.16) represents a typical conceptual approach to calculating a domain score for both formative and reflective models but, in a formative model, this equation also represents an underlying causal relationship. Hence items in the formative scale are not anticipated to correlate and, therefore, analyses such as Cronbach's coefficient alpha for internal consistency reliability and confirmatory factor analysis as part of construct validly are not even recommended by some researchers (de Vet et al. 2011; Fayers and Machin 2016; Mokkink et al. 2010a). In this context, then, the magnitude of the correlation between the items is usually of little relevance, so the standard methods of psychometrics for summated rating scales (internal consistency reliability, construct validation, exploratory factor

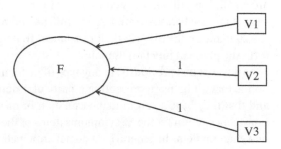

Figure 5.72 Example of the relationships between observed variables and a domain in a formative model.

analysis as well as confirmatory factor analysis) generally do not apply (de Vet et al. 2011; Fayers and Machin 2016; Mokkink et al. 2010a). What is central for a formative model is the inclusion of all important items that measure the construct; missing an important item inevitably means that the construct is not measured comprehensively.

On the other hand, a reflective model is one in which items of interest being evaluated are manifestations of the same underlying construct being evaluated and hence are expected to be sufficiently correlated and, by implication, certain items may be interchangeable and not all of them may be needed during the development phase. In a reflective model, if the underlying construct changes, all items change in tandem.

At the same time, it would still be prudent to perform a correlation analysis and Cronbach's coefficient alpha to understand relationships between items (but not, as noted above, to support internal consistency reliability or construct validly). Recall from Chapter 4 that, even if items do not correlate well, many of them can still result in a large Cronbach's coefficient alpha, which is especially relevant as formative scales tend to be composed from many multiple items often representing symptoms.

The situation is different when a scale has several domains with some of them being reflective domains and some of them being formative domains. In this case, we need to have a strategy on how we can incorporate formative domains as the part of the confirmatory factor analysis. An illustrative example of this type of scale is the Menopause-Specific Quality of Life (MENQOL) (Bushmakin et al. 2014), which is commonly evaluated in postmenopausal women to assess menopause-related changes in health-related quality of life (HRQOL). The MENQOL scale includes 29-items, which measure the HRQOL impact of menopause across four domains: vasomotor, physical, psychosocial, and sexual functions. The overall or aggregated score is calculated as the mean of the four domain scores.

The first and most important examination of the relationships between items representing a formative domain is the assessment of their correlations. If those correlations are small between many items, then it may suggest as a first general clue that those items represent a formative domain. Note that, even if correlations are small, it is still anticipated that all of them will be positive. Another general suggestion is when there are large number of items representing a domain. From the 29 items on the MENQOL, for instance, 16 items (more than half of all items) form the physical function domain.

As it was stated previously, in any type of factor analysis, an underlying assumption is that all items (representing a particular domain) should "march" together and that they have a substantial correlation in measuring different aspects of the same concept. But for the 16 symptoms items of the physical function domain (and for symptom items in general), we do not anticipate this – for example, one woman could have DIFFICULTY SLEEPING (MENQOL item 14) and NO DRYING SKIN (MenQOL item 19), another one could have DRYING SKIN and NO DIFFICULTY SLEEPING, and another could have DIFFICULTY SLEEPING AND DRYING SKIN. In other words, difficulty sleeping is not necessarily linked to drying skin.

If we were to treat these 16 items as "normal" items from a reflective model, it would be like anticipating that if someone has a little of DIFFICULTY SLEEPING, then this person would also have a little of DRYING SKIN; and, conversely, if someone has a lot of DIFFICULTY SLEEPING, then this person would also have a lot of DRYING SKIN. But from knowledge of the subject matter, supported by the item correlations, we know that is not the case. Instead, we know that a woman may experience some of the symptoms in the physical function domain but not others, and the types of symptoms experienced vary from woman to woman.

Figure 5.73 represents the "hybrid" CFA model for the MENQOL scale. This second-order model represents the measurement model of the MENQOL scale, acknowledging that vasomotor, psychosocial, and sexual functions domains are the reflective domains. But physical function domain is represented by a newly created variable v_{30}, which is calculated as the mean of scores of 16 items (which form the physical function domain). And this variable is used as the manifest variable representing "Physical" domain (see also Section 5.2.3 on the implementation of the CFA model with manifest variable).

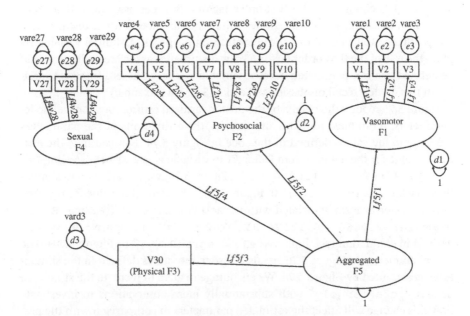

Figure 5.73 The measurement model of the MENQOL scale.

In the previous Section 5.2.4, to demonstrate the implementation of the second-order confirmatory factor analysis model, we "reused" a simulated dataset representing three domains and nine items, which was still acceptable to introduce the second-order model CFA model. But to illustrate the implementation of the model represented by Figure 5.73, we need to simulate the new dataset (see Figure 5.74). This simulated dataset is built to be representative of the MENQOL measurement model.

The first step in the simulation of the data is to create a correlation matrix for the relationships between exogenous variables in the model (the same as in previous data simulations). In this model, the exogenous variables are the second-order factor $F5$ and all the error and disturbance terms. In the second-order model, all exogenous variables are considered to be independent and, as such, all pairwise correlations are equal to zero. The data step "Data _cfa_menqol_;" simulates variables for the procedure CALIS. Note that instead of the variables v_{11}, v_{12}, . . ., v_{25}, v_{26}, we simulate only one new variable v_{30} (in real life, it will be a mean of the 16 items that form the physical function domain).

Figure 5.75 represents the implementation of the CFA model (corresponding to Figure 5.73). The most relevant parts regarding the implementation of the CFA model were described in previous sections. Here we only highlight the important details for modeling of the disturbance terms. In this model, the changes in the second-order factor (factor $F5$ in this example) are considered to be the principal source of the changes in the first-order factors. But, because those first-order latent factors $F1$, $F2$, and $F4$ are unitless, then the variances of their disturbances are postulated to be equal to 1 for identification purposes. Although variable v_{30} plays the role of the first-order factor $F3$, the disturbance associated with it should be defined as a free parameter, because variable v_{30} functions as a manifest variable in this model (recall discussion in Section 5.2.3 on this topic).

Figure 5.76 reports the results of the unstandardized estimations for the model parameters. As in most previous simulations, the estimations of the parameters are close to the values defined in the code in Figure 5.74. For example, the estimated value for the loading from factor $F1$ to variable v_1 is 1.1748 (see line "v1 = 1.1748(**) f1 + 1.0000 e1" in Figure 5.76) vs. 1.2 defined in simulation (see line "Lf1v1 = 1.2;" in Figure 5.74). The estimated value for the variance of the error term associated with variable v_1 is 2.06607 (see line "Error e1 var e1 2.06607 0.17174 12.0302 <.0001" in Figure 5.76) vs. 2.5 defined in simulation (see line "vare1 = sqrt(2.5);" in Figure 5.74). The other parameters in Figure 5.76 are also close to the values defined in the simulations represented by Figure 5.74. We encourage readers to recreate the simulated dataset "_cfa_menqol_" with substantially more observations to investigate how this change will affect the estimated parameters in comparison with the predefined values in the simulation.

```
data _corr_(type=corr);
input _TYPE_ $ _NAME_ $ F5 e1 e2 e3 e4 e5 e6 e7 e8 e9 e10 e27 e28 e29 d1 d2 d3 d4;
datalines;
CORR F5   1   0 0 0 0 0 0 0 0 0 0  0  0  0  0 0 0 0
CORR e1   0   1 0 0 0 0 0 0 0 0 0  0  0  0  0 0 0 0
CORR e2   0   0 1 0 0 0 0 0 0 0 0  0  0  0  0 0 0 0
CORR e3   0   0 0 1 0 0 0 0 0 0 0  0  0  0  0 0 0 0
CORR e4   0   0 0 0 1 0 0 0 0 0 0  0  0  0  0 0 0 0
CORR e5   0   0 0 0 0 1 0 0 0 0 0  0  0  0  0 0 0 0
CORR e6   0   0 0 0 0 0 1 0 0 0 0  0  0  0  0 0 0 0
CORR e7   0   0 0 0 0 0 0 1 0 0 0  0  0  0  0 0 0 0
CORR e8   0   0 0 0 0 0 0 0 1 0 0  0  0  0  0 0 0 0
CORR e9   0   0 0 0 0 0 0 0 0 1 0  0  0  0  0 0 0 0
CORR e10  0   0 0 0 0 0 0 0 0 0 1  0  0  0  0 0 0 0
CORR e27  0   0 0 0 0 0 0 0 0 0 0  1  0  0  0 0 0 0
CORR e28  0   0 0 0 0 0 0 0 0 0 0  0  1  0  0 0 0 0
CORR e29  0   0 0 0 0 0 0 0 0 0 0  0  0  1  0 0 0 0
CORR d1   0   0 0 0 0 0 0 0 0 0 0  0  0  0  1 0 0 0
CORR d2   0   0 0 0 0 0 0 0 0 0 0  0  0  0  0 1 0 0
CORR d3   0   0 0 0 0 0 0 0 0 0 0  0  0  0  0 0 1 0
CORR d4   0   0 0 0 0 0 0 0 0 0 0  0  0  0  0 0 0 1
MEAN  .   0   0 0 0 0 0 0 0 0 0 0  0  0  0  0 0 0 0
STD   .   1   1 1 1 1 1 1 1 1 1 1  1  1  1  1 1 1 1
N     .   500 500 500 500 500 500 500 500 500 500 500 500 500 500 500 500 500 500
;

run;
Proc simnormal data=_corr_ out=_sim_ds numreal=500 seed=345;
var F5 e1 e2 e3 e4 e5 e6 e7 e8 e9 e10 e27 e28 e29 d1 d2 d3 d4;
run;

Proc Corr Data=_sim_ds; Run;
Data _cfa_menqol_; Set _sim_ds;
/* Step 1: Setting values of loadings for latent factors */
Lf1v1 = 1.2; Lf1v2 = 1.4; Lf1v3 = 1.3;
Lf2v4 = 2.1; Lf2v5 = 1.9; Lf2v6 = 1.7; Lf2v7 = 1.9; Lf2v8 = 1.8; Lf2v9 = 2.0; Lf2v10 = 2.2;
Lf4v27= 1.5; Lf4v28= 1.6; Lf4v29= 1.4;
Lf5f1= 1.7; Lf5f2= 1.6; Lf5f3= 1.8; Lf5f4= 1.9;
/* Step 2: Setting values of variances for error terms and disturbance*/
vare1 = sqrt(2.5); vare2 = sqrt(1.5); vare3 = sqrt(2.0);
vare4 = sqrt(2.2); vare5 = sqrt(1.9); vare6 = sqrt(1.8); vare7 = sqrt(2.2); vare8 = sqrt(2.2); vare9 = sqrt(2.3); vare10 = sqrt(1.7); vare10=
sqrt(2.1);
vare27= sqrt(2.3); vare28= sqrt(1.7); vare29= sqrt(2.1);
vard3 = sqrt(1.8);
/* Step 3: Creating factor F1, F2, F4, and variable v30 */
F1 = Lf5f1*F5 + d1; F2 = Lf5f2*F5 + d2; v30= Lf5f3*F5 + vard3*d3; F4 = Lf5f4*F5 + d4;
/* Step 4: Creating variable v1, v2, v8, v9, v27, v28, v29 */
v1 = Lf1v1*F1 + vare1*e1; v2 = Lf1v2*F1 + vare2*e2; v3 = Lf1v3*F1 + vare3*e3;
v4 = Lf2v4*F2 + vare4*e4; v5 = Lf2v5*F2 + vare5*e5; v6 = Lf2v6*F2 + vare6*e6; v7 = Lf2v7*F2 + vare7*e7;
v8 = Lf2v8*F2 + vare8*e8; v9 = Lf2v9*F2 + vare9*e9; v10= Lf2v10*F2 + vare10*e10;
v27= Lf4v27*F4 + vare27*e27; v28 = Lf4v28*F4 + vare28*e28; v29 = Lf4v29*F4 + vare29*e29;
Keep v1 v2 v3 v4 v5 v6 v7 v8 v9 v10 v27 v28 v29 v30;
Run;
```

Figure 5.74 Simulating a dataset representing a measurement model for the MENQOL scale.

```
Proc Calis COV data=_cfa_menqol_  G4=200 GCONV=1E-10 Method=ML ALL;
LINEQS
   v1    = lf1v1 f1 + e1,   v2    = lf1v2 f1 + e2,   v3    = lf1v3 f1 + e3,
   v4    = lf2v4 f2 + e4,   v5    = lf2v5 f2 + e5,   v6    = lf2v6 f2 + e6,
   v7    = lf2v7 f2 + e7,   v8    = lf2v8 f2 + e8,   v9    = lf2v9 f2 + e9,
   v10   = lf2v10 f2 + e10,
   v27   = lf4v1 f4 + e27,  v28   = lf4v2 f4 + e28,  v29 = lf4v3 f4 + e29,
   f1    = lf5f1 f5 + d1,   f2    = lf5f2 f5 + d2,   v30 = lf5f3 f5 + d3,
   f4    = lf5f4 f5 + d4;
VARIANCE
f5=1,
d1=1, d2=1, d3=vard3, d4=1,
e1=vare1, e2=vare2, e3=vare3,
e4=vare4, e5=vare5, e6=vare6, e7=vare7,e8=vare8, e9=vare9, e10=vare10,
e27=vare27, e28=vare28, e29=vare29;
Bounds
 vare1-vare10 > 1.0e-8,   vare27-vare29 > 1.0e-8,   vard3 > 1.0e-8;
Run;
```

Figure 5.75 Implementation of the second-order CFA model with a manifest variable playing role of a first-order factor.

```
          Linear Equations
v1  =     1.1748(**) f1 +   1.0000 e1
v2  =     1.3228(**) f1 +   1.0000 e2
v3  =     1.2537(**) f1 +   1.0000 e3
v4  =     2.2882(**) f2 +   1.0000 e4
v5  =     2.1131(**) f2 +   1.0000 e5
v6  =     1.8698(**) f2 +   1.0000 e6
v7  =     2.1069(**) f2 +   1.0000 e7
v8  =     1.9592(**) f2 +   1.0000 e8
v9  =     2.1492(**) f2 +   1.0000 e9
v10 =     2.3536(**) f2 +   1.0000 e10
v27 =     1.3941(**) f4 +   1.0000 e27
v28 =     1.5420(**) f4 +   1.0000 e28
v29 =     1.3028(**) f4 +   1.0000 e29
f1  =     1.5855(**) f5 +   1.0000 d1
f2  =     1.3077(**) f5 +   1.0000 d2
v30 =     1.7703(**) f5 +   1.0000 d3
f4  =     2.0013(**) f5 +   1.0000 d4
```

Estimates for Variances of Exogenous Variables

Variable Type	Variable	Parameter	Estimate	Standard Error	t Value	Pr > |t|
Latent	f5		1.00000			
Disturbance	d1		1.00000			
	d2		1.00000			
Error	d3	vard3	1.57381	0.13277	11.8540	<.0001
Disturbance	d4		1.00000			
Error	e1	vare1	2.06607	0.17174	12.0302	<.0001
	e2	vare2	1.61407	0.16681	9.6763	<.0001
	e3	vare3	2.10931	0.18235	11.5672	<.0001
	e4	vare4	1.92658	0.14701	13.1049	<.0001
	e5	vare5	1.88619	0.14019	13.4548	<.0001
	e6	vare6	1.79855	0.12960	13.8772	<.0001
	e7	vare7	2.38978	0.17115	13.9632	<.0001
	e8	vare8	2.19734	0.15613	14.0733	<.0001
	e9	vare9	1.94751	0.14479	13.4503	<.0001
	e10	vare10	2.04099	0.15570	13.1086	<.0001
	e27	vare27	2.42988	0.20343	11.9445	<.0001
	e28	vare28	1.40572	0.17635	7.9714	<.0001
	e29	vare29	2.32129	0.18853	12.3127	<.0001

Figure 5.76 Estimation of the parameters for the second-order CFA model with manifest variable.

5.2.6 Bifactor Model

The purpose of CFA as a part of the validation of a scale is to examine whether the measurement model of a scale fits the data. This is very important point – the CFA model should be as close as possible to the measurement model. In the previous Section 5.2.4, the second-order CFA model was introduced for scales that have first-order domains and an overall factor. For this type of scale, an auxiliary CFA model is also proposed, namely, a bifactor model. It is crucial to be aware of what this model represents and, even more importantly, what it does not represent as a part of the quantitative validation of a scale.

Consider a scale with three latent domains (factors $F1$, $F2$, and $F3$) measured by nine items and one aggregated domain (factor $F4$), which generally is calculated as a mean (or a sum) of the three-domain scores (the same example discussed in Section 5.2.4.1 and illustrated by Figure 5.60). If a bifactor model is employed for this scale, then Figure 5.77 represents the general relationships among items, domains, and error terms for this type of model. The first difference from the model depicted by Figure 5.60 is that now all latent factors are represented by first-order exogenous variables at the same level.

Previously it was noted that one of the main assumptions when testing the measurement model of a scale is that every item represents one and only one latent attribute. If an item loads on (or measures) two or more factors, then this item is generally considered a flawed item, which can be deleted (as discussed in Section 5.1.3.4). But in the bifactor model every item measures simultaneously two independent latent factors: an overall factor (usually referenced as a general factor) and a nuisance factor (also called a group factor). For example, in Figure 5.77, item 1 (represented by variable V_1) is affected by factor $F1$ (a nuisance factor), factor $F4$ (a general factor), and, as previously noted, by a latent exogenous latent variable representing the error term e_1.

Note that in bifactor model every item can be affected by only one general factor and by only one (nuisance) factor. This difference is the first important one from the general understanding regarding the behavior of an item – an item manifests the changes in the particular underlining latent attribute (domain or factor), not the changes in the two (or more) latent attributes. This distinction is based on a simple concept that if two or more latent factors simultaneously affect an item, then we do not know why the item is changed or not changed. Those latent factors can affect an item differently. For example, if loading Lf_1v_1 is negative and loading Lf_4v_1 is positive, then it is possible that the observed measurement variable V_1 will stay the same if both attributes represented by factors $F1$ and $F2$ are changed. In another situation, however, when factor $F1$ is changing but factor $F4$ is not, we will not know why the measurement variable V_1 has changed.

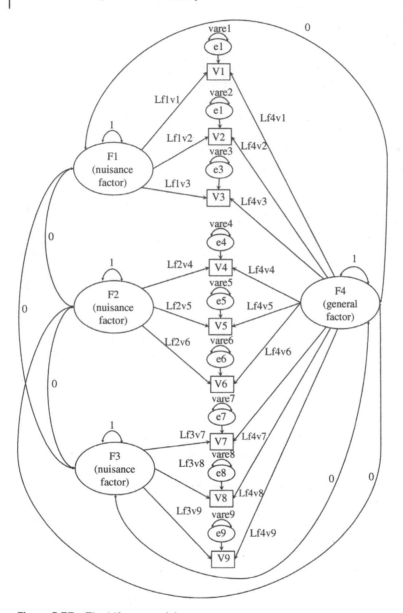

Figure 5.77 The bifactor model.

The second difference from the second-order CFA model is even more concerning – this is the assumption that *all* latent factors are independent. As previously stated, the curved two-headed arrows represent covariances between latent domains *F*1, *F*2, *F*3, and *F*4. But in the bivariate model those covariances are postulated to be zero. It is difficult to rationalize this assumption of independence of latent factors as a part of the measurement model for a scale. First of all, for vast majority of multi-domain PRO scales, latent factors usually measure related (but not the same) attributes and, as such, it is difficult to imagine that the covariance between those factors can be zero. If, in Figure 5.77, the general factor *F*4 is calculated as the mean of domain scores (or as a sum of all items), then, just because of only this aggregation, the general factor will have a notable correlation with factors *F*1, *F*2, and *F*3. Factors *F*1, *F*2, and *F*3 are fundamental parts of the general factor *F*4, and thus they (*F*1, *F*2, *F*3) will naturally covary.

From the above discussion, it should be clear that the bifactor model does not represent the measurement model of a scale with several domains and an overall (aggregated or total) factor. Then the question arises what does the bifactor model actually represent and what kind of questions can we answer with this model? Before we answer this question, let's illustrate the implementation of this model and then discuss its results.

Figure 5.78 represents the implementation of the bifactor model for the simulated scale discussed in Section 5.2.4.1. To showcase differences in results, we use and run this bifactor model with the same simulated dataset "_cfa_1" produced by the code from Figure 5.39. As before, under the section titled LINEQS (Figure 5.78), the causal relationships between observed variables, latent factors, and error terms are described. Note that now three exogenous latent factors (instead of only two) affect every observed variable. For example, in this equation

```
v1 = lf4v1 f4 + lf1v1 f1 + e1
```

variable V_1 is affected simultaneously by latent factors *F*4 and *F*1 and by the error term e_1 (as stated earlier, error terms in CFA modeling are always considered as exogenous latent factors).

```
Proc Calis COV data=_cfa_1 G4=200 GCONV=1E-10 Method=ML  ALL;
LINEQS
v1=lf4v1 f4 + lf1v1 f1 + e1, v2=lf4v2 f4 + lf1v2 f1 + e2, v3=lf4v3 f4 + lf1v3 f1 + e3,
v4=lf4v4 f4 + lf2v4 f2 + e4, v5=lf4v5 f4 + lf2v5 f2 + e5, v6=lf4v6 f4 + lf2v6 f2 + e6,
v7=lf4v7 f4 + lf3v7 f3 + e7, v8=lf4v8 f4 + lf3v8 f3 + e8, v9=lf4v9 f4 + lf3v9 f3 + e9;
VARIANCE
f4=1, f1=1, f2=1, f3=1,
e1=vare1, e2=vare2, e3=vare3, e4=vare4, e5=vare5, e6=vare6, e7=vare7, e8=vare8,
e9=vare9;
Cov
f1 f2 = 0 , f1 f3 = 0 , f1 f4 = 0 , f2 f3 = 0 , f2 f4 = 0 , f3 f4 = 0 ;
Bounds
vare1-vare9 > 1.0e-8;
Run;
```

Figure 5.78 Implementation of the bifactor model (represented by Figure 5.77).

The next part in the description of the model is the section VARIANCE. This section follows the previously described pattern: (i) variances for latent factors $F1$, $F2$, $F3$, and $F4$ are predefined and postulated to be equal to 1 (see Figure 5.77), and (ii) variances for error terms are needed to be estimated.

In the section titled COV, the covariances between latent factors $F1$, $F2$, $F3$, and $F4$ are defined, as was done previously. But in the bifactor model those covariances are not free parameters that need to be estimated – all of them are postulated to equal zero (which means that we postulate that factors $F1$–$F4$ are independent or orthogonal).

This model still fits the data well (Figure 5.79) according to Bentler's CFI, which equals 0.9916. Nevertheless, the results for estimated loadings and variances of the error terms (Figures 5.80 and 5.81) are somewhat puzzling: all loadings for general factor $F4$ are negative, whereas loadings for factor $F1$ are positive, for factor $F2$ are negative, and for factor $F3$ are positive (and not significant). This set of directionality means, for example, that a positive change in the general factor

Modeling Info	Number of Observations	500
	Number of Variables	9
	Number of Moments	45
	Number of Parameters	27
	Number of Active Constraints	0
	Baseline Model Function Value	2.0861
	Baseline Model Chi-Square	1040.9440
	Baseline Model Chi-Square DF	36
	Pr > Baseline Model Chi-Square	<.0001
Absolute Index	Fit Function	0.0530
	Chi-Square	26.4398
	Chi-Square DF	18
	Pr > Chi-Square	0.0901
	Elliptic Corrected Chi-Square	26.5530
	Pr > Elliptic Corr. Chi-Square	0.0878
	Z-Test of Wilson & Hilferty	1.3418
	Hoelter Critical N	545
	Root Mean Square Residual (RMR)	0.0966
	Standardized RMR (SRMR)	0.0210
	Goodness of Fit Index (GFI)	0.9884
Parsimony Index	Adjusted GFI (AGFI)	0.9710
	Parsimonious GFI	0.4942
	RMSEA Estimate	0.0307
	RMSEA Lower 90% Confidence Limit	0.0000
	RMSEA Upper 90% Confidence Limit	0.0541
	Probability of Close Fit	0.9064
	ECVI Estimate	0.1634
	ECVI Lower 90% Confidence Limit	0.1472
	ECVI Upper 90% Confidence Limit	0.1995
	Akaike Information Criterion	80.4398
	Bozdogan CAIC	221.2342
	Schwarz Bayesian Criterion	194.2342
	McDonald Centrality	0.9916
Incremental Index	Bentler Comparative Fit Index	0.9916
	Bentler-Bonett NFI	0.9746
	Bentler-Bonett Non-normed Index	0.9832
	Bollen Normed Index Rho1	0.9492
	Bollen Non-normed Index Delta2	0.9917
	James et al. Parsimonious NFI	0.4873

Figure 5.79 Bifactor model: fit summary.

```
            Linear Equations
v1 =    -0.5789(**) f4  +   0.7752(**) f1  +   1.0000 e1
v2 =    -0.6961(**) f4  +   1.2793(**) f1  +   1.0000 e2
v3 =    -0.7146(**) f4  +   1.1255(**) f1  +   1.0000 e3
v4 =    -1.3180(**) f4  +  -1.6393(**) f2  +   1.0000 e4
v5 =    -1.2213(**) f4  +  -1.2915(**) f2  +   1.0000 e5
v6 =    -1.0341(**) f4  +  -1.1665(**) f2  +   1.0000 e6
v7 =    -0.9972(**) f4  +   0.0700(ns) f3  +   1.0000 e7
v8 =    -0.9966(**) f4  +   1.5339(ns) f3  +   1.0000 e8
v9 =    -1.3573(**) f4  +   0.0658(ns) f3  +   1.0000 e9
```

		Estimates for Variances of Exogenous Variables				
Variable				Standard		
Type	Variable	Parameter	Estimate	Error	t Value	Pr > |t|
Error	e1	vare1	2.78551	0.19865	14.0223	<.0001
	e2	vare2	1.44875	0.26371	5.4936	<.0001
	e3	vare3	1.65332	0.21771	7.5940	<.0001
	e4	vare4	2.69800	0.40259	6.7017	<.0001
	e5	vare5	3.56775	0.31982	11.1554	<.0001
	e6	vare6	3.02034	0.26543	11.3790	<.0001
	e7	vare7	2.36810	0.20961	11.2974	<.0001
	e8	vare8	0.05045	116.95095	0.000431	0.9997
	e9	vare9	2.05534	0.23916	8.5939	<.0001

Figure 5.80 Bifactor model: unstandardized loading and variances of error terms.

```
      Standardized Results for Linear Equations
v1 =    -0.3001(**) f4  +   0.4018(**) f1  +   1.0000 e1
v2 =    -0.3684(**) f4  +   0.6771(**) f1  +   1.0000 e2
v3 =    -0.3858(**) f4  +   0.6077(**) f1  +   1.0000 e3
v4 =    -0.4938(**) f4  +  -0.6143(**) f2  +   1.0000 e4
v5 =    -0.4709(**) f4  +  -0.4979(**) f2  +   1.0000 e5
v6 =    -0.4429(**) f4  +  -0.4997(**) f2  +   1.0000 e6
v7 =    -0.5434(**) f4  +   0.0382(ns) f3  +   1.0000 e7
v8 =    -0.5408(**) f4  +   0.8323(ns) f3  +   1.0000 e8
v9 =    -0.6871(**) f4  +   0.0333(ns) f3  +   1.0000 e9
```

		Standardized Results for Variances of Exogenous Variables				
Variable				Standard		
Type	Variable	Parameter	Estimate	Error	t Value	Pr > |t|
Error	e1	vare1	0.74848	0.04163	17.9778	<.0001
	e2	vare2	0.40582	0.07471	5.4321	<.0001
	e3	vare3	0.48191	0.06372	7.5624	<.0001
	e4	vare4	0.37880	0.05774	6.5601	<.0001
	e5	vare5	0.53033	0.04682	11.3281	<.0001
	e6	vare6	0.55416	0.04731	11.7129	<.0001
	e7	vare7	0.70323	0.05540	12.6939	<.0001
	e8	vare8	0.01485	34.43438	0.000431	0.9997
	e9	vare9	0.52676	0.06081	8.6628	<.0001

Figure 5.81 Bifactor model: standardized loading and variances of error terms.

causes negative changes in the observed variables V_1, V_2, and V_3, but a positive change in the factor $F1$ causes positive changes in the same observed variables.

To come to terms with those results for this bifactor model, it is important to stress again that general factor $F4$ has nothing to do with the total score calculated as a sum or a mean of the variables V_1, V_2, ..., V_8, V_9. And the same can be said about factor $F1$ – it has nothing to do with what we usually consider as a factor with a score calculated as a sum or a mean of the variables V_1, V_2, and V_3. These results stem from the assumption that every variable is affected by two independent (orthogonal) factors. In fact, those factors should be considered as new concepts, which are weakly connected to the original measurement model of a scale. Note also that the variance for the error term associated with variable V_8 is very small (0.05045) compared with other variances and not significant – this type of behavior with an unexplainable very small estimation for the variance can also occasionally be observed.

At that point, it should be clear that the bifactor model does not represent the measurement model of a scale. Then a natural question arises on what this model can and should be used for. Moreover, what kind of conclusions can we draw based on the results of this model? The answer is that the results of this model can corroborate the dimensionality of the scale. The logic behind this interpretation is based on whether a scale should be represented by just one total factor or a more intricate multidimensional structure. How can results of the bifactor modeling help us to answer this question? The answer lies in the relationship between the loadings associated with general factor and the loadings associated with group/nuisance factors.

In the bifactor model, we analyze the relative impact of the general factor (factor $F4$ in our example) and group/nuisance factors (factors $F1$, $F2$, and $F3$) on every item. If factor loadings are high (in absolute value) for the general factor and low on the group/nuisance factors, then it should be interpreted that this scale is unidimensional, and we should consider only the general factor (i.e., it makes little sense to create subscales). If factor loadings are high for both the general factor and the group/nuisance factors, then this scale should be considered as multidimensional or multi-domain.

We are not aware of any established guidelines on the relative impact of factor loadings on every item, a subject worthy of research. The standardized loading for the path from factor $F1$ to variable V_1 is 0.4018, and the standardized loading for the path from factor $F4$ to variable V_1 is -0.3001 (Figure 5.81). The relative impact reflects the ratio (%) between the absolute value of loading from the group/nuisance factors to an item and the absolute value of loading from the general factor to the same item. Thus, for variable V_1 this relative impact is 134% ($1.34=|0.4018|/|-0.3001|$), which is substantial by any standard. In our example, the absolute values of standardized loadings for the paths from factors $F1$, $F2$, and $F3$ to observed variables are generally larger than absolute values of standardized loadings for the paths from general factor $F4$ (except for variables V_7 and V_9), which should be interpreted that a one common factor model is not adequate for this scale.

If, say, all standardized loading for the paths from general factor $F4$ to observed variables V_1, V_2, . . ., V_8, V_9 were larger in absolute values than standardized loadings for the paths from factors $F1$, $F2$, and $F3$ to the same set of observed variables, and the relative impacts of those factors $F1$, $F2$ and $F3$ for all items were small (say, less than 20%), then one common factor model for this scale could be considered.

One of the most critical requirements for this type of model is the independence of all latent factors. This condition allows us to interpret results in a certain way. As the group/nuisance factors are essentially playing the role of disturbances relative to the general factor, the comparison of estimated path coefficients quantifies the independent (orthogonal) unexplained by the general factor variance associated with those group/nuisance factors. Yet the orthogonality requirement is not only based on the theoretical bifactor model framework. It is also rooted in the simple necessity to have this assumption. In fact, if we allow for factors to covary, this model will not be identifiable, and hence a unique solution cannot be generated. To highlight this, let's replace in Figure 5.78 the part of the description of the model under COV statement with the following code:

```
Cov
f1 f2 = covf1f2 ,
f1 f3 = covf1f3 ,
f1 f4 = covf1f4 ,
f2 f3 = covf2f3 ,
f2 f4 = covf2f4 ,
f3 f4 = covf3f4 ; .
```

The above change will define covariances between latent factors as free parameters and force the model to estimate them instead of assuming the zero covariances between latent factors. After running this code (code from Figure 5.78 with above change), the log file will display the following message:

ERROR: LEVMAR Optimization cannot be completed.
NOTE: LEVMAR needs more than 50 iterations or 500 function calls.
NOTE: Due to optimization failure, statistics in the Fit Summary table might not be appropriate.
NOTE: Due to optimization failure, standard error estimates are not computed.

As noted previously, it is important to check log file every time. Note that, even if we see the error in the log file, SAS still produces estimations of all parameters in the model based on the results of the last iteration (which would be obviously incorrect). SAS also informs us that the iteration process may be successful by relaxing some default parameters. Let's therefore change/add parameters in the first line of the CALIS procedure as shown below:

Proc Calis COV data=_cfa_1 G4=**2000** MAXITER=**10000** GCONV=**1E-10** Method=ML ALL; .

The above change allowed the iteration process to converge as shown below (log file) but several WARNING messages persist:

NOTE: Convergence criterion (ABSGCONV=0.00001) satisfied.
NOTE: The Moore-Penrose inverse is used in computing the covariance matrix for parameter estimates.

WARNING: Standard errors and t values might not be accurate with the use of the Moore-Penrose inverse.
WARNING: Although all predicted variances for the latent factors are positive, the corresponding predicted covariance matrix is not positive definite. It has one negative eigenvalue.
WARNING: Although all predicted variances for the observed variables and latent factors are positive, the corresponding predicted covariance matrix is not positive definite. It has one negative eigenvalue.

Recall (Section 5.2.4.2) that we recommended to always take a look at the output part titled as "Covariance Structure Analysis: Optimization" and specifically to check Convergence Status and Linear Dependence (if present). This part of the output is presented below:

Convergence criterion (ABSGCONV=0.00001) satisfied.
NOTE: The Moore-Penrose inverse is used in computing the covariance matrix for parameter estimates.
WARNING: Standard errors and t values might not be accurate with the use of the Moore-Penrose inverse.
NOTE: Covariance matrix for the estimates is not full rank.
NOTE: The variance of some parameter estimates is zero or some parameter estimates are linearly related to other parameter estimates as shown in the following equations:
lf3v9 = -1.919388 - 0.017580*lf4v7 - 0.021839*lf3v7
+ 0.059606*lf4v8 + 0.074046*lf3v8 - 0.506750*lf4v9 -
0.074557*covf1f3 - 0.160472*covf2f3 + 0.261579*covf3f4
covf1f4 = -1.706421 + 0.195120*lf4v1 + 0.134762*lf1v1
+ 0.319988*lf4v2 + 0.221004*lf1v2 + 0.333852*lf4v3 +
0.230579*lf1v3 + 0.069129*covf1f2 + 0.165591*covf1f3
covf2f4 = -2.449433 - 0.427595*lf4v4 - 0.036606*lf2v4
- 0.345405*lf4v5 - 0.029570*lf2v5 - 0.545274*lf4v6 -
0.046680*lf2v6 + 0.397034*covf1f2 + 0.669105*covf2f3

The above results show that the parameters of a model are not identifiable. And linear dependences between parameters in the model is the manifestation of this alongside with the notes that "The Moore-Penrose inverse is used in computing the covariance matrix for parameter estimates" and "Covariance matrix for the estimates is not full rank."

This illustration is a good example to showcase a situation that one of the main requirements for a model to be identifiable – namely, the `Number of Parameters` to be estimated (which is 33 for this model) should be less than the `Number of Moments` for this model (45) (as described in Section 5.2.2) – is not a sufficient condition in some models.

5.2.7 Confirmatory Factor Analysis Using Polychoric Correlations

In Chapter 4 (Section 4.2.2), scales with dichotomous items were discussed. It was shown how polychoric correlations can be used in the assessment of internal consistency reliability. In this section, we demonstrate how those polychoric correlations can be used to investigate the measurement structure of a scale. The simulated dataset "`_sim_ds1`" with binary variables was created by using, first, SAS code from Figure 4.64 (simulating a scale with 10 continuous items) and then SAS code from Figure 4.66 (simulating binary responses). The same dataset "`_sim_ds1`" will be used in this section as a starting point to (i) produce a dataset with polychoric correlations and then (ii) use this new dataset to perform a confirmatory factor analysis. Before readers continue with this section, we recommend reviewing Section 4.2.2, as all assumptions about the continuous nature of the items, even if responses to those items are presented to subjects in the form of a binary choice, are also applicable for the confirmatory factor analyses.

The first step in this analysis is to create the input file for the CALIS procedure with polychoric correlations. As noted earlier, instead of the dataset with subject-level data, the input for the CALIS procedure can be a dataset representing pair-wise correlations. Figure 5.82 shows how CORR procedure can be used to produce such a dataset by simply adding the option "`POLYCHORIC.`" As the process to generate polychoric correlations is iterative, we also need to define additional parameters defining convergence status (`CONVERGE = 1e-10`), maximum allowed number of iterations (`MAXITER = 10 000`), and number of categories (in this example it is two [binary variables], but we also can make this code more general and define this parameter as `NGROUPS = ALL`). Option `OUTPLC` directs CORR procedure to create dataset "`_polychoric_`" with a special structure representing a correlation matrix (the same structure of the data we use frequently as a starting point to generate simulated datasets; see, for example, Figure 4.64).

Figure 5.83 represents the implementation of the CFA analysis for a scale with 10 items and one overall domain. As previously mentioned, we request that the

```
Proc Corr Data=_sim_ds1
POLYCHORIC (CONVERGE=1e-10 MAXITER=10000 NGROUPS=ALL) alpha nomiss OUTPLC=_polychoric_;
Var i1-i10;
run;
```

Figure 5.82 Generating dataset "_polychoric_".

```
Proc Calis COV data=_polychoric_ G4=1000 GCONV=1E-10 Method=ML  TECHNIQUE=LEVMAR  ALL;
LINEQS
   i1   = lv01f1 f1 + e01,  i2   = lv02f1 f1 + e02,  i3   = lv03f1 f1 + e03,
   i4   = lv04f1 f1 + e04,  i5   = lv05f1 f1 + e05,  i6   = lv06f1 f1 + e06,
   i7   = lv07f1 f1 + e07,  i8   = lv08f1 f1 + e08,  i9   = lv09f1 f1 + e09,
   i10  = lv10f1 f1 + e10;
STD
f1=1,
e01 = vare01, e02 = vare02, e03 = vare03, e04 = vare04, e05 = vare05, e06 = vare06,
e07 = vare07, e08 = vare08, e09 = vare09, e10 = vare10;
Run;
```

Figure 5.83 Implementation of the CFA model with one domain.

CFA should be performed based on covariances, but the correlation matrix was provided as the input. It is important to note that the correct dataset of the correlation type also should have additional information on the number of observations, means, and standard deviations, and the generated by CORR procedure the dataset " `_polychoric_` " has all this additional information. The CALIS procedure is intelligent enough to recognize that the input file represents correlations and, based on all available data in this dataset " `_polychoric_` ," will generate covariance matrix to be used in the analysis. Here we illustrate this approach for a simple scale with just one latent domain, but the same will work for any multi-domain scale.

After this analysis has been run (Figure 5.83), the usual set of estimated parameters is produced: the fit indexes, loadings, and variances of the error term. For this particular simulated example, it is interesting to compare the results of the CFA based on the polychoric correlations (dataset " `_polychoric_` ", generated by code from Figure 5.63) vs. the initial dataset " `_sim_ds` " (simulated items represented by continuous variables, generated by code from Figure 4.64) and the dataset " `_sim_ds1` " (simulated items represented by binary variables, generated by code from Figure 4.66). Our intent is to show that the CFA results based on the initial dataset " `_sim_ds` " will be close to the CFA results based on the polychoric correlations, whereas the CFA results based on the dataset " `_sim_ds1` " will be perceptibly different from those two sets of results.

To run those analyses, we can use exactly the same code presented by Figure 5.83 – the only change needed is in replacing ". . .data=_poly-choric_..." by "...data=_sim_ds..." or "...data=_sim_ds1...". Figure 5.84 summarizes the results of those analyses. As we can see, the CFIs for the models based on the polychoric correlations and continuous data are close to each other (0.8995 vs. 0.9093), whereas the CFI for the model which used binary data is noticeably different (0.9439). And the same pattern is observed for the standardized loadings and even variances of the error terms.

As in Chapter 4, it should be noted that the CFA analysis by itself is a modeling, which should be based on the large number of well-distributed observations. When using polychoric correlations this requirement is even more

CFA based on the polychoric correlations (dataset "_polychoric_")

```
Bentler Comparative Fit Index          0.8995

Standardized Results for Linear Equations
i1  = 0.7616(**) f1 +    1.0000 e01
i2  = 0.7457(**) f1 +    1.0000 e02
i3  = 0.7738(**) f1 +    1.0000 e03
i4  = 0.7840(**) f1 +    1.0000 e04
i5  = 0.7885(**) f1 +    1.0000 e05
i6  = 0.7671(**) f1 +    1.0000 e06
i7  = 0.7762(**) f1 +    1.0000 e07
i8  = 0.7780(**) f1 +    1.0000 e08
i9  = 0.8010(**) f1 +    1.0000 e09
i10 = 0.7918(**) f1 +    1.0000 e10

Standardized Results for Variances of
Exogenous Variables
                           Standard
Parameter   Estimate       Error       Pr > |t|
vare01      0.41990        0.01269     <.0001
vare02      0.44394        0.01307     <.0001
vare03      0.40123        0.01238     <.0001
vare04      0.38538        0.01209     <.0001
vare05      0.37831        0.01197     <.0001
vare06      0.41152        0.01255     <.0001
vare07      0.39757        0.01231     <.0001
vare08      0.39475        0.01226     <.0001
vare09      0.35837        0.01159     <.0001
vare10      0.37310        0.01187     <.0001
```

CFA based on the dataset "_sim_ds" (simulated items represented by continuous variables)

```
Bentler Comparative Fit Index          0.9093

Standardized Results for Linear Equations
i1  = 0.7607(**) f1 +    1.0000 e01
i2  = 0.7521(**) f1 +    1.0000 e02
i3  = 0.7576(**) f1 +    1.0000 e03
i4  = 0.7788(**) f1 +    1.0000 e04
i5  = 0.7738(**) f1 +    1.0000 e05
i6  = 0.7763(**) f1 +    1.0000 e06
i7  = 0.7659(**) f1 +    1.0000 e07
i8  = 0.7821(**) f1 +    1.0000 e08
i9  = 0.7798(**) f1 +    1.0000 e09
i10 = 0.8085(**) f1 +    1.0000 e10

Standardized Results for Variances of Exogenous
Variables
                           Standard
Parameter   Estimate       Error       Pr > |t|
vare01      0.42135        0.01274     <.0001
vare02      0.43427        0.01294     <.0001
vare03      0.42611        0.01281     <.0001
vare04      0.39342        0.01226     <.0001
vare05      0.40120        0.01240     <.0001
vare06      0.39733        0.01233     <.0001
vare07      0.41343        0.01261     <.0001
vare08      0.38830        0.01217     <.0001
vare09      0.39191        0.01224     <.0001
vare10      0.34633        0.01138     <.0001
```

CFA based on the dataset "_sim_ds1" (simulated items represented by binary variables)

```
Bentler Comparative Fit Index          0.9439

Standardized Results for Linear Equations
i1  = 0.6565(**) f1 +    1.0000 e01
i2  = 0.3958(**) f1 +    1.0000 e02
i3  = 0.4658(**) f1 +    1.0000 e03
i4  = 0.6432(**) f1 +    1.0000 e04
i5  = 0.6209(**) f1 +    1.0000 e05
i6  = 0.6286(**) f1 +    1.0000 e06
i7  = 0.6253(**) f1 +    1.0000 e07
i8  = 0.5537(**) f1 +    1.0000 e08
i9  = 0.6427(**) f1 +    1.0000 e09
i10 = 0.6289(**) f1 +    1.0000 e10

Standardized Results for Variances of
Exogenous Variables
                           Standard
Parameter   Estimate       Error       Pr > |t|
vare01      0.56902        0.01609     <.0001
vare02      0.84336        0.01347     <.0001
vare03      0.78307        0.01486     <.0001
vare04      0.58628        0.01614     <.0001
vare05      0.61448        0.01617     <.0001
vare06      0.60483        0.01617     <.0001
vare07      0.60906        0.01617     <.0001
vare08      0.69337        0.01593     <.0001
vare09      0.58691        0.01614     <.0001
vare10      0.60452        0.01617     <.0001
```

Figure 5.84 CFA modeling results based on three different datasets.

important, polychoric correlations can be unstable with a relatively small number of observations, which could lead to the problems with convergence of a CFA model. Note that this simulation has a large number of 3000 observations. Suppose we change the number of simulated observations to 300, as shown in Figure 5.85, which is basically the same combined SAS code from Figures 4.64 and 4.66 but generates datasets with only 300 observations). If we rerun three CFA models based on new datasets with only 300 observations, then the models based on the datasets "_sim_ds" and "_sim_ds1" will converge, but the CFA model based on the dataset "_polychoric_" will not and will give the following error message:

ERROR: The sample covariance or correlation matrix is not positive definite. ML or GLS estimates cannot be computed.

Unfortunately, there is no simple way around this problem as only have substantial number of observations. For any dataset the same type of the simulations can be run to estimate the number of observations. For example, in the above-described simulation, the CFA model based on the dataset "_polychoric_" become stable with around 1500 observations.

```
options nofmterr nocenter nodate nonumber pagesize=2000 linesize=256;
data _corr_(type=corr);
input
_TYPE_ $  _NAME_ $  i1    i2    i3    i4    i5    i6    i7    i8    i9    i10;
datalines;
  CORR      i1       1     .4    .5    .6    .6    .6    .6    .6    .6    .8
  CORR      i2       .4    1     .6    .6    .6    .6    .6    .6    .6    .6
  CORR      i3       .5    .6    1     .6    .6    .6    .6    .6    .6    .6
  CORR      i4       .6    .6    .6    1     .6    .6    .6    .6    .6    .6
  CORR      i5       .6    .6    .6    .6    1     .6    .6    .6    .6    .6
  CORR      i6       .6    .6    .6    .6    .6    1     .6    .6    .6    .6
  CORR      i7       .6    .6    .6    .6    .6    .6    1     .6    .6    .6
  CORR      i8       .6    .6    .6    .6    .6    .6    .6    1     .6    .6
  CORR      i9       .6    .6    .6    .6    .6    .6    .6    .6    1     .6
  CORR      i10      .8    .6    .6    .6    .6    .6    .6    .6    .6    1
  MEAN      .        7     7.8   6.5   7     7.4   7.1   7.2   7.4   6.9   6.8
  STD       .        .5    .6    .5    .5    .8    .5    .5    .5    .5    .5
  N         .        300   300   300   300   300   300   300   300   300   300
;
run;

proc simnormal data=_corr_ out=_sim_ds numreal=300 seed=100;
var i1-i10;
run;

Data _sim_ds1; Set  _sim_ds;
array v{10} i1-i10;
Do k=1 to 10;
If v[k]>=7 Then
    Do;    v[k]=1;    End;
Else
    Do;    v[k]=0;    End;
End;
Run;
```

Figure 5.85 Simulating 300 observations for a scale with 10 continuous items.

5.3 Convergent and Discriminant Validity

5.3.1 Convergent and Discriminant Validity Assessment

As noted previously, construct validity of a scale involves the degree to which the scores of a measurement instrument are consistent with hypotheses (Mokkink et al. 2010a). Included among types of construct validity are convergent validity and discriminant validity (sometimes called divergent validity) (Cappelleri et al. 2013).

Convergent validity addresses how much the target scale relates to other variables or measures to which it is expected to be related, according to the theory postulate. For instance, evidence of convergent validity for an anxiety measure under consideration would occur when patients with higher levels of anxiety also have higher levels of depression and, moreover, when this association is sizable. How sizable in general? While it depends on the nature of the variables or measures being compared, and when they are measured (correlations are expected to be higher following a treatment intervention than at baseline or pretreatment), a correlation between 0.4 and 0.8 between similar health-related measures may be reasonable in most circumstances as evidence for convergent validity for the target scale under consideration. A correlation above 0.8 would be reasonable when the two measures are purported to measure the same construct (trait) such as two measures of anxiety.

On the other hand, discriminate or divergent validity addresses how much the target scale relates to other variables or measures to which it is expected to have a weak or no relation (according to the theory postulated). For example, there is evidence of discriminant validity for an anxiety measure in the absence of a correlation between anxiety scores and shoe size, which are two unrelated constructs. While it depends on the nature of the variables or measures compared, and when they are measured (again, correlations are expected to higher following a treatment intervention than at baseline or pretreatment), a correlation less than 0.30 between dissimilar measures may be reasonable in most circumstances as evidence for discriminant validity for the target scale under consideration. In the majority of circumstances, correlations between 0.30 and 0.40 may fall in the gray zone in the sense of indicating no evidence to dismiss either convergent validity or discriminant (divergent) validity.

As noted previously in this book, a clinical outcome assessment (COA) is a measure that describes or reflects how a patient feels, functions, or survives. The four types of COAs include PRO measures, observer-reported outcome measures, clinician-reported outcome measures, and performance-based outcomes measures. In the updated and expanded FDA (draft) documents, the following is stated: "Construct validity of a COA is determined by evidence that relationships among items, domains, and concepts conform to a priori hypotheses concerning logical relationships that should exist with other related measures or characteristics of patients and patient groups (e.g., a COA intended to measure physical function should have a positive association with another existing physical function measure). FDA reviews the construct validity of a COA to determine whether the documented relationships between results gathered using the current instrument and results gathered using other related measures are consistent with a priori hypotheses concerning those relationships (i.e., discriminant and convergent validity). An example of assessing convergent validity would be to examine the associations between a patient global impression of symptoms severity and the endpoint score of a multi-item symptom measure" (FDA 2019).

Therefore, convergent validity and discriminant validity can be viewed as two interlocking propositions. Convergent validity involves "measures of constructs that theoretically should be related to each other are, in fact, observed to be related to each other" (that is, a correspondence or convergence between similar or the same constructs) and "measures of constructs that theoretically should not be related to each other are, in fact, observed not to be related to each other" (that is, discriminating between dissimilar constructs) (Trochim 2001). We typically use the correlation coefficient to estimate the degree to which any two measures are related to each other and examine the patterns of intercorrelations among measures. Generally, "correlations between theoretically similar measures should be "high," whereas correlations between theoretically dissimilar measures should be 'low'" (Trochim 2001).

5.3.2 Convergent and Discriminant Validity Evaluation in a Clinical Study

When using a clinical study data to examine convergent and discriminant validity, several important points should be considered. First, as pointed out in Chapter 2, for a scale under investigation it will be necessary to identify which other patient or clinician reported outcomes from this study will be used for convergent validity and which will be used for discriminant validity. It is usually difficult to convince a study team to include a scale that is expected to correlate weakly with an instrument we want to validate (to support discriminant validity), as the scale considered for discriminant validity will not be likely to respond to the active treatment in the study. As a result, most of the measures will typically support only convergent validity.

As discussed in Chapter 4, the use of the baseline data can lead to flawed conclusions for internal consistency reliability analyses (Cronbach's coefficient alpha) and, in this chapter, for factor analysis. And the same caution of using only baseline data also applies generally to investigating discriminant validity and convergent validity. To highlight this issue on the use of only baseline data and to illustrate, in general, convergent and discriminant validity analyses, let's simulate a hypothetical example provided in the aforementioned FDA document: "An example of assessing convergent validity would be to examine the associations between a patient global impression of symptoms severity and the endpoint score of a multi-item symptom measure." (FDA 2019). There are two important points in this sentence. First, to assess convergent validity we need ". . . to examine the associations between . . ." scales and, second, ". . . a patient global impression of symptoms severity . . ." can be used for this.

Consider the following simulation. There are two measurements $M1$ and $M2$, with $M1$ being a numeric rating scale (which needs to be validated) represented by integer values from 0 to 10. The $M2$ scale is a global severity scale (see Chapter 2 on discussion of global scales) assumed to be suitable to support convergent validity of the $M1$ scale. For this simulation, $M2$ represents the severity of illness by following four categories: "None" (i), "Mild" (ii), "Moderate" (iii), and "Severe" (iv).

Figure 5.86 represents the first step in the simulation. We assume that scales $M1$ and $M2$ are collected at baseline (represented by variables $M1bl$ and $M2bl$) and during the active treatment phase at week 4 (variables $M1w4$ and $M2w4$) and week 8 (variables $M1w8$ and $M2w8$). It is also assumed that there is an overall improvement – the mean score for $M1$ scale is 4 at week 4 and 3 at week 8 (assuming that a lower score indicates a better outcome). Overall improvement is also taken for the global assessment scale $M2$. Its mean at week 4 is 2 ("Mild") and at week 8 is 1.5 (meaning that subjects largely responded as "None" or "Mild"). Those longitudinal data are generated for 300 subjects.

In addition, we also assume that the correlation between $M1$ and $M2$ scales at baseline is 0.6 and 0.7 at week 4 and week 8. The responses collected for the same

```
data _corr_(type=corr);
input
_TYPE_ $   _NAME_ $    M1bl   M1w4   M1w8   M2bl   M2w4   M2w8;
datalines;
CORR       M1bl         1     .2     .2     .6     0      0
CORR       M1w4        .2      1     .2     0     .7      0
CORR       M1w8        .2     .2      1     0      0     .7
CORR       M2bl        .6      0      0      1     .2     .2
CORR       M2w4         0     .7      0     .2      1     .2
CORR       M2w8         0      0     .7     .2     .2      1
MEAN        .           5      4      3    2.5     2     1.5
STD         .          1.8    1.5    1.7    .8     .8     .7
N           .          300    300    300    300    300    300
;
run;
proc simnormal data=_corr_ out=_sim_ds numreal=300 seed=12345;
var M1bl   M1w4   M1w8   M2bl   M2w4   M2w8;
run;
proc corr data=_sim_ds ;
Var M1bl   M1w4   M1w8   M2bl   M2w4   M2w8;
Run;
```

Figure 5.86 Simulating starting values for the *M1* and *M2* scales at baseline, week 4, and week 8.

scale are usually correlated in time (because they are based on the same set of subjects). In this simulation, we assume that measurements for the scale $M1$ are weakly correlated in time (without loss of generality in messaging); for example, a correlation of 0.2 is defined between the $M1$ measurements at baseline (variable $M1bl$) and the $M1$ measurements at week 4 (variable $M1w4$). At the same time, the measurements based on two different scales separated in time should have even lower correlations. To simplify the simulated example, the correlations between $M1$ measurements at week 4 ($M1w4$) and $M2$ measurements at week 8 ($M2w8$) is defined as 0 (without any notable loss of generality in messaging). Figure 5.87 displays results of the simulation (based on SAS code from Figure 5.86). As expected, correlations, means, and standard deviations are close to the predefined values.

We see from Figure 5.87 that simulated values for $M2$ measurement at, for example, week 4 are from -0.68689 to 4.14664. But we want to simulate the real-life-like data with values for the scales $M1$ and $M2$ represented by integers and within a certain range, as would occur in practice. To do so, we first round all data to the closest integer and then only select observations where the $M1$ scale is represented by integers from 0 to 10 and, similarly, where the $M2$ scale is represented by integers from 1 to 4 (see Figure 5.88). The results of this step are presented by Figure 5.89. From 300 subjects, data on 264 subjects remain available for analysis.

The responses to the measurements $M1$ and $M2$ are now in predefined range from 0 to 10 and from 1 to 4, respectively, and correlations between variables are still close to the predefined values. But the dataset "_sim_ds2" still differs from the real-life situation in one important matter: in a vast majority of clinical studies

Simple Statistics

Variable	N	Mean	Std Dev	Sum	Minimum	Maximum
M1bl	300	4.99156	1.75020	1497	-0.46412	9.02019
M1w4	300	4.02939	1.50883	1209	-1.61241	8.11762
M1w8	300	2.92165	1.67916	876.49650	-1.90521	7.27570
M2bl	300	2.44617	0.78839	733.85014	0.17424	4.95622
M2w4	300	1.98000	0.77737	594.00140	-0.68689	4.14664
M2w8	300	1.44592	0.70409	433.77681	-0.77794	3.56205

Pearson Correlation Coefficients, N = 300
Prob > |r| under H0: Rho=0

	M1bl	M1w4	M1w8	M2bl	M2w4	M2w8
M1bl	1.00000	0.21709	0.19700	0.57782	0.03568	0.02989
		0.0002	0.0006	<.0001	0.5381	0.6061
M1w4	0.21709	1.00000	0.18094	-0.03035	0.69553	-0.01227
	0.0002		0.0016	0.6005	<.0001	0.8324
M1w8	0.19700	0.18094	1.00000	-0.05210	0.01520	0.74061
	0.0006	0.0016		0.3685	0.7932	<.0001
M2bl	0.57782	-0.03035	-0.05210	1.00000	0.19206	0.14101
	<.0001	0.6005	0.3685		0.0008	0.0145
M2w4	0.03568	0.69553	0.01520	0.19206	1.00000	0.19286
	0.5381	<.0001	0.7932	0.0008		0.0008
M2w8	0.02989	-0.01227	0.74061	0.14101	0.19286	1.00000
	0.6061	0.8324	<.0001	0.0145	0.0008	

Figure 5.87 Initial simulation results.

```
Data _sim_ds1; Set _sim_ds;
M1b1=round(M1b1,1); M2b1=round(M2b1,1); M1w4=round(M1w4,1); M2w4=round(M2w4,1);
M1w8=round(M1w8,1); M2w8=round(M2w8,1);
Run;

Data _sim_ds2; Set _sim_ds1;
If M1b1 In (0 1 2 3 4 5 6 7 8 9 10);
If M1w4 In (0 1 2 3 4 5 6 7 8 9 10);
If M1w8 In (0 1 2 3 4 5 6 7 8 9 10);
If M2b1 In (1 2 3 4);
If M2w4 In (1 2 3 4);
If M2w8 In (1 2 3 4);
Run;

proc corr data=_sim_ds2 ;
Var M1b1    M1w4    M1w8  M2b1    M2w4    M2w8;
Run;
```

Figure 5.88 Converting continuous simulated responses into integers.

```
                              Simple Statistics
Variable      N          Mean      Std Dev        Sum       Minimum       Maximum
M1b1         264       5.00758      1.68643       1322             0       9.00000
M1w4         264       4.08712      1.42091       1079       1.00000       8.00000
M1w8         264       3.14394      1.51611     830.00000          0       7.00000
M2b1         264       2.45833      0.73877     649.00000    1.00000       4.00000
M2w4         264       2.05303      0.80222     542.00000    1.00000       4.00000
M2w8         264       1.60227      0.62043     423.00000    1.00000       4.00000
```

		Pearson Correlation Coefficients, N = 264			
		Prob > |r| under H0: Rho=0			
	M1b1	M1w4	M1w8	M2b1	M2w4	M2w8

```
                M1b1          M1w4         M1w8          M2b1          M2w4          M2w8
M1b1         1.00000       0.23615       0.18546       0.51297       0.03343       0.01379
                           0.0001        0.0025        <.0001        0.5887        0.8235

M1w4         0.23615       1.00000       0.15654       0.01977       0.63304      -0.07700
             0.0001                      0.0109        0.7492        <.0001        0.2124

M1w8         0.18546       0.15654       1.00000      -0.08628      -0.02193       0.56637
             0.0025        0.0109                      0.1622        0.7228        <.0001

M2b1         0.51297       0.01977      -0.08628       1.00000       0.17696       0.09229
             <.0001        0.7492        0.1622                      0.0039        0.1348

M2w4         0.03343       0.63304      -0.02193       0.17696       1.00000       0.11129
             0.5887        <.0001        0.7228        0.0039                      0.0710

M2w8         0.01379      -0.07700       0.56637       0.09229       0.11129       1.00000
             0.8235        0.2124        <.0001        0.1348        0.0710
```

Figure 5.89 Results of converting continuous simulated responses into integers.

(which investigate treatment effectiveness), only subjects matching specific entry criteria are present at baseline. And to be eligible to participate in a study, a subject should generally have some level of the condition or of disease severity (e.g., pain in a study on fibromyalgia), which can be assessed in certain situations using a global assessment of severity (like the $M2$ scale here). In our simulation, therefore, we choose that all subjects at baseline should have a score of 3 ("Moderate") or 4 ("Severe") on the measurement scale $M2$ (see Figure 5.90 for SAS code and Figure 5.91 for results).

```
Data _sim_ds3; Set _sim_ds2;
Where M2bl>=3;
Run;
Proc corr data=_sim_ds3;
Var M1bl    M1w4    M1w8    M2bl    M2w4    M2w8;
Run;
```

Figure 5.90 Selection of only "moderate" or "severe" subjects at baseline.

```
                              Simple Statistics

Variable        N        Mean      Std Dev         Sum        Minimum      Maximum

M1bl           128      5.80469    1.44210     743.00000     2.00000      9.00000
M1w4           128      4.14844    1.39792     531.00000     1.00000      7.00000
M1w8           128      3.04688    1.49466     390.00000           0      6.00000
M2bl           128      3.12500    0.33202     400.00000     3.00000      4.00000
M2w4           128      2.19531    0.81384     281.00000     1.00000      4.00000
M2w8           128      1.63281    0.61313     209.00000     1.00000      4.00000
```

```
                 Pearson Correlation Coefficients, N = 128
                         Prob > |r| under H0: Rho=0
             M1bl         M1w4         M1w8         M2bl         M2w4         M2w8
M1bl      1.00000      0.25275      0.35863      0.29807      0.04618      0.22103
                       0.0040       <.0001       0.0006       0.6047       0.0122

M1w4      0.25275      1.0000       0.15869      0.01060      0.67335     -0.07371
          0.0040                    0.0736       0.9054       <.0001       0.4083

M1w8      0.35863      0.15869      1.00000      0.13090      0.01183      0.58602
          <.0001       0.0736                    0.1408       0.8945       <.0001

M2bl      0.29807      0.01060      0.13090      1.00000      0.17120      0.34328
          0.0006       0.9054       0.1408                    0.0533       <.0001

M2w4      0.04618      0.67335      0.01183      0.17120      1.00000      0.06596
          0.6047       <.0001       0.8945       0.0533                    0.4595

M2w8      0.22103     -0.07371      0.58602      0.34328      0.06596      1.00000
          0.0122       0.4083       <.0001       <.0001       0.4595
```

Figure 5.91 Correlations between variables (at baseline, only "moderate" and "severe" subjects are present).

Figure 5.91 shows that only 128 subjects were "selected" to participate in this simulated study. Such a reduction in sample size is a typical situation when a sizable number of subjects are rejected after the screening visit. We also see a drastic change in the correlation between $M1$ and $M2$ scale at baseline – it is now only 0.29807, less than 0.3, and can be considered by some researchers erroneously as the evidence of discriminant validity for the $M1$ scale. We know that the correlation between $M1$ and $M2$ scale at baseline should be substantial, as we originally simulated it this way, but because of the restricted range in data at baseline, this correlation is now attenuated. Note that later in this simulated study, we continue to have substantial correlations (more than 0.4) between $M1$ and $M2$ scales (see Figure 5.91, 0.67335 at week 4 and 0.58602 at week 8). This simulation highlights the importance of using all available data for convergent and discriminant validity and avoiding any conclusions based on only baseline data.

5.4 Known-Groups Validity

According to the FDA draft document (FDA 2019), "FDA also will review evidence that the COA can differentiate among clinically distinct groups hypothesized a priori (i.e., known groups analysis)." Known-groups validity is another test of construct validity and is commonly used to assess the sensitivity of a PRO instrument (and other COA instruments) in relation to established clinical or patient measurements of disease severity.

In Section 5.3, we simulated data for two scales, $M1$ and $M2$, where scale $M1$ was a scale that needed to be validated, while scale $M2$ represented a patient global impression of symptoms severity with four categories: "None" (i), "Mild" (ii), "Moderate" (iii), and "Severe" (iv). Let's assume that the severity scale $M2$ is well known and accepted as a patient measurement of disease severity. The most evident two distinct groups, for which we can reasonably hypothesize that scale $M1$ can differentiate, are represented by the subjects who rated themselves as "None" and subjects who rated themselves as "Severe." Then to establish known-groups validity for scale $M1$, we will need to show that the difference in scores on scale $M1$ is substantial and meaningful between subjects who rated themselves as "None" versus "Severe" on scale $M2$.

For this example, we are using the final dataset "_sim_ds3" from Section 5.3.2 (created in Figure 5.90). However, this approach to investigate known-groups validity will not work if only data at baseline are used – there are simply no subjects who rated themselves as "None" at baseline due to entry criteria. The next logical step would be to use data collected at the end of the study, generally data from the time point associated with the primary endpoint. In a placebo-controlled double-blind trial, there is a high probability that subjects will range on a severity scale from "None" to "Severe." Nonetheless, if an active treatment is efficacious and a placebo effect is considerable (which occurs in many studies like those in pain), the number of "Severe" subjects is expected to be relatively small.

To overcome those challenges, instead of investigating cross-sectional data at baseline or at any other time point in the study, we can unify all available data from the study in one comprehensive and integrated model. Figure 5.92 represents the first step in the implementation of such a model. First, we need to

```
Data _mixed_; Set _sim_ds3;
ID=Rnum;
M1=M1bl; M2=M2bl; Week="bl"; output;
M1=M1w4; M2=M2w4; Week="w4"; output;
M1=M1w8; M2=M2w8; Week="w8"; output;
Keep ID M1 M2 Week;
Run;
```

Figure 5.92 Creating dataset with vertical structure for MIXED procedure.

rearrange the data to create a vertical structure appropriate for the MIXED procedure (analogous to the example from Section 4.1.3, specifically Figure 4.10). Note
that we also need to create a subject identifier (represented by the variable "ID")
to inform the MIXED procedure that a certain set of data belongs to the same
subject. We also need to add a variable representing the time point when data
were collected so that the MIXED procedure will be able to distinguish measurements across time – for this purpose, the variable "Week" is added. In essence, we
are creating a dataset whose structure is close to the structure represented by
Figure 4.11, but now there are three observations per subject (note that the variable "Rnum" is generated as a part of the dataset produced by the SIMNORMAL
procedure and originally uniquely defines simulated observation)

When using all available data to model the relationship between variables $M2$
and $M1$, the longitudinal structure of the data should be accounted for. For every
subject we have in this simulation three observations, and as such those observation cannot be treated as statistically independent. The MIXED procedure allows
us to assess the relationship between variable $M2$ and $M1$ and account for statistical nonindependence of data.

Figure 5.93 represents the implementation of the model using variable $M2$ as a
continuous anchor (using anchor as a continuous variable imposes linear relationship between anchor and outcome). The Model statement defines variable
$M1$ as the outcome and variable $M2$ as the anchor, but it did not provide any information on the longitudinal structure of the data – to do so, the Repeated statement is needed. First, we inform the MIXED procedure that variable Week defines
when measurements for subjects are collected in time (as a part of the Repeated
statement a variable that defines occurrence should be a categorical variable and,
accordingly, should be a part of Class statement). In real life, though, subjects
could have data only at baseline, or data at baseline and at only one postbaseline
observation, or data for all three observations; this implementation accommo-
dates all those situations.

```
Proc Mixed data=_mixed_;
Class Week;
Model M1=M2 / ddfm=kr s;
Repeated Week / Type=UN Subject=ID;
Estimate "Severe vs None" M2 3    /cl;
Estimate "One category  " M2 1    /cl;
Estimate "M2=1" Intercept 1 M2 1 /cl;
Estimate "M2=2" Intercept 1 M2 2 /cl;
Estimate "M2=3" Intercept 1 M2 3 /cl;
Estimate "M2=4" Intercept 1 M2 4 /cl;
Run;
```

Figure 5.93 Implementation of the known-groups validity assessment using all
available data with scale $M2$ as a continuous anchor.

Second, we also need to define which set of observations belongs to a subject – which is also done as part of the `Repeated` statement by including "`Subject=ID`". Lastly, the error terms and relationships between them should be defined (the variance–covariance matrix for error terms). In this example, the most general variance–covariance matrix is postulated, which is unstructured "`Type=UN`". Therefore, the variances of error terms at every time point can be different, and no predefined structure is imposed on covariances between those error terms.

To support the known-groups validity property, we need to assess the difference between "Severe" subjects and subjects without symptoms. The following `Estimate` statement (Figure 5.93)

```
Estimate "Severe vs. None" M2 3 /cl;
```

will calculate a difference in means for the *M*1 scale corresponding to a three-category difference in the *M*2 scale (which is the numerical distance between "None" and "Severe"). The next Estimate statement (`Estimate "One cate-gory...`) generates a difference in means on the *M*1 scale corresponding to a just one-category difference. Because this model imposes a linear relationship between *M*1 and *M*2, this Estimate statement represents a difference in means on *M*1 scores corresponding to a one-category difference on *M*2 scale for any pair of adjacent categories: "None" vs. "Mild," "Mild" vs. "Moderate," or "Moderate" vs. "Severe." The subsequent set of four `Estimate` statements in Figure 5.93 produces least-square means for the *M*1 scale corresponding to the four categories of the *M*2 scale.

The model represented by Figure 5.93 imposes a linear functional relationship between anchor (*M*2 scale) and outcome (*M*1 scale). Figure 5.94 represents a complementary alternative model – one that does not impose any functional relationship between an outcome and an anchor, by treating anchor as a categorical predictor. To accomplish this, variable *M*2 is now included in the `Class` statement and to estimate least-square means for *M*1 scale the `LSMeans` statement is added.

Figures 5.95 and 5.96 show partial outputs produced by those two models. Figure 5.97 depicts relationships between *M*1 and *M*2 scales for *M*2 used as a

```
Proc Mixed data=_mixed_;
Class M2 Week;
Model M1=M2 / ddfm=kr s;
Repeated Week / Type=UN Subject=ID;
LSMeans M2 /diff cl;
Run;
```

Figure 5.94 Implementation of the known-groups validity assessment using all available data with scale *M*2 as a categorical anchor.

Label	Estimate	Standard Error	Pr > |t|	Alpha	Lower	Upper
		Estimates				
Severe vs None	4.6307	0.1962	<.0001	0.05	4.2445	5.0169
One category	1.5436	0.06540	<.0001	0.05	1.4148	1.6723
M2=1	2.2737	0.1129	<.0001	0.05	2.0509	2.4965
M2=2	3.8173	0.08193	<.0001	0.05	3.6551	3.9794
M2=3	5.3608	0.09612	<.0001	0.05	5.1710	5.5507
M2=4	6.9044	0.1426	<.0001	0.05	6.6235	7.1853

Figure 5.95 Estimations of the least-square means for the *M*1 scale based on the model with continuous anchor (partial output for the model represented by Figure 5.93).

Least Squares Means

Effect	M2	Estimate	Standard Error	Pr > |t|	Alpha	Lower	Upper
M2	1	2.2851	0.1351	<.0001	0.05	2.0189	2.5513
M2	2	3.7956	0.1074	<.0001	0.05	3.5838	4.0075
M2	3	5.3976	0.1132	<.0001	0.05	5.1743	5.6208
M2	4	6.8101	0.2493	<.0001	0.05	6.3192	7.3009

Differences of Least Squares Means

Effect	M2	_M2	Estimate	Standard Error	Pr > |t|	Alpha	Lower	Upper
M2	1	2	-1.5105	0.1573	<.0001	0.05	-1.8205	-1.2006
M2	1	3	-3.1125	0.1533	<.0001	0.05	-3.4143	-2.8106
M2	1	4	-4.5250	0.2753	<.0001	0.05	-5.0665	-3.9834
M2	2	3	-1.6019	0.1317	<.0001	0.05	-1.8612	-1.3427
M2	2	4	-3.0144	0.2577	<.0001	0.05	-3.5218	-2.5071
M2	3	4	-1.4125	0.2630	<.0001	0.05	-1.9303	-0.8947

Figure 5.96 Estimations of the least-square means for the *M*1 scale based on the model with a categorical anchor (partial output for the model represented by Figure 5.94).

continuous anchor vs. *M*2 as a categorical anchor. The examination of this graph represents a necessary step as part of known-groups validity assessment. The graph in Figure 5.97 uncovers how we should treat the results from the two models. Note that we a priori do not know whether a relationship between anchor and outcome can be approximated by a linear function. In this simulated example, we can see that both models produced practically the same results, indicating that the first implementation of the model (with a continuous anchor), represented by Figure 5.93, is acceptable. Thus, the value of 4.6307 (Figure 5.95), which represents the difference between "Severe" subjects and subjects without symptoms ("None"), can be used for assessment of known-groups validity.

Nevertheless, if we did not observe good agreement between models, then it would be more logical to use results from the second model (Figure 5.94, with a categorical anchor) for assessment of known-groups validity, as this model is completely general without any assumption regarding the functional relationship between anchor and outcome. Then why not always use this model? The answer to this question lays in the data – in a real-life situation, there is a tendency to have

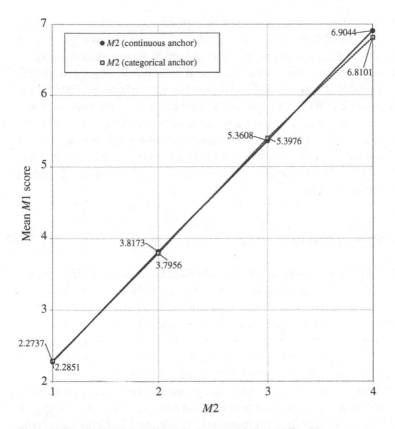

Figure 5.97 Estimated relationship between *M*1 and *M*2 scales.

a smaller number of the subjects who characterize themselves as the extremes, either "Severe" or "None," which could lead to a distorted assessment of known-groups validity. In our example, the difference in means between "Severe" subjects and subjects without symptoms based on the second model is 4.5250 in absolute value ("M2 1 4 -4.5250..."; see Figure 5.96), which is very close to the value of 4.6307 based on the first model.

The results from the first model with anchor as a continuous variable also show that the M1 scale can distinguish not only subjects with "Severe" symptoms vs. subjects with no symptoms, but also "Severe" subjects vs. "Moderate" subjects, "Moderate" subjects vs. "Mild" subjects, and "Mild" subjects vs. subjects with no symptoms. The difference in the mean *M*1 scores between any of those adjacent pairs of severity groups is 1.5436 ("One category 1.5436..."; see Figure 5.95).

The next step in the evaluation of known-groups validity results is the interpretation of the estimated value of 4.6307. Is this difference meaningful? Recall that the $M1$ measurement scale can range from 0 to 10. Hence this difference of 4.6307 represents almost half of the theoretical score range, which can be considered quite sizable. However, if the estimated mean difference in $M1$ scores between subjects with "Severe" symptoms vs. subjects with no symptoms was, say, only one point, then it would be less convincing evidence in support of known-groups validity property for $M1$ scale. If interpretation of the results of analyses is not straightforward, then the standardized effect size of the estimated difference can be calculated and interpreted in the same way introduced in Chapter 4 (specifically in Section 4.1.4.2).

5.5 Criterion Validity

"There is a special type of convergent validity, called the criterion validity, where evidence of validity is established by quantifying the relationship between the scores of a COA and scores of a known gold standard measure of the same concept. If a criterion measure is proposed, sponsors should provide rationale and support that the criterion is an accepted gold standard measure (i.e., relevant, valid, and reliable)" (FDA 2019). Criterion validity involves assessing a PRO (or other COA) instrument against the true value of measurement (from the gold standard criterion measure) or, alternatively, against another standard indicative of the true value of measurement. Criterion validity can be defined as "the degree to which the scores of a PRO instrument are an adequate reflection of a 'gold standard'" (Mokkink et al. 2010b).

To illustrate assessment of criterion validity, we will use the same simulated data from Section 5.4. But now we simply posit that the $M2$ scale represents the gold standard and $M1$ scale represents a new COA measure, which is postulated to measure the same concept as the $M2$ measure. The above FDA definition outlines that the criterion validity should be ". . . established by quantifying the relationship between the scores of a COA and scores of a known gold standard measure of the same concept" (FDA 2019). The most important word in this definition is *quantifying*.

In the previous section the model represented by Figure 5.93 does exactly what is recommended – it quantifies the relationship between the scores of scale $M1$ and scale $M2$ (the results of this modeling are presented in Figure 5.95). To put those results in the context for the evaluation of criterion validity, we need to compare estimated least-square means for the $M1$ scale corresponding to scores of 1, 2, 3, and 4 for the $M2$ scale. If we assume that the $M2$ scale is the gold standard, then ideally the value of 1 on the $M2$ scale should correspond to the value of 0 on the M1 scale, the value of 2 on the M2 scale should correspond to the value of 3.33 on the M1 scale, the value of 2 on the M2 scale should correspond to the value of 6.66 on the M1 scale, and value of 3 on the M2 scale should correspond to the value of 10 on M1 scale. For a given value on the M2 scale, there is a fixed value on the M1 scale that, ideally, indicates complete equivalence between these two scales. Figure 5.98 summarizes the results of the modeling of the relationship between M1 and M2 scales in contrast to their "perfect relationship" if, in fact, the scales are exactly measuring the same concept (despite their being measured on different metrics).

In Figure 5.98, we see that the estimated value of 2.2737 on the M1 scale corresponds to the score of 1 on the M2 scale. This value of 2.2737 represents the difference between the ideal value of 0 and the estimated value (which is the same

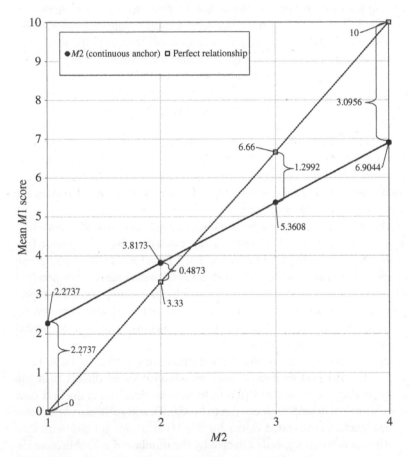

Figure 5.98 Illustration of criterion validity assessment.

value of 2.2737). Preferably, for criterion validity, we want this difference between the estimated value and the ideal value not to be statistically significant (*p*-value >0.05). Nevertheless, it can be affected by many factors – for example, simply by large number of observations. Still, it is important to investigate this. For the *M*2 score of 2, the corresponding estimated value on the *M*1 scale is 3.8173. But we are not interested in the estimated value per se; instead, we are interested in the difference between the estimated value of 3.8173 and the ideal value of 3.33 (which is 3.8173-3.33 = 0.4873). Hence the question becomes, is this value of 0.4873 significantly different from zero?

Unfortunately, if the MIXED procedure and data with scores for *M*1 and *M*2 scale in their original format are used (as in Figure 5.93), the estimation of the differences between ideal score and estimated least-square means is not workable directly. Although the difference between ideal value of 0 and estimated *M*1 score corresponding *M*2 score of 1 gave us the desirable result, we need somehow trick the MIXED procedure to estimate the differences we want. Note that it worked for the point where ideal *M*1 score was zero. For example, to assess the difference between ideal score of 3.33 and estimated *M*1 score corresponding to the *M*2 score of 2, we simply need to remap *M*1 scores in a way that the ideal score of 0 will be in the place of the ideal score of 3.33. To do so, we need simply subtract the value of 3.33 from every *M*1 score and then just rerun the MIXED procedure.

The implementation of the aforementioned analyses is represented by Figure 5.99, and its partial output is represented by Figure 5.100. As depicted in Figure 5.98, the difference of 0.4873 is obtained between the ideal value of 3.33 and the estimated *M*1 score corresponding to the *M*2 score of 2. The results of this revised modeling using the dataset with revised ("new") *M*1 scores also gives the same result ("Ideal 3.33 vs. estimated M1 for M2=2 0.4873..."), as given in Figure 5.100. This strategy on modifying *M*1 score can also be viewed as if we move or shift the horizontal axis (*x*-axis) up by 3.33 points (see Figure 5.101). Note that the graph in Figure 5.101 is technically the same graph found in Figure 5.98, but now the estimated value of the *M*1 scale corresponding to the *M*2 value of 2 is 0.4873, which coincidently (as noted previously) represents the difference between ideal and estimated values for *M*1 scale corresponding to the *M*2 score of 2. Thus, we now achieve the objective of drawing statistical inference (with a *p*-value) for estimating the difference.

From Figure 5.100, we can see that all differences (2.2737, 0.4873, -1.2992, -3.0956) between ideal and estimated values for the *M*1 scale are significantly (having $p < 0.0001$) different from zero. Note that in the best-case scenario, we want all those differences not to be significantly different from zero, implying that ideal and estimated values for the *M*1 scale are not different. But, as noted earlier, *p*-values are greatly affected by the number of available observations for modeling and, in addition, the variability in the data. From clinical

```
Data _mixed_2; Set _mixed_;
M1=M1-3.33;
Run;

Proc Mixed data=_mixed_2;
Class Week;
Model M1=M2 / ddfm=kr s;
Repeated Week / Type=UN Subject=ID;
Estimate "Ideal 3.33 vs estimated M1 for M2=2" Intercept 1 M2 2 /cl;
Estimate "M2=1" Intercept 1 M2 1 /cl;
Estimate "M2=2" Intercept 1 M2 2 /cl;
Estimate "M2=3" Intercept 1 M2 3 /cl;
Estimate "M2=4" Intercept 1 M2 4 /cl;
Run;

Data _mixed_3; Set _mixed_;
M1=M1-6.66;
Run;

Proc Mixed data=_mixed_3;
Class Week;
Model M1=M2 / ddfm=kr s;
Repeated Week / Type=UN Subject=ID;
Estimate "Ideal 6.66 vs estimated M1 for M2=3" Intercept 1 M2 3 /cl;
Run;

Data _mixed_4; Set _mixed_;
M1=M1-10;
Run;

Proc Mixed data=_mixed_4;
Class Week;
Model M1=M2 / ddfm=kr s;
Repeated Week / Type=UN Subject=ID;
Estimate "Ideal 10 vs estimated M1 for M2=4" Intercept 1 M2 4 /cl;
Run;
```

Figure 5.99 Assessment of the differences between ideal and estimated values for the *M1* scale (implementation).

Estimates

Label	Estimate	Standard Error	Pr > |t|	Alpha
Ideal 3.33 vs estimated M1 for M2=2	0.4873	0.08193	<.0001	0.05
M2=1	-1.0563	0.1129	<.0001	0.05
M2=2	0.4873	0.08193	<.0001	0.05
M2=3	2.0308	0.09612	<.0001	0.05
M2=4	3.5744	0.1426	<.0001	0.05

Estimates

Label	Estimate	Standard Error	Pr > |t|	Alpha
Ideal 6.66 vs estimated M1 for M2=3	-1.2992	0.09612	<.0001	0.05

Estimates

Label	Estimate	Standard Error	Pr > |t|	Alpha
Ideal 10 vs estimated M1 for M2=4	-3.0956	0.1426	<.0001	0.05

Figure 5.100 Assessment of the differences between ideal and estimated values for the *M1* scale (partial output based on the SAS code from Figure 5.99).

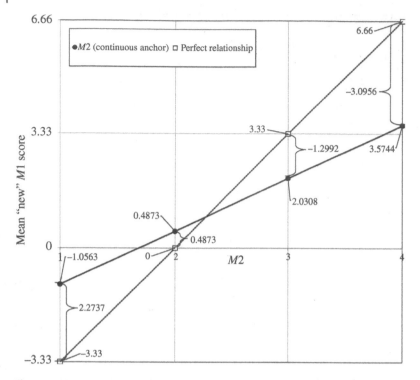

Figure 5.101 Criterion validity assessment using adjusted or "new" M1 scores ("new" M1 scores are equal to the original M1 scores −3.33).

studies with a large number of subjects and with data collected longitudinally at several visits (with varying amounts of variability in outcome scores), it is likely to find statistically significant differences, and thus we may be tempted to conclude that criterion validity is not corroborated. At the same time, though, the opposite situation is even more concerning, since studies with a small number of subjects are likely to assess true differences as being not statistically significant, which would lead to the inaccurate conclusion that criterion validity is upheld. Therefore, while testing of statistical significance differences between estimated and ideal values is important, it is not sufficient evidence to affirm the criterion validity property.

As a result, the test on statistical significance of the differences should be appended by interpretation of these differences. For example, for an M1 scale from 0 to 10, we can assume that if all four differences (absolute value) in our simulated example are less than one point (category), then it may be acceptable to assume that criterion validity is demonstrated. But if a scale range is from 0 to 100, then should acceptability be also one point or should it be, say, five points? Given that scale range differ, should the criterion for equivalence be set at a fixed thresh-old percentage? In the authors' view, perhaps the best tactic is to use standardized effect sizes (see Chapter 4) to interpret those differences. The standard deviations for the M1 scale are 1.44210 at baseline, 1.39792 at week 4, and 1.49466 at week 8 (see Figure 5.91). Generally, we recommend to use baseline standard deviations for calculations of the effect sizes in longitudinal studies, as those standard deviations are not affected by the treatments. However, the smallest standard deviation, which would lead to the largest (most conservative) effect sizes, also can be used in sensitivity analyses.

The effect sizes of the differences (2.2737, 0.4873, −1.2992, −3.0956) between ideal and estimated values for M1 scale are 1.58, 0.34, −0.91, −2.15 (using the baseline standard deviation of 1.44210); for example, 1.58 = 2.2737/1.44210. Being above 0.80 standard deviation units (in absolute value), three estimated effect sizes (1.6, −0.9, −2.1) can be characterized as large. The smallest effect size of 0.34 can be interpreted as "small-to-medium" (0.2 being "small" and 0.5 being "medium"). Based on the same approach to the interpretation of the results introduced in Chapter 4 (specifically Section 4.1.4.2), if all effect sizes of the estimated differences could have been interpreted as, at least, "small," or even better "triv-ial," then we could conclude that the criterion validity had been demonstrated (even if those differences were statistically different from zero). In this simulated example, we only can conclude that the criterion validity for M1 scale was not supported by the data.

5.6 Summary

The first four sections involve aspects or manifestations of construct validity through simulated learning exercises that highlight the methodologies. Instructional detail is given on exploratory factor analysis (Section 5.1) and its implementation, along with evaluation of factor loadings and the number of fac-tors. Next, the confirmatory factor model (Section 5.2) is described visually and analytically, and its implementation is discussed. Special topics on confirmatory factor analysis are addressed: domains represented by only a single item, second-order confirmatory factor analysis, differences between formative and reflective models, the bifactor model, and use of polychoric correlations.

A separate section is given to the assessment of convergent validity and discri-minant validity (Section 5.3) and their evaluation in a clinical study. A thorough assessment of known-groups validity is presented (Section 5.5). Finally, the last section describes via simulated learning the assessment of criterion validity (Section 5.6), a form of validity typically considered distinct from construct valid-ity, when there is a gold standard criterion.

References

Bentler, P.M. and Bonnett, D.G. (1990). Comparative fit indexes in structural models. *Psychological Bulletin* 107: 231–246.

Brown, T.A. (2015). *Confirmatory Factor Analysis for Applied Research*, 2e. New York: The Guilford Press.

Bushmakin, A.G., Abraham, L., Pinkerton, J.V. et al. (2014). Evaluation of the measurement model and clinically important differences for menopause-specific quality of life associated with bazedoxifene/conjugated estrogens. *Menopause* 21: 815–822.

Canjur, S. and Ercan, I. (2015). Comparison of model fit indices used in structural equation modeling under multivariate normality. *Journal of Modern Applied Statistical Methods* 14: 152–167.

Cappelleri, J.C., Bushmakin, A.G., Baker, C.L. et al. (2005). Revealing the multidimensional framework of the Minnesota nicotine withdrawal scale. *Current Medical Research and Opinion* 21: 749–760.

Cappelleri, J.C., Zou, K.H., Bushmakin, A.G. et al. (2013). *Patient-Reported Outcomes: Measurement, Implementation and Interpretation*. Boca Raton, FL: Chapman & Hall/CRC Press.

Chen, F., Curran, P.J., Bollen, K.A. et al. (2008). An empirical evaluation of the use of fixed cutoff points in RMSEA test statistic in structural equation models. *Sociological Methods & Research* 36: 462–494.

Cook, K.F., Kallen, M.A., and Amtmann, D. (2009). Having a fit: impact of number of items and distribution of data on traditional criteria for assessing IRT's unidimensionality assumption. *Quality of Life Research* 18: 447–460.

DeVellis, R.F. (2017). *Scale Development: Theory and Applications*, 4e. Thousand Oaks, CA: SAGE Publications, Inc.

Fan, X. and Sivo, S.A. (2005). Sensitivity of fit indexes to misspecified structural or measurement model components: rationale of the two-index strategy revisited. *Structural Equation Modeling* 12: 343–367.

Fayers, P.M. and Machin, D. (2016). *Quality of Life: The Assessment, Analysis and Reporting of Patient-Reported Outcomes*, 3e. Chichester, UK: Wiley.

FDA (Food and Drug Administration) (2009). Guidance for industry on patient-reported outcome measures: use in medical product development to support labeling claims. *Federal Register* 74 (235): 65132–65133.

FDA (Food and Drug Administration) (2019). Patient-focused drug development guidance series for enhancing the incorporation of the patient's voice in medical product development and regulatory decision making. Draft Guidance Documents. https://www.fda.gov/drugs/development-approval-process-drugs/fda-patient-focused-drug-development-guidance-series-enhancing-incorporation-patients-voice-medical (accessed 15 April 2020).

Gonzales, D., Rennard, S.I., Nides, M. et al. (2006). Varenicline, an α4β2 nicotinic acetylcholine receptor partial agonist, vs. sustained-release bupropion and placebo for smoking cessation: a randomized controlled trial. *JAMA* 296: 47–55.

Hooper, D., Coughlan, J., and Mullen, M. (2008). Structural equation modelling: guidelines for determining model fit. *Electronic Journal of Business Research Method* 6: 53–60.

Jackson, D.L. (2003). Revisiting sample size and number of parameter estimates: some support for the N:q hypothesis. *Structural Equation Modeling* 10: 128–141.

Jorenby, D.E., Hays, J.T., Rigotti, N.A. et al. (2006). Efficacy of varenicline, an α4β nicotinic acetylcholine receptor partial agonist, vs. placebo or sustained-released bupropion for smoking cessation: a randomized controlled trial. *JAMA* 296: 56–63.

Kline, R.B. (2011). *Principles and Practice of Structural Equation Modeling*, 3e. New York: The Guilford Press.

Kyriazos, T.A. (2018). Applied psychometrics: sample size and sample power considerations in factor analysis (EFA, CFA) and SEM in general. *Psychology* 9: 2207–2230.

Marsh, H., Hau, H.T., and Wen, Z. (2004). In search of golden rules: comment on hypothesis testing approaches to setting cutoff values for fit index and dangers in overgeneralizing Hu and Bentler's (1999) findings. *Structural Equation Modeling* 11: 320–341.

Mokkink, L.B., Terwee, C.B., Knol, D.L. et al. (2010a). The COSMIN checklist for evalating the methodological quality of studies on measurement properties: a clarification of its content. *BMC Medical Research Methodology* 10: 22.

Mokkink, L.B., Terwee, C.B., Patrick, D.L. et al. (2010b). The COSMIN study reached internatioanl consensus on taxonomy, terminology, and definitions of measurement properties for health-related patient-reported outcomes. *Journal of Clinical Epidemiology* 63: 737–745.

O'Rourke, N. and Hatcher, L. (2013). *A Step-by-Step Approach to Using SAS for Factor Analysis and Structural Equation Modeling*, 2e. Cary, NC: SAS Institute Inc.

Stevens, J. (2009). *Applied Multivariate Analysis*, 5e. New York: Taylor & Francis Group.

Streiner, D.L., Norman, G.R., and Cairney, J. (2015). *Health Measurement Scales: A Practical Guide to Their Development and Use*, 5e. Oxford, UK: Oxford Univeristy Press.

Trochim, W.M.K. (2001). *The Research Methods Knowledge Base*, 2e. Cincinnati, OH: Atomic Dog Publishing.

de Vet, H.C.W., Terwee, C.B., Mokkink, L.B., and Knol, D.L. (2011). *Measurement in Medicine*. Cambridge, UK: Cambridge University Press.

West, S.G., Taylor, A.B., and Wu, W. (2012). Chapter 13: Model fit and model selection in structural equation modeling. In: *Handbook of Structural Equation Modeling* (ed. R.H. Hoyle), 2009–2031. Guildford Press.

Yuan, K.H. (2005). Fit indices versus test statistics. *Multivariate Behavioral Research* 40: 115–148.

6

Responsiveness and Sensitivity

The responsiveness and sensitivity of a patient-reported outcome (PRO) measure or, more generally, other types of clinical outcome assessments (COA) are the twin themes of this chapter; responsiveness and sensitivity are aspects of the validity of a measurement scale. Responsiveness – or the ability to detect the change (Section 6.1) – of a PRO or COA scale involves quantifiable evidence that such a measurement scale can identify differences in scores over time in individuals or groups who have changed with respect to the measurement concept. Data of within-patient change are necessary to evaluate the ability to detect change on a measurement scale and to establish a clinically meaningful within-patient change threshold. A related psychometric entity is sensitivity – specifically, sensitivity to treatment effects (Section 6.2) – that reflects the ability of the measurement scale to detect treatment effects and to discriminate between treatment and control groups.

A measurement scale is futile for patient monitoring unless it can reflect changes in a patient's condition over time and be sensitive to treatment effects. An establishment of measurement properties on a PRO (or COA) scale is intended to reduce unwanted random error or noise in its responses and to support responsive to change and sensitivity to detect treatment benefits. Like other measurement properties (content validity, reliability, construct validity, and criterion validity), responsiveness and sensitivity are specific to the measurement application and cannot be necessarily assumed to be relevant in all measurement situations or circumstances in which the instrument is used.

A Practical Approach to Quantitative Validation of Patient-Reported Outcomes: A Simulation-Based Guide Using SAS, First Edition. Andrew G. Bushmakin and Joseph C. Cappelleri.

6.1   Ability to Detect Change

6.1.1   Definitions and Concepts

In its updated and expanded (draft) guidance, the United Stated Food and Drug Administration (FDA) provides insight and guidance on the ability to detect change for COA, which include PRO tools as well as clinician-reported outcome, observer-reported outcome, and performance-based outcome tools. Specifically, the FDA defines the ability to detect change as follows: "FDA reviews a COA's ability to detect change using data that compares change in COA scores to change in other similar measures that indicate that the patient's state has changed with respect to the concept of interest. A review of the ability to detect change includes evidence that the instrument is sensitive to gains and losses in the measurement concept and to change across the entire range expected for the target patient population" (FDA 2019).

The above description provides a clear and direct path for the assessment of the ability to detect the change, which advances three key points. First, this description specifies that we need to compare "change in COA scores to change in other similar measures." It is important to highlight the assumption that those other similar measures should be known a priori, or it should be evident from previous research that they are sensitive to the change in patient state ("other similar measures that indicate that the patient's state has changed with respect to the concept of interest"). If an anchor scale itself (selected to support the ability to detect change for a COA under investigation) is not responsive to the change in a patient's health status, then an erroneous conclusion will follow.

The second key point is that "the ability to detect change includes evidence that the instrument is sensitive to gains and losses in the measurement concept." This clearly stipulates that it should be shown that improvement in scores of the anchoring scale corresponds to improvement in scores of the COA under investigation and deterioration in scores of the anchoring scale scores corresponds to worsening of scores of the COA.

The third point is that those "gains and losses" should be investigated for the entire possible range ("change across the entire range expected for the target patient population"), not just a part of the distribution. Consider, hypothetically, a numeric rating scale (NRS) with scores from 0 to 10. Its entire (theoretical) range for change from baseline is from -10 to 10, but it is not always possible. To achieve this full range depends on many factors, the most important one being whether the scale of interest is used as a part of the entry criteria in the study. In this case, generally, only subjects who are exhibiting a certain level of severity will become eligible for the study. As discussed previously, for this type of the NRS scale, it is not uncommon, if not typical, to define subjects as "moderate" with scores of 4, 5, or 6 and as "severe" with scores 7, 8, 9, or 10. If we want to have only "moderate" or "severe" subjects at baseline, then the possible range will be from −10 (assuming that we have subjects with score of 10 at baseline who improved at some point in the study to have score of 0) to 6 (subjects with baseline score of 4 cannot worsen more than six points). In practice even this range may be considered more extreme than that observed.

On the other hand, if a scale is not used as a part of entry criteria for a clinical study, then a larger range is likely to be present. In Chapter 5 (see Section 5.3.2), the dataset "_sim_ds3" was simulated to illustrate convergent validity. In this dataset, the $M2$ measure, taken as a global severity anchor scale to support the convergent validity of the $M1$ scale under investigation, was "used" as a part of the entry criteria (see Figure 5.91) and at baseline only subjects with scores of 3 or 4 for the $M2$ scale were selected for the study. But for the $M1$ scale the range of values was still large from 2 to 9 (with theoretical range from 0 to 10). This situation illustrates a relevant realization: If a measurement scale of interest (like $M1$) is not used as a part of entry criteria, and even if for a study only a subset of subjects with a certain severity is selected (based on a different distinct scale like $M2$), the measurement scale of interest at baseline can still have a substantial range of responses from "mild" to "severe" (based on this scale being taken in isolation from other measures).

Let's continue with the FDA description on ability to detect change property: "When patient experience of a concept changes, the value(s) for the COA measuring that concept also should change. If there is clear evidence that patient experience relative to the concept has changed, but the value(s) of the COA do not change accordingly, then either the ability to detect change is inadequate or the COA's content and/or construct validity should be questioned. Conversely, if there is evidence that value(s) of the COA are affected by changes that are not specific to the concept of interest, the COA's content and/or construct validity may be questioned." (FDA 2019).

There are several focal points in the aforementioned text. One is "When patient experience of a concept changes, the value(s) for the COA measuring that concept also should change." Note that the context here pertains to a new (or modified) scale whose measurement properties have not been established yet. This point reiterates the utmost importance for selection of the additional scales needed to be included in the study, which can be used to establish that the "patient experience of a concept changes."

Now consider the next sentence in the FDA text, namely, "If there is clear evidence that patient experience relative to the concept has changed, but the value(s) of the COA do not change accordingly, then either the ability to detect change is inadequate or the COA's content and/or construct validity should be questioned." This sentence, in principal, provides some clues to a researcher why "the ability to detect change is inadequate" if the "value(s) of the COA do not change" when "the concept has changed." For instance, some items in a multi-item domain may not change when the underlying concept of interest has changed and, as a result, the change in the domain score (calculated as a mean or as a sum of scores of items from this domain) will be attenuated.

Another situation is when the ceiling effect for a considerable number of items is present at baseline (assuming that larger score corresponds to a better health state), which prevents observing improvement in the domain score (these items do not have an opportunity to change, as they already had the largest possible score at baseline). In this situation, "the COA's content and/or construct validity should be questioned," which would requiring taking a closer look at those particular items and maybe exclude them from a domain or reformulate them (note that in this case, an additional qualitative study should be done, along with another psychometric assessment). Alternatively, there may be a need to change how the items are scored.

From the same FDA text, its last sentence "Conversely, if there is evidence that value(s) of the COA are affected by changes that are not specific to the concept of interest, the COA's content and/or construct validity may be questioned" describes another undesirable situation. This description seems obvious. After all, if the changes in the scale of interest for validation have a strong relationship with changes in another scale, which is not related to the measured concept, then this result shows that the scale under consideration has issues. And we, therefore, need to reassess the construct and/or content validity of this scale. But, while obvious, this interpretation of the result should be always investigated, because in clinical studies this situation can be observed.

Consider a clinical study to investigate a drug to treat nerve pain associated with fibromyalgia, and we want to validate a new pain scale. Suppose we observe a noticeable relationship between changes in pain (as measured by proposed pain scale) and changes in a scale measuring sleep disturbance. Given that these two scales are measuring distinct concepts, does the aforementioned noticeable relationship indicate that the content validity of the pain scale needs to be reassessed? The answer is "it depends."

In our illustrative example a quite plausible explanation is that improvements in fibromyalgia pain will lead to reduction in sleep disturbance. Many patients may believe their pain is disruptive to their sleep. Improvement in pain also can lead to reductions in number of awakenings and improvements in sleep continuity (Russell et al. 2009).

This example highlights the importance of the subject matter and the examination of the interrelationships between measurements in a study beyond just considering the concepts they represent. Nevertheless, if after careful consideration, no plausible clinical explanation exists on how one of those two variables (each measuring a different concept) can affect another one, then the statement "Conversely, if there is evidence that value(s) of the COA are affected by changes that are not specific to the concept of interest" is relevant and apt.

6.1.2 Ability to Detect Change Analysis Implementation

As discussed in the previous section on the ability to detect change property for a scale, we need (i) to have in a study at least one additional scale which measures a similar concept and (ii) "that the instrument is sensitive to gains and losses in the measurement concept and to change across the entire range expected for the target patient population." As such, we need to quantify the relationship between changes in scores of a scale we are validating and changes in scores of the additional anchor scale.

Consider the following simulation. There are two measurement scales, $M1$ and $M2$, collected as a part of a longitudinal study. $M1$ is a scale to be validated, while $M2$ measures a similar concept and is known a priori to be sensitive to the change in the patient's state with respect to the concept of interest. We assume that scales $M1$ and $M2$ are collected at baseline and at weeks 2, 4, and 8. It is also assumed that there is an overall improvement – the mean change from baseline in the score for the $M2$ scale is 1 at week 2, 2 at week 4, and 2.5 at week 8 (positive change in both scales represents improvement in this simulated example). We also assume that changes from baseline in the $M2$ scale are correlated over time. For example, the correlation between change from baseline at week 8 (represented by variable M2W8 in Figure 6.1) and change from baseline at week 4 (variable M2W4) is 0.4. These longitudinal data are generated for 500 subjects.

Figure 6.1 represents the corresponding implementation: the dataset "_m2" has the "standard" vertical structure with just three columns (i) representing subject

```
data _corr_m2 (type=corr);
input
_TYPE_ $   _NAME_ $   M2W2     M2W4      M2W8;
datalines;
 CORR      M2W2       1        .4        .2
 CORR      M2W4       .4       1         .4
 CORR      M2W8       .2       .4        1
 MEAN      .          1        2         2.5
 STD       .          1        1         1
 N         .          500      500       500
;
run;
Proc simnormal data=_corr_m2 out=_sim_m2 numreal=500 seed=345;
var M2W2  M2W4  M2W8 ;
run;
Proc Transpose data=_sim_m2 out=_sim_m2_tr;
var M2W2  M2W4  M2W8 ;
By Rnum;
Run;
Data _m2;
Set _sim_m2_tr;
ID=Rnum;
chgM2=COL1;
If _NAME_="M2W2" Then Week="W2"; If _NAME_="M2W4" Then Week="W4";
If _NAME_="M2W8" Then Week="W8";
Keep ID chgM2 Week;
Run;
```

Figure 6.1 Simulating longitudinal values for the anchor scale.

ID (variable "`ID`"), (ii) time point in a study ("`Week`"), and (iii) change from baseline in the $M2$ scale score ("`chgM2`"), as these three variables are kept (see Keep statement in Figure 6.1). It is basically the same structure represented by Figure 4.11 in Chapter 4, with now the additional variable representing time when data are collected.

The model for quantifying relationship between changes in anchor scale $M2$ and changes in target scale $M1$ assumes that this relationship can be represented by the following equation:

$$Y_{ij} = a + bX_{ij} + e_{ij} \qquad (6.1)$$

where

Y_{ij} is the change from baseline on the $M1$ scale for subject i ($i = 1, 2, \ldots, 500$) at postbaseline measurement j ($j =$ Week 2, Week 4, Week 8)

X_{ij} is the change from baseline on the $M2$ scale for subject i at post-baseline measurement j

e_{ij} is the error term [assumed to be from a normal distribution with mean 0 and variance σ_j^2, i.e., $e_{ij} \sim N(0, \sigma_j^2)$]

a is the intercept

b is the slope associated with variable X_{ij}.

There are two important assumptions associated with Eq. (6.1). First, we assume that the true relationship between changes in $M1$ and $M2$ scales is the same at any time point in a study and differs only by a random error term, which is consistent with good measurement. But, at the same time, the error term variance is allowed to be different at every measurement occasion. Second, as represented by Eq. (6.1), a linear relationship is imposed between the anchor (X_{ij}) and outcome (Y_{ij}), represented by the slope parameter b and, correspondingly, the anchor is used as a continuous variable. Later we relax this second assumption by treating the anchor as a categorical predictor.

There is an additional detail worth noting. In model 6.1, the intercept will be defined empirically by the data. The $M1$ and $M2$ scales are measuring similar concepts (but not the *same* concept), and, as such, we do not anticipate that zero change on the anchor scale ($M2$) will correspond to zero change in the target $M1$ scale; the intercept term is not expected to be zero. This effect for relationships between changes in scales was also discussed earlier in Section 4.1.4.2 (specifically, the discussion of results presented by Figure 4.24 in Chapter 4).

The second step to complete data simulation for the analysis is to model error terms and then to define the relationship between changes in scores for the two measurement scales. Figure 6.2 represents implementation of this second step. The data for the same subjects over time cannot be assumed to be independent and, as

```
Data _corr_e (type=corr);
input
_TYPE_ $   _NAME_ $   eW2        eW4        eW8;
datalines;
  CORR       eW2        1          .3         .2
  CORR       eW4        .3         1          .3
  CORR       eW8        .2         .3         1
  MEAN       .          0          0          0
  STD        .          2.5        1.7        3
  N          .          500        500        500
;
run;
Proc simnormal data=_corr_e out=_sim_e numreal=500 seed=678;
var eW2 eW4 eW8;
run;
Proc Corr Data=_sim_e COV;
var eW2 eW4 eW8;
Run;
Proc Transpose data=_sim_e out=_sim_e_tr;
var eW2 eW4 eW8;
By Rnum;
Run;
Data _err; Set _sim_e_tr;
ID=Rnum; err=COL1;
If _NAME_="eW2" Then Week="W2"; If _NAME_="eW4" Then Week="W4";
If _NAME_="eW8" Then Week="W8";
Keep ID err Week;
Run;
Proc Sort Data=_m2 out=m2;    By ID Week; Run;
Proc Sort Data=_err out=err;  By ID Week; Run;
Data _mixed_ds;
Merge m2 err;
chgM1=1+2*chgM2+err;
By ID Week;
Run;
Proc Print data=_mixed_ds NOOBS;
Var ID Week chgM1 chgM2;
Where ID<=3;
Run;
```

Figure 6.2 Simulating error terms and defining relationship between score changes in *M*1 and *M*2 scales.

such, the simulated error terms are assumed to covary across time. For example, the correlation between the error term at week 2 (represented by variable eW2 in Figure 6.2) and the error term at week four (variable eW4) is 0.3. Note that variances for the error terms are also different at every week (standard deviation of 2.5 at week 2, 1.7 at week 4, and 3 at week 8). It is also assumed that, on average, a zero change in *M*2 scale score corresponds to a change of one point in *M*1 scale score, and a one-point change in *M*2 scale score corresponds to a change of two points in *M*1 scale score (as defined by following code line "chgM1=1+2*chgM2+err;" in Figure 6.2). The structure of the final dataset and simulated data for the first three subjects are represented by Figure 6.3.

In the final dataset "_mixed_ds" the changes for *M*1 and *M*2 scales are represented by variables chgM1 and chgM2. In Figure 6.4, the first data step

ID	Week	chgM1	chgM2
1	W2	1.82795	0.72751
1	W4	6.53398	1.56725
1	W8	6.99809	2.09136
2	W2	-4.67316	-0.36559
2	W4	7.03009	3.11412
2	W8	7.10490	2.78327
3	W2	1.74747	1.56990
3	W4	0.72125	0.54618
3	W8	8.61059	4.17714

Figure 6.3 Example of the dataset structure for the ability to detect change analysis (data for the first three subjects are shown).

```
Data _mixed_ds; Set _mixed_ds;
cat_chgM2=round(chgM2,1);
By ID Week;
Run;
Proc Means Data=_mixed_ds;
Var chgM1 chgM2 cat_chgM2;
Run;
Proc Mixed Data=_mixed_ds;
Class ID Week;
Model chgM1=chgM2 / solution ddfm=kr;
Repeated Week / Subject=ID Type=UN R;
Estimate "chgM2=-3" Intercept 1 chgM2 -3 /cl;
Estimate "chgM2=-2" Intercept 1 chgM2 -2 /cl;
Estimate "chgM2=-1" Intercept 1 chgM2 -1 /cl;
Estimate "chgM2= 0" Intercept 1 chgM2 0 /cl;
Estimate "chgM2= 1" Intercept 1 chgM2 1 /cl;
Estimate "chgM2= 2" Intercept 1 chgM2 2 /cl;
Estimate "chgM2= 3" Intercept 1 chgM2 3 /cl;
Estimate "chgM2= 4" Intercept 1 chgM2 4 /cl;
Estimate "chgM2= 5" Intercept 1 chgM2 5 /cl;
Run;
```

Figure 6.4 Modeling the relationship between changes in scores in *M*1 and *M*2 scales using *M*2 scale as a continuous anchor.

("Data _mixed_ds;...") adds the additional variable cat_chgM2 based on rounding the variable chgM2 to the closest integer. In a real-life circumstance, change in both variables (i.e., change scores in *M*1 and *M*2 scales) more likely to be represented by a continuous variable. A multi-item domain score, calculated as a mean of the items, or a visual analog scale on a continuous metric are examples of such continuous variables. The implications of using *M*2 scale scores as a categorical variable (represented by cat_chgM2) are enormously important in the assessment of the ability to detect change and will be discussed at length later in this section and the next section.

Before implementing the model to assess the relationship between changes in scores in *M*1 and *M*2 scales, we need to know the range of their changes, specifically the range for the *M*2 anchor scale (Figure 6.5 provides this information, which is produced by "Proc Means Data=_mixed_ds;..." in Figure 6.4). From this figure we can identify the range for changes in *M*2 scale to be from −3 to 5 (as represented by variable cat_chgM2). From this information, the series of

Variable	N	Mean	Std Dev	Minimum	Maximum
chgM1	1500	4.6054358	3.4427263	-6.8301127	15.6156666
chgM2	1500	1.8220016	1.2004988	-2.6614946	5.2550763
cat_chgM2	1500	1.8306667	1.2351829	-3.0000000	5.0000000

Figure 6.5 Means and range for simulated scores.

`Estimate` statements is added to the PROC MIXED to calculate least-square means for a change in $M1$ target scale corresponding to a change of $-3, -2, \ldots, 4,$ 5 change in the $M2$ anchor scale (see Figure 6.6 for partial output produced by "`Proc Mixed Data=_mixed_ds;...`" in Figure 6.4).

The output represented by Figure 6.6 contains several parts. One part represents the estimation of the variance–covariance matrix for error terms (represented by e_{ij} in Eq. (6.1)). When those error terms were simulated (see Figure 6.2), the variance–covariance matrix was also estimated (produced by "`Proc Corr Data=_sim_e COV; ...`" in Figure 6.2) and represented by Figure 6.7 before modeling with Proc Mixed. As we can see, the estimated variance–covariance matrix

```
         Estimated R Matrix for ID 1
Row      Col1      Col2      Col3
 1      6.0219    1.3009    1.4712
 2      1.3009    2.8824    1.4379
 3      1.4712    1.4379    8.9112

Covariance Parameter Estimates
Cov Parm   Subject   Estimate
UN(1,1)    ID         6.0219
UN(2,1)    ID         1.3009
UN(2,2)    ID         2.8824
UN(3,1)    ID         1.4712
UN(3,2)    ID         1.4379
UN(3,3)    ID         8.9112

              Solution for Fixed Effects
                      Standard
Effect      Estimate   Error     DF    t Value   Pr > |t|
Intercept    0.8956   0.1119    858      8.00     <.0001
chgM2        2.0275   0.04836  1186     41.93     <.0001

                          Estimates
                Standard
Label      Estimate  Error    DF   t Value  Pr > |t|  Alpha    Lower     Upper
chgM2=-3   -5.1869   0.2432  1136  -21.32   <.0001    0.05   -5.6641   -4.7097
chgM2=-2   -3.1594   0.1973  1096  -16.01   <.0001    0.05   -3.5466   -2.7722
chgM2=-1   -1.1319   0.1530  1016   -7.40   <.0001    0.05   -1.4320   -0.8317
chgM2= 0    0.8956   0.1119   858    8.00   <.0001    0.05    0.6759    1.1153
chgM2= 1    2.9231   0.07960   611   36.72   <.0001    0.05    2.7668    3.0794
chgM2= 2    4.9506   0.06944   504   71.29   <.0001    0.05    4.8142    5.0870
chgM2= 3    6.9781   0.08936   678   78.09   <.0001    0.05    6.8027    7.1536
chgM2= 4    9.0056   0.1258   864   71.59   <.0001    0.05    8.7587    9.2525
chgM2= 5   11.0331   0.1684   974   65.53   <.0001    0.05   10.7027   11.3635
```

Figure 6.6 Partial output of the modeled relationship between changes in $M1$ scale scores and changes in $M2$ scale scores using the change in $M2$ scale as a continuous anchor.

```
          Covariance Matrix, DF = 499
              eW2           eW4           eW8
eW2      6.033636784   1.303232408   1.467889076
eW4      1.303232408   2.882289746   1.436293830
eW8      1.467889076   1.436293830   8.905769273
```

Figure 6.7 Covariance matrix using original simulated error terms.

(represented by Estimated R Matrix for ID 1 in Figure 6.6, this matrix being the same for all individuals) and calculated using original error terms (Figure 6.7) are numerically very close. For example, the estimated variance of the error term at week two is 6.0219 (see Figure 6.6), and the calculated variance for eW2 is 6.033636784 (see Figure 6.7). Note that, in Figure 6.6, the part "Covariance Parameter Estimates" of the output is the same Estimated R Matrix for ID 1 but is not represented as a matrix.

The next section of the output shows the estimated intercept and slope (represented respectively by a and b in Eq. (6.1)) and are defined correspondingly as 1 and 2 in the simulation. Again, we see that estimated values of 0.8956 and 2.0275 are close to the predefined simulation values of $a = 1$ and $b = 2$, respectively. The last section "Estimates" in Figure 6.6 gives least-square means for the changes in $M1$ target scale scores corresponding to a change of $-3, -2, \ldots, 4$, 5 in $M2$ anchor scale scores.

As discussed earlier, modeling the relationship between changes in $M1$ and $M2$ scale scores, when change in the $M2$ scale is used as a categorical predictor, is an important part of the assessment on the ability to detect change property for the PRO measure of interest (here taken as the $M1$ scale). In this section, we simulated this relationship as linear and, as a result, we do not anticipate any surprises from this analysis. Nonetheless, we still need to compare and interpret results from both models. The paramount importance of this second analysis, with change in the $M2$ scale taken as a categorical predictor, will become evident from the set of analyses and examples described in the next section of this chapter.

Figure 6.8 shows the implementation of the longitudinal model using change in the $M2$ scale as a categorical anchor. The most important property of this model is that we do not impose any functional relationships between anchor (variable cat_chgM2) and outcome (the same variable chgM1 used when the anchor is continuous). Note that now the variable cat_chgM2 should be part of the Class statement and, to produce least-square means for the changes in the $M1$ scale scores corresponding to changes of $-3, -2, \ldots, 4, 5$ in the $M2$ scale scores, we need only "LSMeans cat_chgM2" to be added.

Figure 6.9 displays results for the estimated least-square means on the change in $M1$ scale scores, and Figure 6.10 summarizes the estimated results from both

```
Proc Mixed Data=_mixed_ds;
Class ID Week cat_chgM2;
Model chgM1=cat_chgM2 / solution ddfm=kr;
Repeated Week / Subject=ID Type=UN R;
LSMeans cat_chgM2;
Run;
```

Figure 6.8 Modeling the relationship between score changes in $M1$ and $M2$ scales using the $M2$ scale as a categorical anchor.

Effect	cat_ chgM2	Estimate	Least Squares Means Standard Error	Pr > |t|	Alpha	Lower	Upper
cat_chgM2	-3	-5.5671	2.4136	0.0215	0.05	-10.3094	-0.8248
cat_chgM2	-2	-1.7144	1.1865	0.1488	0.05	-4.0428	0.6141
cat_chgM2	-1	-1.0462	0.3849	0.0068	0.05	-1.8020	-0.2903
cat_chgM2	0	1.0051	0.1826	<.0001	0.05	0.6466	1.3635
cat_chgM2	1	2.9933	0.1147	<.0001	0.05	2.7682	3.2184
cat_chgM2	2	4.9961	0.1048	<.0001	0.05	4.7905	5.2017
cat_chgM2	3	6.7395	0.1257	<.0001	0.05	6.4928	6.9862
cat_chgM2	4	8.7855	0.2375	<.0001	0.05	8.3194	9.2515
cat_chgM2	5	10.0441	0.5993	<.0001	0.05	8.8681	11.2201

Figure 6.9 Estimated least-square means for the score changes in the *M1* scale (modeled with change in the *M2* scale as a categorical anchor).

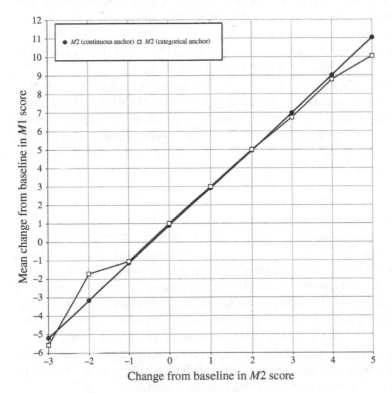

Figure 6.10 Relationship between score changes in *M1* and *M2* scales.

models (models with change in the *M2* scale as a continuous vs. as a categorical anchor). As we can see, the results of the modeling using change in *M2* as a categorical anchor are numerically very close to the results of the modeling using change in *M2* as a continuous anchor, supporting the assumption that the relationship between score changes in those two scales can be considered linear.

Note that even in this simulated example, where it is known that the true relationship between score changes on *M1* and *M2* scales is linear, we observe some visible dissimilarities between results from the two models for largest and smallest changes on the anchor, which occur generally due to the smaller overall number of observations present for those changes on the anchor. We have often observed this type of divergence from linearity for "extreme" anchor values in analyses with real data.

It is important to determine how the relationship between change scores between $M1$ and $M2$ scales can be characterized. Is it linear or something else? After all, unlike with simulated data, with real study data, we do not know what kind of relationship exists between score changes on two scales (which may not be necessarily linear). Because we established in this simulation that the relationship between change in anchor scale and change in scale under investigation is approximately linear, then we are close to conclude ". . . that the instrument is sensitive to gains and losses in the measurement concept . . .."

The next step is to show that a meaningful change in the anchor corresponds to the meaningful change in the scale under validation. If a change in such a scale of interest corresponding to a meaningful change in the anchor is small or negligible, even if empirical evidence exists for a linear relationship between score changes on the two scales, we cannot posit that the ability to detect change has been demonstrated on the PRO measure under validation ($M1$ in our case).

First, we need to establish what represents a meaningful change in an anchor scale ($M2$ in our case). In Section 5.4, in Chapter 5, the global impression of symptoms severity with four categories was used as the anchor measure. If a change in this scale would be used as an anchor, then it is reasonable to assume that a one-category change can be viewed as a meaningful change. A different situation would be if another COA or PRO measure is used as an anchor. In this case, if a meaningful change was established previously for the anchor scale, then this value can be used. For example, for the Physical Functioning domain of the SF-36 scale using normed-based scoring, the value of 3.5 points is established by the scale developers as a "clinically important change" (Ware et al. 2007). Thus, if this domain is used as the anchor, then the value of 3.5 points can be used as the basis for the meaningful score change in the anchor in order to assess the ability to detect change property on the PRO scale under validation.

There is also the possibility that there is no meaningful change threshold determined for an anchor measure. In this case, standardized effect sizes can help to approximate meaningful change for an anchor. Changes corresponding to a "small" effect size or a "medium" effect size (e.g., a change score on the anchor corresponding to a half a standard deviation on the anchor at baseline) can be suggestive of meaningful change on the anchor (Farivar et al. 2004; Norman et al. 2004).

Second, after establishing a meaningful change in an anchor, the corresponding value for a change in a scale under consideration needs to be interpreted.

Is this change negligible and inconsequential or is it large enough to be considered as supportive of the ability to detect change properly? The most straightforward approach to interpret results will be, again, the estimation of the effect size of the change. We anticipate that those changes in terms of the effect sizes should be interpreted as at least "small" or "medium." If the change can only be interpreted as "trivial" (i.e., less than 0.20 standard deviation units in absolute value), then it is likely that the analysis does not support the ability to detect change properly.

6.1.3 Correlation Analysis to Support Ability to Detect Change

Correlations between score changes from baseline on two measures is often used to support evidence of the ability to detect change on the PRO measure of attention (de Boer et al. 2006; Husted et al. 2000; Mokkink et al. 2010; Vincent et al. 2013). Correlation analysis, while having merit, by itself may not be enough to provide evidence of "COA's ability to detect change" and may play only a supportive role as, methodologically, correlations provide only evidence of overall tendency and may not fully support "evidence that the instrument is sensitive to gains and losses in the measurement concept."

To illustrate this potential insufficiency, let's first calculate correlations between score changes in M1 and M2 scales introduced in the previous section. Figure 6.11 demonstrates the calculation of the correlations using data from final dataset "_ mixed_ds" (the same dataset used in analyses represented by Figure 6.4). Figure 6.12 shows partial output where we see sizable correlations of 0.67048, 0.76228, and 0.51052 between score changes (from baseline) in M1 and M2 scales, respectively, at weeks 2, 4, and 8.

As noted above, analyses should support the "evidence that the instrument is sensitive to gains and losses in the measurement concept." In the previous section, we simulated the relationship between score changes in M1 and M2 scales as linear, which deliberately corroborates that M1 scale (the target PRO measure of interest) is sensitive to gains and losses in the measurement concept. But what will happen if the relationship is not linear? What will happen if we a priori simulate a relationship between score changes in M1 and M2 scales where the M1 scale will be sensitive only to some gains and not sensitive at all to losses?

```
Proc Sort Data=_mixed_ds out=_mixed_ds_sort; By Week; Run;
Proc Corr data= _mixed_ds_sort Pearson Spearman;
Var chgM1 chgM2;
By Week;
Run;
```

Figure 6.11 Estimation of correlations.

```
                       Week=W2
Pearson Correlation Coefficients, N = 500
          Prob > |r| under HO: Rho=0
                  chgM1            chgM2
chgM1           1.00000          0.67048
                                 <.0001

                       Week=W4
Pearson Correlation Coefficients, N = 500
          Prob > |r| under HO: Rho=0
                  chgM1            chgM2
chgM1           1.00000          0.76228
                                 <.0001

                       Week=W8
Pearson Correlation Coefficients, N = 500
          Prob > |r| under HO: Rho=0
                  chgM1            chgM2
chgM1           1.00000          0.51052
                                 <.0001
```

Figure 6.12   Partial correlation output.

For example, Figure 6.13 represents a hypothetical overall relationship between score changes in $M1$ and $M2$ scales. It shows that, for changes in the $M2$ scale score of more than one, the relationship between score changes in $M1$ and $M2$ scales is represented by a linear function (a one-point change in the $M2$ scale score corresponds to a two-point change in the $M1$ scale score) but, for changes in the $M2$ scale score of less than one, the relationship between score changes in $M1$ and $M2$ scales is represented by a horizontal flat line (any change in the $M2$ scale score corresponds to the same score change of three points in the $M1$ scale).

To implement simulation based on the hypothetical relationship presented by Figure 6.13, we can use the same SAS code represented by Figures 6.1, 6.2, 6.4, 6.8, and 6.11. The only change is in the code that simulates the relationship between score changes in $M1$ and $M2$ scales. In Figure 6.2 the following code

```
Data _mixed_ds;
Merge m2 err;
chgM1=1+2*chgM2+err;
By ID Week;
Run;
```

should be replaced by

```
Data _mixed_ds;
Merge m2 err;
If chgM2>1 Then
Do;
chgM1=1+2*chgM2+err;
End;
Else
```

```
Do;
chgM1=3+err;
End;
By ID Week;
Run;
```

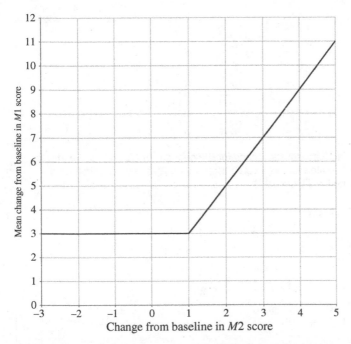

Figure 6.13 The hypothetical overall relationship between change scores in *M*1 and *M*2 scales.

Figures 6.14–6.16 represent results for the estimated relationships and correlations between score changes in *M*1 and *M*2 scales after running SAS code from Figures 6.1, 6.2 (replaced with the previously noted data step code), 6.4, 6.8, and 6.11. Figure 6.17 graphically summarizes results from Figures 6.14 and 6.15.

Figure 6.17 shows that a predefined simulated relationship and, separately, a modeled relationship when change in the *M*2 scale is used as a categorical anchor. Both relationships are close. But the results of the modeling with change in *M*2 scale as a continuous anchor are, as expected, notably different from those of the predefined simulated relationship. These results show that in this simulation, we cannot conclude that the *M*1 scale is "sensitive to gains and losses in the measurement concept" and, as a result, ability to detect change properly for the *M*1 scale is not confirmed.

		Estimates						
Label	Estimate	Standard Error	DF	t Value	Pr > |t|	Alpha	Lower	Upper
chgM2=-3	-2.4652	0.2540	1148	-9.70	<.0001	0.05	-2.9637	-1.9668
chgM2=-2	-0.9394	0.2061	1106	-4.56	<.0001	0.05	-1.3437	-0.5351
chgM2=-1	0.5864	0.1596	1025	3.67	0.0003	0.05	0.2732	0.8996
chgM2= 0	2.1122	0.1165	866	18.13	<.0001	0.05	1.8835	2.3408
chgM2= 1	3.6380	0.08225	617	44.23	<.0001	0.05	3.4764	3.7995
chgM2= 2	5.1637	0.07103	501	72.70	<.0001	0.05	5.0242	5.3033
chgM2= 3	6.6895	0.09173	675	72.92	<.0001	0.05	6.5094	6.8697
chgM2= 4	8.2153	0.1299	869	63.24	<.0001	0.05	7.9604	8.4703
chgM2= 5	9.7411	0.1744	986	55.85	<.0001	0.05	9.3988	10.0834

Figure 6.14 Estimated least-square means for the change in *M1* scale scores (model with change in the *M2* scale score as a continuous anchor, based on the simulated relationship represented by Figure 6.13).

		Least Squares Means				
Effect	cat_chgM2	Estimate	Standard Error	DF	t Value	Pr > |t|
cat_chgM2	-3	1.8461	2.3715	494	0.78	0.4367
cat_chgM2	-2	3.4238	1.1735	939	2.92	0.0036
cat_chgM2	-1	2.7020	0.3787	609	7.13	<.0001
cat_chgM2	0	2.8290	0.1802	862	15.70	<.0001
cat_chgM2	1	3.1811	0.1138	1043	27.96	<.0001
cat_chgM2	2	4.9896	0.1042	903	47.91	<.0001
cat_chgM2	3	6.7431	0.1251	957	53.90	<.0001
cat_chgM2	4	8.7822	0.2365	985	37.14	<.0001
cat_chgM2	5	10.0445	0.5968	991	16.83	<.0001

Figure 6.15 Estimated least-square means for the changes in *M1* scale score (model with change in the *M2* scale score as a categorical anchor, based on the simulated relationship represented by Figure 6.13).

```
                    Week=W2
    Pearson Correlation Coefficients, N = 500
          Prob > |r| under H0: Rho=0
                  chgM1             chgM2
    chgM1       1.00000           0.40500
                                  <.0001

    Spearman Correlation Coefficients, N = 500
          Prob > |r| under H0: Rho=0
                  chgM1             chgM2
    chgM1       1.00000           0.37228
                                  <.0001

                    Week=W4
    Pearson Correlation Coefficients, N = 500
          Prob > |r| under H0: Rho=0
                  chgM1             chgM2
    chgM1       1.00000           0.70040
                                  <.0001

    Spearman Correlation Coefficients, N = 500
          Prob > |r| under H0: Rho=0
                  chgM1             chgM2
    chgM1       1.00000           0.68861
                                  <.0001

                    Week=W8
    Pearson Correlation Coefficients, N = 500
          Prob > |r| under H0: Rho=0
                  chgM1             chgM2
    chgM1       1.00000           0.48702
                                  <.0001

    Spearman Correlation Coefficients, N = 500
          Prob > |r| under H0: Rho=0
                  chgM1             chgM2
    chgM1       1.00000           0.48218
                                  <.0001
```

Figure 6.16 Correlations (based on the simulated relationship represented by Figure 6.13).

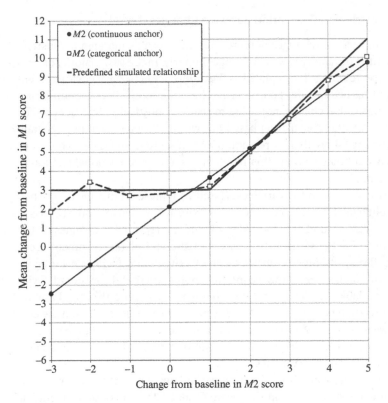

Figure 6.17 Relationships between score changes in M1 and M2 scales (based on the simulated relationship represented by Figure 6.13).

Yet if only correlations are used to support the ability to detect change properly for the $M1$ scale, then we still observe sizable (Pearson) correlations of `0.40500`, `0.70040`, and `0.48702` between score changes in $M1$ and $M2$ scales at weeks 2, 4, and 8, respectively, despite the fact that the estimated relationship between score changes in $M1$ and $M2$ scales shows that the $M1$ scale is not sensitive to gains and losses in the measurement concept (as uncovered by the model with change in $M2$ scale scores as a categorical anchor). While Pearson correlation coefficients assume a linear relationship between variables, Spearman correlation coefficients, which merely assume a monotonic relationship, nevertheless also give similar (but slightly smaller) correlation values (see Figure 6.16).

This simulated example accentuates the immense importance of the analyses using anchor as a categorical variable and highlights the fact that correlations can only serve as supplementary evidence of the ability to detect change properly.

6.1.4 Deconstructing Correlation Between Changes

In the previous sections, changes in scores for scales were simulated to illustrate the assessment of the ability to detect change properly. In the vast majority of real-life cases, the score change is calculated as the difference between a post-treatment observation at particular time point and the baseline score. The relevant philosophical nuance is that change, not being measured holistically, does not exist by itself – it is an "artificial" construct based on two measurements at two separate occasions. Here we show that correlation between score changes between a pair of variables is a complicated function based on a set of cross-sectional and longitudinal correlations.

Consider two scales X and Y. Variables $X1$ and $Y1$ represent outcomes of the two scales at baseline for 1050 subjects. The mean score at baseline for both scales is 0, with standard deviation of 0.5. Variables $X2$ and $Y2$ represent outcomes of the same two scales for the same 1050 subjects at the end of the treatment. Let's assume that all subjects improve on both scales by five points, giving a mean score of five points for both scales at the second time point and that the standard deviation of both variables at the second time point is 1. Suppose that the baseline (Pearson) correlation between $X1$ and $Y1$ is small with a value of 0.1, and the correlation between $X2$ and $Y2$ at the end of the treatment (the second time point) is substantial with a value of 0.6 (owing, say, to more variation in scale scores stemming from an efficacious treatment).

Assuming that data come from the multivariate normal distribution, we additionally need to define correlations between $X1$ and $X2$ (value of 0.11 in simulation), $Y1$ and $Y2$ (value of 0.12 in simulation), $X1$ and $Y2$ (value of 0.09 in simulation), and $X2$ and $Y1$ (value of 0.2 in simulation). The small values of the correlations between $X1$ and $X2$ ($Y1$ and $Y2$) would be representative, for instance, of the situation when baseline and end of treatment measurements are separated by a considerable time period. Figure 6.18 represents the aforementioned simulation. Figure 6.19 shows that the correlation between score changes in X and Y scales is equal to 0.38132.

Now let's redefine some of the correlations in the simulation as follows. Correlations between $X1$ and $X2$ is 0.51; $Y1$ and $Y2$, 0.52; $X1$ and $Y2$, 0.39; and $X2$ and $Y1$, 0.42. The larger values of the correlations between $X1$ and $X2$ ($Y1$ and $Y2$) would be representative of the situation when baseline and end of treatment are separated by a relatively small time period. To run this second simulation, we need to replace the first data step (**data** `_cov_ (type=corr; . . .`) in Figure 6.18 by the data step represented in Figure 6.20.

Figure 6.21 shows that (in this second simulation) the correlation between score changes for X and Y scales now gives a smaller value of 0.27, compared with the slightly larger value of 0.38 from the prior simulation, despite being based on

```
data _cov_(type=corr);
input
_TYPE_ $   _NAME_ $   x1        y1        x2        y2        ;
datalines;
 CORR      x1         1         0.1       0.11      0.09
 CORR      y1         0.1       1         0.2       0.12
 CORR      x2         0.11      0.2       1         0.6
 CORR      y2         0.09      0.12      0.6       1
 MEAN      .          0         0         5         5
 STD       .          0.5       0.5       1         1
 N         .          1050      1050      1050      1050
;
run;
Proc Simnormal data=_cov_ out=xy_sim numreal=1050 seed=10000;
var x1 y1 x2 y2;
run;
Proc Corr data=xy_sim; Var x1 y1 x2 y2; Run;
Data change_sim; Set  xy_sim;
Change1=x2 - x1; Change2=y2 - y1;
Keep Change1 Change2;
Run;
Proc Corr data=change_sim;
Var Change1 Change2;
Run;
```

Figure 6.18   Simulating score change and estimating correlation (simulation 1).

```
                        Simple Statistics
Variable       N        Mean      Std Dev    Sum      Minimum    Maximum
Change1        1050     4.98057   1.07933    5230     1.85869    9.24720
Change2        1050     4.96664   1.06770    5215     2.04726    8.05387


Pearson Correlation Coefficients, N = 1050
       Prob > |r| under H0: Rho=0

               Change1        Change2

Change1        1.00000        0.38132
                              <.0001

Change2        0.38132        1.00000
               <.0001
```

Figure 6.19   Correlation between score changes for two scales based on simulation from Figure 6.18.

```
data _cov_(type=corr);
input
_TYPE_ $   _NAME_ $   x1        y1        x2        y2    ;
datalines;
 CORR      x1         1         0.1       0.51      0.39
 CORR      y1         0.1       1         0.42      0.52
 CORR      x2         0.51      0.42      1         0.6
 CORR      y2         0.39      0.52      0.6       1
 MEAN      .          0         0         5         5
 STD       .          0.5       0.5       1         1
 N         .          1050      1050      1050      1050
;
run;
```

Figure 6.20   Initial correlation structure for the data simulation (simulation 2).

```
                              Simple Statistics

Variable         N          Mean       Std Dev      Sum      Minimum     Maximum
Change1        1050       4.99632      0.88189      5246     2.21460     7.91308
Change2        1050       4.98578      0.86230      5235     2.64065     7.44223


Pearson Correlation Coefficients, N = 1050
         Prob > |r| under H0: Rho=0


                 Change1         Change2

Change1        1.00000         0.27159
                               <.0001

Change2        0.27159         1.00000
                <.0001
```

Figure 6.21 Correlation between score changes (based on the correlation data from Figure 6.20).

a majority of pairwise correlations being considerably larger than in the prior simulation (the first simulation).

As shown and supported by the methodological literature (Cohen et al. 2003; Cronbach and Furby 1970; Griffin et al. 1999), the correlation between score changes is a complicated function of the six pairwise correlations between scores of the two scales at two time points. This correlation is highly affected by, and confounded with, three sets of correlations: (i) the correlation between scores of the two measures at each time point (between $X1$ and $Y1$, between $X2$ and $Y2$); (ii) the correlation between scores of the same measure at two different time points (between $X1$ and $X2$, between $Y1$ and $Y2$); and (iii) the correlation between scores of the two measures at two different time points (between $X1$ and $Y2$, $X2$ and $Y1$). The above examples show that correlations between score changes do not have a straightforward interpretation and, as such, reinforce the conclusion from the previous Section 6.1.3 that correlations between score changes may serve only as supplementary evidence of the ability to detect change property.

6.2 Sensitivity to Treatment

6.2.1 What Is the Sensitivity to Treatment?

During the validation of a measurement scale, there is no specific property such as sensitivity to treatment, which needs to be evaluated to support psychometric validity of the scale. Then, what do we actually mean by "the sensitivity to treatment?" There are several key points researchers need to investigate to ensure that a scale will be successful in the measurement of the treatment effects. Some of those points should be examined earlier in the development of the instrument. For example, the recall period should be "based on the instrument's purpose and intended use; the variability, duration, frequency, and intensity of the concept measured; the disease or condition's characteristics; and the study treatment" (FDA 2019).

Suppose we want to measure the effect of the treatment for (say) erectile dysfunction, a chronic condition. Then "the recall period should be long enough to capture the event or experience of interest, but not so long that the respondent is unable to adequately recall the information, because this can lead to measurement error and potentially a limitation to the responsiveness or sensitivity of the treatment effect" (FDA 2019). Consider the International Index of Erectile Function (IIEF) for men with erectile dysfunction (Rosen et al. 1997, 2002). In assessing sexual function over the four-week period prior to completing the questionnaire, the IIEF provides researchers or clinicians with a reliable measure of the erectile function concept. The four-week time period was selected as a relatively standard period of assessment in sexual function studies, one deemed long enough for patients to have an opportunity to engage in sexual activity.

Another issue is when measurements should be taken. For example, the following statements describe the situation when quality of life can be affected by the treatment: "Concepts related to treatment safety, tolerability, or burden may also be measured by COAs . . .. When assessing treatment safety, tolerability, or burden with a PRO, sponsors should select symptomatic adverse events and other topics in an unbiased manner." (FDA 2019). Those statements raise at least two important points.

The first point is that when measuring treatment safety, tolerability, or burden, symptomatic adverse events and other topics should be selected in an unbiased manner. Therefore, we should not select or develop a scale that emphasizes or understates some adverse events or symptoms over others based on the likely treatment adverse event profile. As a matter of fact, a scale should be treatment agnostic to be a valid measurement scale (i.e., it should not be associated with any particular treatment or intervention).

The second point, related to the first, concerns at which time points a scale measuring safety, tolerability, or burden should be collected. Consider a treatment applied in four week cycles where, after the treatment, it is anticipated that a subject will have a worsening of some symptoms, which levels out in two to three weeks thereafter. Should the subject's symptomology be measured shortly after treatment administration or be delayed by three weeks? Using either approach in isolation will give a misleading picture of the treatment burden. Collecting data only shortly after treatment administration will give the worst overall result on treatment burden. But waiting three weeks is not any better, as it will lead to the most favorable overall result on treatment burden. In this case, an accurate and a balanced overall representation of symptomology would be to collect data at both time points. It is important not to choose a particular timing that will systematically bias the results.

The frequency of assessments should correspond appropriately to the natural history of disease and the likelihood of changes in outcome within that period (Fairclough 2010). Assessments should be frequent enough to capture meaningful change but not so frequent as to be incongruent with the recall period of the assessment. In a renal cell carcinoma study, for instance, patients were self-assessed, in part, using the Functional Assessment of Cancer Therapy-Kidney Symptom Index-15-item (FKSI-15) questionnaire (Cella et al. 2008). Patients were asked to complete the questionnaires before any clinical activities during visits to the study clinics at screening, on days 1 and 28 of each 42-day treatment cycle, and at the end of treatment or study withdrawal. Within-group changes over time from baseline in the post-baseline scores indicated that there were sharp decreases (more severe symptoms and concerns) in FKSI-15 scores after the first cycle of treatment; the initial decreases were more pronounced for the control group than the experimental group. After the initial decreases, however, FKSI-15 scores for both groups remained essentially unchanged thereafter at subsequent cycles.

The decisions made in the aforementioned situations are typically made at the design stage while the study is being planned. Decisions made at the design stage of what items to include and how they are grouped and scored directly affect the validation of the scale and the sensitivity of the scale to effective treatment. What we can do during the validation is implied by the following sentence: "It would be disadvantageous to use a measure with items that include activities irrelevant to the target population. Doing so would miss the opportunity to assess a symptom or impact of importance to patients and may also yield a *bias toward the null*, or a tendency to show no effect of treatment, even if the treatment were effective. In such cases, a negative response (or indication of little to no activity) is not useful" (FDA 2019).

An extension or variation of this draft guidance (FDA 2019) (as of this writing) is that, even if the items include activities relevant to the target population, the measurement of a treatment effect can go awry when the items in a scale are not appropriately grouped and scored. In Chapter 5, the Minnesota Nicotine Withdrawal Scale was discussed to highlight some important features of the exploratory factor analysis (see Section 5.1.3.4). At the same time, this scale is also a good example to illustrate a *bias toward the null* with respect to treatment effect. Recall that the nine-item MNWS contains two multi-item domains Negative Affect with four items (depressed mood; irritability, frustration, or anger; anxiety; difficulty concentrating) and Insomnia with two items (difficulty going to sleep, difficulty staying asleep) and three individual items (Craving, Restlessness, Increased Appetite). This measurement structure was supported by exploratory factor analysis in one Phase II clinical trial and confirmatory factor analyses in two independent Phase II clinical trials (Cappelleri et al. 2005).

When this scale was used in the clinical study to investigate a new drug for smoking cessation, it was important to understand how the described domains and items of the MNWS would be affected. Each of its nine items is relevant in measuring nicotine withdrawal symptoms in the target population of smokers in a smoking cessation trial involving active and control treatments (Gonzales et al. 2006; Jorenby et al. 2006). There exists an interesting dilemma. Should the total score be analyzed and considered as the primary outcome or should individual domains and manifest variables be the key outcomes?

Consider a drug for smoking cessation that reduces cravings and blocks the rewarding effects of smoking. As a result of using this drug, patients are more likely to stop smoking, because the drug removes one of most burdensome withdrawal symptoms, which is urge to smoke (or craving) and, at the same time, also eliminates satisfaction from smoking. But if the drug only affects cravings and rewarding effects of smoking, the other withdrawal symptoms, such as restlessness, irritability, increased appetite, sleeplessness still will be there after patients stop smoking and these other symptoms are likely to worsen. This means that if we were to use the MNWS total score as the measure of the effect of the drug as a part of a clinical study, the results will be *biased toward the null*, because items will not "march" together. The item representing craving will show improvement, but the other two domains and the four individual items will likely show worsening or no change. This example demonstrates the danger of using total scores when a drug can improve some attributes of a scale and concurrently not affect or worsen other attributes.

Another important decision regards the suitable time point for analysis. Let's continue with the smoking cessation example. When should MNWS be collected? Suppose the study is eight weeks in duration. Should we just collect MNWS at baseline and at the end of the study at week 8? Given that certain withdrawal symptoms are expected to generally manifest themselves shortly after the last cigarette is consumed earlier in a study and then start to subside by week 4–5, postbaseline MNWS measurements only at week 8 will miss all the changes and experiences required to evaluate the full patient experience over time (in a sense it can also be characterized as *bias toward the null*). Instead, it would be more sensible to collect this scale at least weekly to capture changes over time in withdrawal symptoms associated with the effect of the drug and, at the same time, the separate effects of possible smoking abstinence.

6.2.2 Concurrent Estimation of the Treatment Effects for a Multi-Domain Scale

6.2.2.1 Assessment of the Treatment Effect for a Single Domain

As pointed out in previous section, we do not have a specific "sensitivity to treatment" property to assess as a part of an ongoing validation of a scale. But for a new scale to be used in a clinical study we recommend to investigate how this scale will respond to a treatment intervention. Ideally, this investigation should be a part of Phase 2 in a clinical program for a new drug. The main purpose of this analysis will be to understand which domains of a multi-item scale will respond (or not) and in which way (showing improvement or worsening) to an intervention. Simply stated, we need to assess the treatment effect (active treatment vs. control treatment) of a drug as measured by a scale under investigation.

As an introductory example, consider a simple multi-item scale with just one domain. This fictitious scale is used in a longitudinal study where subjects are given an experimental treatment or a placebo. The following equation will represent one of several possible models to estimate treatment effect, generally referenced here as a longitudinal repeated measures model (Cappelleri et al. 2013; Fairclough 2010; Fitzmaurice et al. 2011; Singer and Willett 2003):

$$Y_{ijk} = a + b \times x_i + t_j + d_k + r_{jk} + e_{ijk} \tag{6.2}$$

where

Y_{ijk} is the domain score for subject i at measurement occasion j on treatment k ($i = 1, 2, \ldots, N_s$; $j = 1, 2, \ldots, N_t$; $k = 1, 2, \ldots, N_d$; N_s is number of subjects in the study, N_t is number of time points when this scale was collected, and N_d is number of treatments);

a is the unknown fixed effect intercept;

x_i is a baseline domain score for subject i, and b is the corresponding regression coefficient (slope) for this covariate;

t_j is the fixed time effect at time point j;

d_k is the fixed effect of the treatment k;

r_{jk} is the interaction effect between drug k and time point j;

e_{ijk} is the error term associated with scale score measurement Y_{ijk} for subject i on treatment k at time point j.

For any subject i at time point j on treatment k it is assumed that the error term e_{ijk} is taken from a normal distribution with mean 0 and variance σ_j^2, that is, $e_{ijk} \sim N(0, \sigma_j^2)$. Error terms are independent between subjects, meaning that covariance of error terms for any two different subjects i_1 and i_2 at any two time points j_1 and j_2 (which can be the same time points) and on any treatments k_1 and k_2 (which can be the same treatment) is zero, that is, $\mathrm{cov}(e_{i_1 j_1 k_1}, e_{i_2 j_2 k_2}) = 0$. It is also assumed that measurements from the same subject are not independent, which means that error terms covary over time within a subject – the error at time point j_1 covaries with error at time point j_2 (for time point $j_1 = 1, 2, \ldots, N_t$; $j_2 = 1, 2, \ldots,$ N_t; $j_1 \neq j_2$) with covariance $\mathrm{cov}(e_{ij_1 k}, e_{ij_2 k}) = \sigma_{j_1 j_2}$ for any subject i and treatment k.

This simulated example assumes that measurements are collected at baseline (baseline scores are part of the model) and at four post-baseline occasions. There are only two treatments: active treatment and placebo. And, overall, 600 subjects from the population of interest were "recruited" for this simulated study (300 subjects per treatment arm).

The SAS code in Figure 6.22 represents the first step for the data simulation and is based on the Eq. (6.2) but simulating only the "true/perfect" part of the variable Y_{ijk} based on the following equation without error term:

$$Y_{ijk} = a + b \times x_i + t_j + d_k + r_{jk}. \tag{6.3}$$

The following fragment

```
a=3;  /* the intercept */
```

from Figure 6.22 specifies the overall mean for the simulated Y_{ijk} and corresponds to the parameter a in Eq. (6.3). The next code line

```
b=0.07;  /* baseline slope */
```

defines the slope for the baseline and corresponds to the $b \times x_i$ term in Eq. (6.3). Moreover, the one-dimensional array of the data

```
Array t{1:4}  (-0.25 -0.50 -0.75 0);
```

defines the time effect for every time point.

There is one important detail associated with this array of values. Since we are going to use the MIXED procedure to estimate all those parameters, we define the

```
/* For this example, there are 600 subjects (NumberOfSubjectsPerTreatment * NumberOfTreatments).
For every subject there are 4 visits (NumberOfVisits = 4;).
There are also 2 treatments arms (NumberOfTreatments = 2;)*/
options nofmterr nocenter pagesize=2000 linesize=256;

%Let NumberOfSubjectsPerTreatment = 300;
%Let NumberOfVisits       = 4;
%Let NumberOfTreatments = 2;

data mixed_ds;
Retain seed1 1  ;
a=3;    /* the intercept */
b=0.07; /* baseline slope */
Array t{1:4} (-0.25 -0.50 -0.75  0 ); /*the time effect at time point j=1,2,3,4*/
Array d{1:2} (-1.00 0); /*the effect of the treatments k=1,2*/
Array r{1:2,1:4} (
-0.1 -0.2 -0.3 0 /*interaction effect between drug 1 and time point j (j=1, 2, 3, 4)*/
  0    0    0    0 /*interaction effect between drug 2 and time point j (j=1, 2, 3, 4)*/
);
        ID=0;
        Do k=1 to &NumberOfTreatments;
        Do i=1 To &NumberOfSubjectsPerTreatment;
        ID=ID+1;
        Call rannor(seed1,e);
        x = 4 + sqrt(0.1)*e;
            Do j=1 To &NumberOfVisits;
            Y      = a + b*x + t[j] + d[k] +  r[k,j];
            Visit = j; Treatment = k; Baseline = x;
            Output;
            End;
        End;
        End;
Keep Y Baseline ID Visit Treatment;
run;

Proc Print data=mixed_ds NOOBS; Where ID In (1 2 3); Run;
```

Figure 6.22 Generating a dataset with "true/perfect" outcomes.

last category of the categorical variables (time is the categorical variable in this model) as zero to simplify the comparison of the estimated values with the values defined in the simulation. The rationale for this simplification is to address the over-parameterizing done by the MIXED procedure. The time effects are represented by the categorical variable (CLASS variable in the MIXED procedure) corresponding to time effects at four post-baseline time points. This means that it will be sufficient to have the three binary (0/1) variables to describe the time effects in analyses. Nonetheless, the MIXED procedure will create internally four binary variables to define time effects and automatically will assign zero value to the last variable, which is used as a reference category. These inserted zero effects can be spotted in the outputs by the lack of any estimated values for statistics, such as standard errors and p-values, generally associated with the estimated effects (as later shown in Figure 6.27).

The treatment effects are defined by the following array

```
Array d{1:2} (-1.00 0);
```

with the second (last) category serving as the reference treatment.

The last two-dimensional array defines the treatment-by-time interaction effects

```
Array r{1:2,1:4}
(-0.1 -0.2 -0.3 0
 0  0  0  0 );
```

Because of overparameterization in this two-dimensional array, the last categories in both dimensions are defined as zeros.

Running the SAS code from Figure 6.22 generates a dataset with 2400 observations. Figure 6.23 represents a fragment of this dataset to highlight the standard (in SAS) structure of the dataset to be used by the MIXED procedure (recall that the same vertical structure was used previously; for example, see Figure 4.11 in Chapter 4 and Figure 6.3 in this chapter). The data for the first three subjects are shown. Note that, in this dataset, the values of the variable Y (corresponds to the Y_{ijk} in Eq. (6.3)) can be considered as the "true" subject scores (i.e., error-free scores), as we have not yet simulated the error term e_{ijk}.

ID	Y	Visit	Treatment	Baseline
1	1.96995	1	1	4.57074
1	1.61995	2	1	4.57074
1	1.26995	3	1	4.57074
1	2.31995	4	1	4.57074
2	1.92823	1	1	3.97473
2	1.57823	2	1	3.97473
2	1.22823	3	1	3.97473
2	2.27823	4	1	3.97473
3	1.93878	1	1	4.12541
3	1.58878	2	1	4.12541
3	1.23878	3	1	4.12541
3	2.28878	4	1	4.12541

Figure 6.23 Example of the dataset structure for the analyses with the MIXED procedure.

Previously in this chapter, we introduced the approach of how error terms for longitudinal data can be generated (see specifically Figure 6.2). First, to generate error terms, the dataset with correlation information ("corr" type) was generated and then used by SIMNORMAL procedure to simulate random error terms for every subject at every time point. Note that this approach is used throughout the book in many different simulations. But, for this particular simulated example, we will slightly change this approach by generating a dataset with covariance information ("cov" type) and then using it as the input for SIMNORMAL procedure.

To generate the variance–covariance matrix for error terms, we start with defining correlations between error terms and standard deviations for those errors at every time point. Figure 6.24 shows the implementation of this procedure using the IML procedure. The first matrix corr defines correlations. For example, the value of 0.5 corresponds to the correlation between errors at time point $j = 1$ and time point $j = 2$, that is, *corr* $(e_{j = 1}, e_{j = 2}) = 0.5$. Vector SD represents standard deviations of the error terms at every time point. Now, based on this information the variance–covariance matrix is calculated (see Figure 6.25 for estimated covariances). Now this estimated variance is simply used to create the SAS dataset of covariance structure with a specific structure (see Figure 6.26; specifically data step "**data** _cov_(type=cov);").

As previously noted, this dataset is then used as the input for the SIMNORMAL procedure, which is intelligent enough to recognize the type of the input dataset and simulate data accordingly. Note that the code in Figure 6.26 assumes that the dataset "mixed_ds" created earlier (by code from Figure 6.22) is present. The datastep "**Data** mixed_ds1;" combines previously generated "exact" outcome Y and just generated error terms to create the variable Yijk (see code line "Yijk=Y+Eijk;") which corresponds to variable Y_{ijk} in Eq. (6.2).

```
Proc IML;
corr = {1          0.5          0.4          0.3,
          0.5        1            0.5          0.4,
          0.4        0.5          1            0.5,
          0.3        0.4          0.5          1  };
SD = {0.2    0.3    0.25    0.15};
cov=diag(SD)*corr*diag(SD);
print cov;
Quit;
```

Figure 6.24 Calculations of the variance–covariance matrix.

	cov		
0.04	0.03	0.02	0.009
0.03	0.09	0.0375	0.018
0.02	0.0375	0.0625	0.01875
0.009	0.018	0.01875	0.0225

Figure 6.25 Estimated variance–covariance matrix.

```
data _cov_ (type=cov);
input _TYPE_ $  _NAME_ $  COL1      COL2      COL3      COL4;
datalines;
  COV        COL1      0.04      0.03      0.02      0.009
  COV        COL2      0.03      0.09      0.0375    0.018
  COV        COL3      0.02      0.0375    0.0625    0.01875
  COV        COL4      0.009     0.018     0.01875   0.0225
  MEAN        .        0         0         0         0
  N           .        600       600       600       600
;
run;
Proc Simnormal data=_cov_ out=err_sim numreal=600 seed=12345; var Col1-Col4; Run;
Proc Corr data=err_sim COV ; Var Col1-Col4; Run;
Proc Transpose data=err_sim out=err_sim_tr; Var Col1-Col4; By Rnum; Run;
Data _errors_; Set err_sim_tr;
ID= Rnum; Eijk=Col1;
Keep ID Eijk;
Run;
Data mixed_ds1;
Merge mixed_ds _errors_;
Yijk=Y+Eijk;
By ID;
Keep Yijk Baseline ID Visit Treatment;
Run;
Proc Mixed data=mixed_ds1;
Class Visit Treatment ID ;
Model Yijk = Baseline Visit Treatment Visit*Treatment / solution ddfm=kr;
Repeated Visit / Subject=ID Type=UN R rcorr;
LSMeans Treatment Visit*Treatment / cl diff;
Run;
```

Figure 6.26 Creating final simulated dataset and estimating parameters by using the MIXED procedure.

Figure 6.27 represents partial output for parameters used to simulate data (produced by the MIXED procedure). Comparing estimated covariance matrix from Figure 6.27 (titled **Estimated R Matrix for ID 1**) with covariance matrix from Figure 6.25, we can see that the estimated covariance matrix is numerically very close to the values used to generate error terms. Note that the same can be said about the correlation matrix from Figure 6.27 (titled **Estimated R Correlation Matrix for ID 1**) and initial correlation matrix corr from Figure 6.24.

The last section in Figure 6.27 is titled Solution for Fixed Effects. The first estimated effect is "Intercept 3.0887...", which corresponds to the "a=3; /* the overall mean */" in Figure 6.22. The value for the effect "Baseline" is estimated as 0.04948, which in the simulation is defined as 0.07 (b = 0.07; /* baseline slope */; see Figure 6.22). The next two effects ("Treatment") correspond to the vector "Array d{1:2} (-1.00 0); /*the effect of the treatments k=1,2*/" in Figure 6.22. The estimated value for the first element is -1.0233, which is practically the same value of -1.00 defined in the simulation. Note that the second value for the "Treatment" effect is 0, and it is not estimated (there is no any statistical appraisal such as "**Standard Error**" or "**t Value**" attached to this zero value) but rather used as a reference category. Note that the same pattern of results is observed for other effects in the model: Numerical values of the estimated effects

```
           Estimated R Matrix for ID 1
Row      Col1        Col2        Col3        Col4
 1     0.03817     0.02837     0.02000     0.009430
 2     0.02837     0.08388     0.03544     0.01684
 3     0.02000     0.03544     0.06231     0.01824
 4     0.009430    0.01684     0.01824     0.02180

        Estimated R Correlation Matrix for ID 1
Row      Col1        Col2        Col3        Col4
 1     1.0000      0.5014      0.4101      0.3269
 2     0.5014      1.0000      0.4902      0.3938
 3     0.4101      0.4902      1.0000      0.4949
 4     0.3269      0.3938      0.4949      1.0000
```

Effect	Visit	Treatment	Estimate	Standard Error	DF	t Value	Pr > |t|
Intercept			3.0887	0.07134	600	43.29	<.0001
Baseline			0.04948	0.01764	597	2.80	0.0052
Visit	1		-0.2491	0.01171	598	-21.28	<.0001
Visit	2		-0.5031	0.01549	598	-32.48	<.0001
Visit	3		-0.7464	0.01260	598	-59.23	<.0001
Visit	4		0	.	.	.	.
Treatment		1	-1.0233	0.01207	597	-84.81	<.0001
Treatment		2	0	.	.	.	.
Visit*Treatment	1	1	-0.09437	0.01656	598	-5.70	<.0001
Visit*Treatment	1	2	0	.	.	.	.
Visit*Treatment	2	1	-0.1966	0.02191	598	-8.97	<.0001
Visit*Treatment	2	2	0	.	.	.	.
Visit*Treatment	3	1	-0.3088	0.01782	598	-17.33	<.0001
Visit*Treatment	3	2	0	.	.	.	.
Visit*Treatment	4	1	0	.	.	.	.
Visit*Treatment	4	2	0	.	.	.	.

Figure 6.27 Partial results of the modeling of data using the MIXED procedure.

are close to the values originally defined in simulation, and reference categories are automatically assigned zero values by the MIXED procedure.

6.2.2.2 Assessment of the Treatment Effects for a Multi-Domain Scale

Often a multi-item scale is represented by several related but distinct aspects of a measured concept. For example, health-related quality of life concepts can be represented by several domains measuring, for example, emotional, mental, physical, and social aspects of a patient's health situation. In this case, if analyses of treatment effects are done separately for every domain, those analyses are treated typically as statistically independent. In this section, however, we will show how several domains of a scale collected repeatedly in a study can be evaluated using one unified multi-domain longitudinal model, thereby increasing the efficiency of the analyses (Bushmakin et al. 2013).

For this simulated example consider a multi-domain scale, which is used in a longitudinal study where subjects are given investigative treatments or placebo. The following equation will represent a model to estimate treatment effects simultaneously for several domains (the extension of Eq. (6.2)):

$$Y_{mijk} = a_m + b_m \times x_{mi} + t_{mj} + d_{mk} + r_{mjk} + e_{mijk} \tag{6.4}$$

where

Y_{mijk} is the (observed) domain score for domain m for subject i at measurement occasion j on treatment k ($m = 1, 2, \ldots, N_f; i = 1, 2, \ldots, N_s; j = 1, 2, \ldots, N_t; k = 1,$

2, . . ., N_d; N_f is number of domains or factors; N_s is number of subjects in the study, N_t is number of time points when this scale was collected, and N_d is number of treatments);

a_m is the intercept for the domain m;

x_{mi} is a baseline domain score for domain m for subject i and b_m is the corresponding regression coefficient (slope) for this covariate;

t_{mj} is the fixed time effect on domain m at time point j;

d_{mk} is the fixed effect of the treatment k on domain m;

r_{mjk} is the interaction effect between drug k and time point j on domain m;

e_{mijk} is the error term associated with measurement Y_{mijk} for domain m for subject i on treatment k at time point j.

For a domain m and subject i at time point j on treatment k, it is assumed that error term e_{mijk} is taken from a normal distribution with mean 0 and variance σ_{mj}^2, that is, $e_{mijk} \sim N(0, \sigma_{mj}^2)$. Error terms are independent between subjects, meaning that covariance of error terms for any two different subjects i_1 and i_2 at any two time points j_1 and j_2 (can be the same time points), on any treatments k_1 and k_2 (can be the same treatment), and for any two domains m_1 and m_2 (can be the same domains) is zero. Hence $\operatorname{cov}(e_{m_1 i_1 j_1 k_1}, e_{m_2 i_2 j_2 k_2}) = 0$. It is also assumed that measurements in a subject are not independent, which means that error terms covary over time and domains within a subject. Therefore, the error for domain m_1 at time point j_1 covaries with the error for domain m_2 at time point j_2 (for domain $m_1 = 1$, 2, . . ., N_f; $m_2 = 1, 2, \ldots, N_f$; for time point $j_1 = 1, 2, \ldots, N_t$; $j_2 = 1, 2, \ldots, N_t$; if $j_1 = j_2$ then $m_1 \neq m_2$; if $m_1 = m_2$ then $j_1 \neq j_2$) with covariance $\operatorname{cov}(e_{im_1 j_1 k}, e_{im_2 j_2 k}) = \sigma_{m_1 m_2 j_1 j_2}$ for any subject i and treatment k.

To illustrate the implementation of the model to assess treatment differences simultaneously for all domains of a multi-domain scale, we will extend the simulated example from the previous Section 6.2.2.1 to include several domains. Now we assume that a scale has three domains and is collected, as previously, at baseline and at four post-baseline occasions. There are two treatments: active treatment and placebo. Overall, 600 subjects from the population of interest are "recruited" with 300 subjects per treatment arm.

The first step in the previous section was to generate "true" values (without error terms) for the outcome (see Figure 6.22). Now we need to do the same but run this code from Figure 6.22 three times (we have three domains) using different initial parameters to simulate different effects of the drug and time on those three domains. To minimize and simplify SAS code, the code from Figure 6.22 was converted into a function as a part of the earlier introduced LUA language (see Figure 6.28). The first run of the LUA procedure ("`proc lua` restart; . . .") defines the function, which is just a code from Figure 6.22 but made to be more general. The only difference is that most parameters that were hard coded

```
/* The first run of the LUA procedure */
proc lua restart;
submit;
--[[
Function CreateDomainScores simulates dataset with scores for a domain
ds                          - string variable representing the name of the output
dataset
UDomainID                   - string variable to identify a domain
NumberOfSubjectsPerTreatment - string variable representing number of subjects per
treatment arm
NumberOfVisits              - string variable representing number of visits
NumberOfTreatments          - string variable representing number of treatment
a                           - string variable representing intercept
d                           - string variable representing slope coefficient for
baseline value
TimeEffect                  - string variable representing array of the time
effects at week j=1,2,3,4
TreatmentEffect             - string variable representing array of the effect of
the treatments k=1,2
InteractionEffect           - string variable representing two-dimensial array of
the interaction effects between drugs and weeks
--]]

function CreateDomainScores(ds, UDomainID, NumberOfSubjectsPerTreatment,
NumberOfVisits, NumberOfTreatments, a, d, blmean, blvar, blseed, TimeEffect,
TreatmentEffect, InteractionEffect)

sas.submit[[
data @ds@;
Retain seed1 @blseed@ ;
Array b{1:4} (@TimeEffect@);
Array r{1:2} (@TreatmentEffect@);
Array g{1:2,1:4}
(
@InteractionEffect@
);

    ID=0;
    Do k=1 to @NumberOfTreatments@;
    Do i=1 To @NumberOfSubjectsPerTreatment@;
    ID=ID+1;
    Call rannor(seed1,e);
    x = @blmean@ + sqrt(@blvar@)*e;
        Do j=1 To @NumberOfVisits@;
        Y1     = @a@ + @d@*x + b[j] + r[k] +  g[k,j];
        Visit = j ; Treatment = k; Baseline = x;
        DomainID=@UDomainID@;
        Output;
        End;
    End;
    End;
Keep Y1 Baseline ID Visit Treatment DomainID;
run;
]]
end
endsubmit;
run;
```

Figure 6.28 Generating dataset with "true" outcomes for three domains at four time points.

```
/* The second run of the LUA procedure */
proc lua;
submit;
ds="Domain_1"
UDomainID="1"
NumberOfSubjectsPerTreatment="300"
NumberOfVisits="4"
NumberOfTreatments="2"
a="3"
d="0.07"
blmean="4"
blvar="0.1"
blseed="1"
TimeEffect="-0.25 -0.50 -0.75 0"
TreatmentEffect="-1.00 0"
InteractionEffect=
[[-0.10 -0.20 -0.30  0
   0.0   0.0   0.0   0.0]]
CreateDomainScores (ds, UDomainID,
NumberOfSubjectsPerTreatment, NumberOfVisits, NumberOfTreatments,
a, d, blmean, blvar, blseed,
TimeEffect, TreatmentEffect, InteractionEffect)

ds="Domain_2"
UDomainID="2"
NumberOfSubjectsPerTreatment="300"
NumberOfVisits="4"
NumberOfTreatments="2"
a="4"
d="0.05"
blmean="6"
blvar="0.2"
blseed="2"
TimeEffect="-0.45 -0.80 -0.8 0.0"
TreatmentEffect="-2.00 0.0"
InteractionEffect=
[[-0.15 -0.25 -0.35  0
   0.0   0.0   0.0   0.0]]
CreateDomainScores (ds, UDomainID,
NumberOfSubjectsPerTreatment, NumberOfVisits, NumberOfTreatments,
a, d, blmean, blvar, blseed,
TimeEffect, TreatmentEffect, InteractionEffect)

ds="Domain_3"
UDomainID="3"
NumberOfSubjectsPerTreatment="300"
NumberOfVisits="4"
NumberOfTreatments="2"
a="2"
d="0.02"
blmean="3"
blvar="0.1"
blseed="3"
TimeEffect="-0.3 -0.3 -0.4 0.0"
TreatmentEffect="-1.5 0.0"
InteractionEffect=
[[-0.2 -0.2 -0.3  0
   0.0  0.0  0.0  0.0]]

CreateDomainScores (ds, UDomainID,
NumberOfSubjectsPerTreatment, NumberOfVisits, NumberOfTreatments,
a, d, blmean, blvar, blseed,
TimeEffect, TreatmentEffect, InteractionEffect)
endsubmit;
Run;

Data Domains; Set Domain_1 Domain_2 Domain_3; Run;
Proc Sort Data=Domains; By ID DomainID Visit; Run;
Proc Print data=Domains NOOBS; Where ID=1;    Run;
```

Figure 6.28 *(Continued)*

ID	Y1	Visit	Treatment	Baseline	Domain ID
1	1.96995	1	1	4.57074	1
1	1.61995	2	1	4.57074	1
1	1.26995	3	1	4.57074	1
1	2.31995	4	1	4.57074	1
1	1.72933	1	1	6.58667	2
1	1.27933	2	1	6.58667	2
1	1.17933	3	1	6.58667	2
1	2.32933	4	1	6.58667	2
1	0.06580	1	1	3.29009	3
1	0.06580	2	1	3.29009	3
1	-0.13420	3	1	3.29009	3
1	0.56580	4	1	3.29009	3

Figure 6.29 Structure of the dataset for the simultaneous assessments of the multiple domains in longitudinal studies.

are now defined as input parameters. The additional variable DomainID is added into the output dataset to have an ability to identify a domain later in the analyses.

The second run of the LUA procedure ("**proc lua**; . . .") invokes the function CreateDomainScores three times with different input parameters (those parameters were discussed in the previous section; note that for the first domain we even kept the same parameters). The datastep "**Data** Domains;" summarizes simulated data for every domain into one dataset, and the SORT procedure ("**Proc Sort** Data=Domains; . . .") reorders data to position all data related to the same subject as one continuous block. After the code from Figure 6.28 is run, the dataset Domains (see Figure 6.29) will have the structure suitable for the MIXED procedure (data for the subject with *ID* = 1 are shown). Note that the data for the first domain are the same as in Figure 6.23.

As in the previous section, now we need to create a variance–covariance matrix to simulate error terms. But, for this particular case, we should first introduce a special type of variance–covariance matrix available as a part of the MIXED procedure. This type is UN@UN, which should be the part of the Repeated statement (Type= UN@UN; this symbolizes Kronecker product of two matrices). In our simulation this overall variance–covariance matrix is created by taking the Kronecker product of two variance–covariance matrixes: the first one models covariance across domains and the second one models covariance across time.

Figure 6.30 shows how an overall variance–covariance matrix is created based on the two matrices. In the previous section, we demonstrated how the variance–covariance matrix can be calculated based on the correlation matrix and an accompanying vector with standard deviations. Here, though, two variance–covariance matrixes (matrix cov1 and matrix cov2) are created based on the correlation matrixes corr1 and corr2 and standard deviation vectors SD1 and SD2. The first matrix cov1 corresponds to the three domains, and the second matrix cov2 is tied to the time structure of the data. It is important to note that these two matrices by themselves do not represent relationships between error terms but rather serve as building blocks to create overall

```
Proc IML;
corr1 = {1         0.6        0.7,
            0.6      1          0.8,
            0.7      0.8        1 };
SD1 = {0.2   0.3   0.25};
cov1=diag(SD1)*corr1*diag(SD1);

corr2 = {1         0.5        0.4        0.3,
            0.5      1          0.5        0.4,
            0.4      0.5        1          0.5,
            0.3      0.4        0.5        1 };
SD2 = {0.2       0.3        0.25       0.15};
cov2=diag(SD2)*corr2*diag(SD2);

cov_Kronecker = cov1@cov2; corr_Kronecker = corr1@corr2;
print cov1; print cov2; print corr_Kronecker; print cov_Kronecker;
Quit;
```

Figure 6.30 Creating an overall variance–covariance matrix.

variance–covariance matrices with a certain structure (Galecki 1994). Figure 6.31 shows the resultant individual covariance matrices (cov1, cov2), as well as the overall correlation matrix corr_Kronecker and the overall variance–covariance matrix cov_Kronecker.

Now we can finalize the simulated dataset (see Figure 6.32). It is practically the same code as in Figure 6.26, but now the covariance matrix in the first datastep ("**data** _cov_(type=cov);...") is taken from the Figure 6.31. As a result, the SIMNORMAL procedure will generate 12 random errors for every subject: the first four errors are associated with the first domain at four postbaseline time points, the second four errors are associated with the second domain, and the last four errors are associated with the third domain. The structure of this final dataset is the same as presented by Figure 6.29 with variable Ymijk representing simulated measurement scores for the three domains.

The final step in this simulated example is the modeling of those data using the MIXED procedure to unravel the parameters of the model. Figure 6.33 represents the implementation of the model. In the previous Section 6.2.2.1 (Figure 6.26), the Model statement for one domain was expressed as follows:

```
Model Yijk = Baseline Visit Treatment Visit*Treatment /
solution ddfm=kr; .
```

To estimate a different set of parameters for every domain, though, we need to have an additional term in the Model statement with DomainID as the fixed effect. And all other terms in the Model statement are now represented as interaction terms with variable DomainID.

Another distinction is that the NOINT option is now added as a part of the Model statement (Figure 6.33). This NOINT option excludes the fixed-effect intercept from the modeling. Generally, it is not recommended to exclude the intercept term from regression models (which sometimes can be done if there are some

cov1

$$
\begin{array}{ccc}
0.04 & 0.036 & 0.035 \\
0.036 & 0.09 & 0.06 \\
0.035 & 0.06 & 0.0625
\end{array}
$$

cov2

$$
\begin{array}{cccc}
0.04 & 0.03 & 0.02 & 0.009 \\
0.03 & 0.09 & 0.0375 & 0.018 \\
0.02 & 0.0375 & 0.0625 & 0.01875 \\
0.009 & 0.018 & 0.01875 & 0.0225
\end{array}
$$

corr_Kronecker

$$
\begin{array}{cccccccccccc}
1 & 0.5 & 0.4 & 0.3 & 0.6 & 0.3 & 0.24 & 0.18 & 0.7 & 0.35 & 0.28 & 0.21 \\
0.5 & 1 & 0.5 & 0.4 & 0.3 & 0.6 & 0.3 & 0.24 & 0.35 & 0.7 & 0.35 & 0.28 \\
0.4 & 0.5 & 1 & 0.5 & 0.24 & 0.3 & 0.6 & 0.3 & 0.28 & 0.35 & 0.7 & 0.35 \\
0.3 & 0.4 & 0.5 & 1 & 0.18 & 0.24 & 0.3 & 0.6 & 0.21 & 0.28 & 0.35 & 0.7 \\
0.6 & 0.3 & 0.24 & 0.18 & 1 & 0.5 & 0.4 & 0.3 & 0.8 & 0.4 & 0.32 & 0.24 \\
0.3 & 0.6 & 0.3 & 0.24 & 0.5 & 1 & 0.5 & 0.4 & 0.4 & 0.8 & 0.4 & 0.32 \\
0.24 & 0.3 & 0.6 & 0.3 & 0.4 & 0.5 & 1 & 0.5 & 0.32 & 0.4 & 0.8 & 0.4 \\
0.18 & 0.24 & 0.3 & 0.6 & 0.3 & 0.4 & 0.5 & 1 & 0.24 & 0.32 & 0.4 & 0.8 \\
0.7 & 0.35 & 0.28 & 0.21 & 0.8 & 0.4 & 0.32 & 0.24 & 1 & 0.5 & 0.4 & 0.3 \\
0.35 & 0.7 & 0.35 & 0.28 & 0.4 & 0.8 & 0.4 & 0.32 & 0.5 & 1 & 0.5 & 0.4 \\
0.28 & 0.35 & 0.7 & 0.35 & 0.32 & 0.4 & 0.8 & 0.4 & 0.4 & 0.5 & 1 & 0.5 \\
0.21 & 0.28 & 0.35 & 0.7 & 0.24 & 0.32 & 0.4 & 0.8 & 0.3 & 0.4 & 0.5 & 1
\end{array}
$$

cov_Kronecker

$$
\begin{array}{cccccccccccc}
0.0016 & 0.0012 & 0.0008 & 0.00036 & 0.00144 & 0.00108 & 0.00072 & 0.000324 & 0.0014 & 0.00105 & 0.0007 & 0.000315 \\
0.0012 & 0.0036 & 0.0015 & 0.00072 & 0.00108 & 0.00324 & 0.00135 & 0.000648 & 0.00105 & 0.00315 & 0.0013125 & 0.00063 \\
0.0008 & 0.0015 & 0.0025 & 0.00075 & 0.00072 & 0.00135 & 0.00225 & 0.000675 & 0.0007 & 0.0013125 & 0.0021875 & 0.0006563 \\
0.00036 & 0.00072 & 0.00075 & 0.0009 & 0.000324 & 0.000648 & 0.000675 & 0.00081 & 0.000315 & 0.00063 & 0.0006563 & 0.0007875 \\
0.00144 & 0.00108 & 0.00072 & 0.000324 & 0.0036 & 0.0027 & 0.0018 & 0.00081 & 0.0024 & 0.0018 & 0.0012 & 0.00054 \\
0.00108 & 0.00324 & 0.00135 & 0.000648 & 0.0027 & 0.0081 & 0.003375 & 0.00162 & 0.0018 & 0.0054 & 0.00225 & 0.00108 \\
0.00072 & 0.00135 & 0.00225 & 0.000675 & 0.0018 & 0.003375 & 0.005625 & 0.0016875 & 0.0012 & 0.00225 & 0.00375 & 0.001125 \\
0.000324 & 0.000648 & 0.000675 & 0.00081 & 0.00081 & 0.00162 & 0.0016875 & 0.002025 & 0.00054 & 0.00108 & 0.001125 & 0.00135 \\
0.0014 & 0.00105 & 0.0007 & 0.000315 & 0.0024 & 0.0018 & 0.0012 & 0.00054 & 0.0025 & 0.001875 & 0.00125 & 0.0005625 \\
0.00105 & 0.00315 & 0.0013125 & 0.00063 & 0.0018 & 0.0054 & 0.00225 & 0.00108 & 0.001875 & 0.005625 & 0.0023438 & 0.001125 \\
0.0007 & 0.0013125 & 0.0021875 & 0.0006563 & 0.0012 & 0.00225 & 0.00375 & 0.001125 & 0.00125 & 0.0023438 & 0.0039063 & 0.0011719 \\
0.000315 & 0.00063 & 0.0006563 & 0.0007875 & 0.00054 & 0.00108 & 0.001125 & 0.00135 & 0.0005625 & 0.001125 & 0.0011719 & 0.0014063
\end{array}
$$

Figure 6.31 Matrices produced by the IML procedure (from Figure 6.30).

```
data _cov_ (type=cov);
input
_TYPE_ $ _NAME_ $ COL1 ... COL12;
datalines;
```

TYPE	_NAME_	COL1	COL2	COL3	COL4	COL5	COL6	COL7	COL8	COL9	COL10	COL11	COL12
COV	COL1	0.0016	0.0012	0.0008	0.00036	0.00144	0.00108	0.00072	0.000324	0.0014	0.00105	0.0007	0.000315
COV	COL2	0.0012	0.0036	0.0015	0.00072	0.00108	0.00324	0.00135	0.000648	0.00105	0.00315	0.0013125	0.00063
COV	COL3	0.0008	0.0015	0.0025	0.00075	0.00072	0.00135	0.00225	0.000675	0.0007	0.0013125	0.0021875	0.0006563
COV	COL4	0.00036	0.00072	0.00075	0.0009	0.000324	0.000648	0.000675	0.00081	0.000315	0.00063	0.0006563	0.0007875
COV	COL5	0.00144	0.00108	0.00072	0.000324	0.0036	0.0027	0.0018	0.00081	0.0024	0.0018	0.0012	0.00054
COV	COL6	0.00108	0.00324	0.00135	0.000648	0.0027	0.0081	0.003375	0.00162	0.0018	0.0054	0.00225	0.00108
COV	COL7	0.00072	0.00135	0.00225	0.000675	0.0018	0.003375	0.005625	0.0016875	0.0012	0.00225	0.00375	0.001125
COV	COL8	0.000324	0.000648	0.000675	0.00081	0.00081	0.00162	0.0016875	0.002025	0.00054	0.00108	0.001125	0.00135
COV	COL9	0.0014	0.00105	0.0007	0.000315	0.0024	0.0018	0.0012	0.00054	0.0025	0.001875	0.00125	0.0005625
COV	COL10	0.00105	0.00315	0.0013125	0.00063	0.0018	0.0054	0.00225	0.00108	0.001875	0.005625	0.0023438	0.001125
COV	COL11	0.0007	0.0013125	0.0021875	0.0006563	0.0012	0.00225	0.00375	0.001125	0.00125	0.0023438	0.0039063	0.0011719
COV	COL12	0.000315	0.00063	0.0006563	0.0007875	0.00054	0.00108	0.001125	0.00135	0.0005625	0.001125	0.0011719	0.0014063
MEAN	.	.	.	.	.	0	0	0	0	0	0	0	0
N	.	600	600	600	600	600	600	600	600	600	600	600	600

```
;
run;
Proc Simnormal data=_cov_ out=err_sim numreal=600 seed=12345; var Col1-Col12; Run;
proc corr data=err_sim COV ; Var Col1-Col12;Run;
Proc Transpose data=err_sim out=err_sim_tr; Var Col1-Col12; By Rnum; Run;
Data _errors_; Set err_sim_tr;
ID= Rnum; E1=Col1;
Keep ID E1;
Run;
Data mixed_ds1;
Merge Domains _errors_;
Ymijk=Y1+E1;
By ID;
Keep Ymijk Baseline ID Visit Treatment DomainID;
Run;
```

Figure 6.32   Generating simulated dataset with three domains and four time points.

```
Proc Mixed data=mixed_ds1;
Class Visit Treatment ID DomainID;
Model Ymijk = DomainID DomainID*Baseline DomainID*Visit DomainID*Treatment
DomainID*Visit*Treatment / solution NOINT ddfm=kr;
Repeated DomainID Visit / Subject=ID Type=UN@UN R rcorr;
LSMeans DomainID*Treatment DomainID*Treatment DomainID*Visit*Treatment / cl diff;
Run;
```

Figure 6.33 Model implementation for the simultaneous assessment of the several domains in longitudinal studies.

theoretical reasons for it; however, note also that model parameters will likely be biased). For this model, we can actually keep this overall fixed-effect intercept (by not adding NOINT option) or we can add the NOINT option and, as a result, be able to simplify comparison of the simulated vs. estimated parameters. As such, we choose to do the later here (add the NOINT option) because we, in fact, included fixed-effect intercepts for the domains as part of the regression models, which are represented by the variable DomainID as the first term of the Model statement.

Special attention should be paid to the Repeated statement. The two variables DomainID and Visit are included to describe repeated effects. Their relative position can be important in certain situations and should correspond to the Type option. For example, for this model, we use Type = UN@UN and for current Repeated statement

Repeated DomainID Visit / Subject=ID Type=UN@UN R rcorr;

the order of repeated effects is not important because the variance–covariance matrix is represented by UN@UN. But the MIXED procedure also has two additional more simple structures, which are also based on the Kronecker product of two matrices: UN@AR(1) and UN@CS. If either of these structures is considered, then the first repeated effect (as a part of the Repeated statement) should always represent domains and the second should always represent time. In other words, the matrix associated with domains should always be represented by the unstructured variance–covariance matrix, while the matrix associated with time can vary.

Figures 6.34 and 6.35 represent partial outputs with the results generated by the model from Figure 6.33. The first matrix (titled "**Estimated R Matrix for ID 1**") in Figure 6.34 shows the estimated variance–covariance; the second matrix (titled "**Estimated R Correlation Matrix for ID 1**") shows the estimated correlation matrix. Comparing those two matrices with the matrix "**cov_Kronecker**" and "**corr_Kronecker**" from Figure 6.31, we can see that the estimated matrixes are numerically close to the matrices used to simulate data. The third part of the output in Figure 6.34 (titled "**Covariance Parameter Estimates**") shows the estimated covariances corresponding to domains and

Estimated R Matrix for ID 1

Row	Col1	Col2	Col3	Col4	Col5	Col6	Col7	Col8	Col9	Col10	Col11	Col12
1	0.001647	0.001197	0.000867	0.000396	0.001512	0.001099	0.000796	0.000364	0.001446	0.001051	0.000761	0.000348
2	0.001197	0.003461	0.001493	0.000683	0.001099	0.003178	0.001371	0.000627	0.001051	0.003038	0.001310	0.000599
3	0.000867	0.001493	0.002580	0.000751	0.000796	0.001371	0.002368	0.000690	0.000761	0.001310	0.002264	0.000659
4	0.000396	0.000683	0.000751	0.000901	0.000364	0.000627	0.000690	0.000827	0.000348	0.000599	0.000659	0.000791
5	0.001512	0.001099	0.000796	0.000364	0.003798	0.002761	0.001999	0.000914	0.002496	0.001814	0.001313	0.000601
6	0.001099	0.003178	0.001371	0.000627	0.002761	0.007981	0.003443	0.001574	0.001814	0.005244	0.002262	0.001034
7	0.000796	0.001371	0.002368	0.000690	0.001999	0.003443	0.005949	0.001733	0.001313	0.002262	0.003909	0.001138
8	0.000364	0.000627	0.000690	0.000827	0.000914	0.001574	0.001733	0.002077	0.000601	0.001034	0.001138	0.001365
9	0.001446	0.001051	0.000761	0.000348	0.002496	0.001814	0.001313	0.000601	0.002545	0.001850	0.001339	0.000612
10	0.001051	0.003038	0.001310	0.000599	0.001814	0.005244	0.002262	0.001034	0.001850	0.005347	0.002306	0.001054
11	0.000761	0.001310	0.002264	0.000659	0.001313	0.002262	0.003909	0.001138	0.001339	0.002306	0.003986	0.001161
12	0.000348	0.000599	0.000659	0.000791	0.000601	0.001034	0.001138	0.001365	0.000612	0.001054	0.001161	0.001392

Estimated R Correlation Matrix for ID 1

Row	Col1	Col2	Col3	Col4	Col5	Col6	Col7	Col8	Col9	Col10	Col11	Col12
1	1.0000	0.5015	0.4205	0.3254	0.6045	0.3032	0.2542	0.1967	0.7061	0.3541	0.2969	0.2298
2	0.5015	1.0000	0.4996	0.3865	0.3032	0.6045	0.3020	0.2337	0.3541	0.7061	0.3528	0.2729
3	0.4205	0.4996	1.0000	0.4929	0.2542	0.3020	0.6045	0.2980	0.2969	0.3528	0.7061	0.3480
4	0.3254	0.3865	0.4929	1.0000	0.1967	0.2337	0.2980	0.6045	0.2298	0.2729	0.3480	0.7061
5	0.6045	0.3032	0.2542	0.1967	1.0000	0.5015	0.4205	0.3254	0.8028	0.4026	0.3376	0.2612
6	0.3032	0.6045	0.3020	0.2337	0.5015	1.0000	0.4996	0.3865	0.4026	0.8028	0.4011	0.3103
7	0.2542	0.3020	0.6045	0.2980	0.4205	0.4996	1.0000	0.4929	0.3376	0.4011	0.8028	0.3957
8	0.1967	0.2337	0.2980	0.6045	0.3254	0.3865	0.4929	1.0000	0.2612	0.3103	0.3957	0.8028
9	0.7061	0.3541	0.2969	0.2298	0.8028	0.4026	0.3376	0.2612	1.0000	0.5015	0.4205	0.3254
10	0.3541	0.7061	0.3528	0.2729	0.4026	0.8028	0.4011	0.3103	0.5015	1.0000	0.4996	0.3865
11	0.2969	0.3528	0.7061	0.3480	0.3376	0.4011	0.8028	0.3957	0.4205	0.4996	1.0000	0.4929
12	0.2298	0.2729	0.3480	0.7061	0.2612	0.3103	0.3957	0.8028	0.3254	0.3865	0.4929	1.0000

Covariance Parameter Estimates

Cov Parm		Subject	Estimate
DomainID	UN(1,1)	ID	0.001647
	UN(2,1)	ID	0.001512
	UN(2,2)	ID	0.003798
	UN(3,1)	ID	0.001446
	UN(3,2)	ID	0.002496
	UN(3,3)	ID	0.002545
Visit	UN(1,1)	ID	1.0000
	UN(2,1)	ID	0.7269
	UN(2,2)	ID	2.1014
	UN(3,1)	ID	0.5263
	UN(3,2)	ID	0.9064
	UN(3,3)	ID	1.5662
	UN(4,1)	ID	0.2407
	UN(4,2)	ID	0.4144
	UN(4,3)	ID	0.4562
	UN(4,4)	ID	0.5469

Figure 6.34 Estimated covariance and correlation matrices.

Solution for Fixed Effects								
Effect	Visit	Treatment	Domain ID	Estimate	Standard Error	DF	t Value	Pr > |t|
DomainID			1	2.9959	0.01035	1210	289.53	<.0001
DomainID			2	3.9853	0.01386	1217	287.53	<.0001
DomainID			3	2.0093	0.007419	1287	270.82	<.0001
Baseline*DomainID			1	0.07121	0.002541	1187	28.03	<.0001
Baseline*DomainID			2	0.05243	0.002276	1180	23.04	<.0001
Baseline*DomainID			3	0.01756	0.002341	1192	7.50	<.0001
Visit*DomainID	1		1	-0.2510	0.002419	1231	-103.75	<.0001
Visit*DomainID	1		2	-0.4499	0.003674	1197	-122.45	<.0001
Visit*DomainID	1		3	-0.3024	0.003007	1205	-100.57	<.0001
Visit*DomainID	2		1	-0.5047	0.003162	1208	-159.59	<.0001
Visit*DomainID	2		2	-0.8063	0.004802	1218	-167.90	<.0001
Visit*DomainID	2		3	-0.3049	0.003930	1197	-77.58	<.0001
Visit*DomainID	3		1	-0.7491	0.002569	1194	-291.60	<.0001
Visit*DomainID	3		2	-0.7992	0.003901	1180	-204.86	<.0001
Visit*DomainID	3		3	-0.4001	0.003193	1176	-125.29	<.0001
Visit*DomainID	4		1	0	.	.	.	.
Visit*DomainID	4		2	0	.	.	.	.
Visit*DomainID	4		3	0	.	.	.	.
Treatment*DomainID		1	1	-1.0013	0.002453	1190	-408.23	<.0001
Treatment*DomainID		1	2	-1.9985	0.003724	1214	-536.66	<.0001
Treatment*DomainID		1	3	-1.5012	0.003049	1224	-492.35	<.0001
Treatment*DomainID		2	1	0	.	.	.	.
Treatment*DomainID		2	2	0	.	.	.	.
Treatment*DomainID		2	3	0	.	.	.	.

Figure 6.35 Estimated model parameters (partial output).

time points. The first set of estimated covariances (from Figure 6.34) associated with domains can be expressed as a 3×3 matrix:

$$D = \begin{bmatrix} 0.001647 & 0.001512 & 0.001446 \\ 0.001512 & 0.003798 & 0.002496 \\ 0.001446 & 0.002496 & 0.002545 \end{bmatrix}.$$

The second set of estimated covariances (from Figure 6.34) corresponds to the time structure of the data and can be expressed as a 4×4 matrix:

$$T = \begin{bmatrix} 1.0000 & 0.7269 & 0.5263 & 0.2407 \\ 0.7269 & 2.1014 & 0.9064 & 0.4144 \\ 0.5263 & 0.9064 & 1.5662 & 0.4562 \\ 0.2407 & 0.4144 & 0.4562 & 0.5469 \end{bmatrix}.$$

If we perform a direct (Kronecker) multiplication of the matrices D and T (see Figure 6.36 for the IML procedure code), the resultant matrix will be identical to

```
Proc IML;
cov1 = {0.001647 0.001512 0.001446,
        0.001512 0.003798 0.002496,
        0.001446 0.002496 0.002545};
cov2 = {1.0000 0.7269 0.5263 0.2407,
        0.7269 2.1014 0.9064 0.4144,
        0.5263 0.9064 1.5662 0.4562,
        0.2407 0.4144 0.4562 0.5469};
cov_Kronecker = cov1@cov2;
print cov_Kronecker;
Quit;
```

Figure 6.36 Estimating the direct product based on the "**Covariance Parameter Estimates**".

the estimated variance–covariance matrix in Figure 6.34 (as it should). Then the "logical assumption" is that those estimated matrices D and T should be numerically close to the initial matrixes "`cov1`" and "`cov2`" in Figure 6.31, but they do not. This result highlights an important property of the direct product of two matrixes: There are an infinite number of different two matrixes that can produce exactly the same direct product.

For that reason, to make the model identifiable, the MIXED procedure sets the upper left value in the second matrix to be equal to 1 (as it was done for estimated matrix T). The important consequence is that those "`Covariance Parameter Estimates`" should not be overinterpreted. They are simply building blocks to create a variance–covariance matrix with a specific structure, with the understanding that those two estimated matrices separately do not provide numerically pertinent information on domains or time points. In other words, the MIXED procedure was not able to decipher two matrices we used to simulate data. And the same can be said for real-life analyses.

Figure 6.35 displays the partial output for the other parameters of the model – all those estimated parameters are numerically close to the values we use to simulate data. For example, in Figure 6.28 the following line was used to define the time effect for the first domain:

```
TimeEffect="-0.25 -0.50 -0.75 0".
```

In Figure 6.35 the estimated values for the time effect are represented by the interaction effect "`Visit*DomainID`" with two additional descriptors "`Visit`" and "`DomainID`". For the first domain associated with the four time points, those respective estimated parameters are represented (in time order) by following the values $-0.2510, -0.5047, -0.7491, 0$, which are nearly identical to the initial values used in the simulation.

Earlier we mentioned that there are two additional more simple variance–covariance structures available for the analyses. The UN@UN structure is more general and can and should be used when data are collected at uneven intervals, but it also requires more parameters to estimate, which in turn can lead to the convergence criteria being not met. For example, in the above simulation 16 covariance parameters need to be estimated (number of unique elements in both matrixes D and T). In a case of a sizable number of the post-baseline observations and a scale with many domains, the number of covariance parameters can grow very rapidly. To overcome this, the structure UN@AR(1) can be used if data are collected frequently and at the same intervals. In the above simulation defining the option Type=UN@AR(1), added as a part of the Repeated statement, will lead to the need to estimate only seven covariance parameters (number of unique elements in the matrix D, which is 6, and just one parameter needed to define the AR(1) structure).

In the above simulation, the eventual variance–covariance structure (repre-sented by matrix "`cov_Kronecker`" in Figure 6.31) is based on the assumption that we can simplify modeling of relationships among domains and time through the direct product of the two distinct matrixes. The completely general approach can be also considered where there are no predefined assumptions about the variance–covariance matrix. To implement this model, we need to create an iden-tifier for every unique combination of domain and time, which will be used as a part of the `Repeated` statement. Recall that in the simulation the variable `Visit` is represented by integers from 1 to 4, and the variable `DomainID` is represented by integers from 1 to 3. Hence the new variable `DomainVisit` can be created as:

$$DomainVisit = DomainID \times 10 + Visit.$$

For example, observations for the first domain and first visit will be then identi-fied by `DomainVisit=11`.

Figure 6.37 represents implementation of the completely general model. The first datastep ("`Data mixed_ds2;...`") adds the variable `DomainVisit` into the dataset to uniquely identify domain and time point using only one variable. To construct this model with the MIXED procedure, the newly created variable `DomainVisit` is used as a part of the `Repeated` statement to specify the repeated effect. (Note that `DomainVisit` is added in the `Class` statement also, since only categorical variables can be used to define repeated effects.)

For this general model, only one option for the variance–covariance matrix can be used, which is unstructured and given by `Type=UN`. The use of any other vari-ance–covariance structures will be inappropriate, since we model domains and time simultaneously. Note that in this example, the number of covariance param-eters needed to be estimated is 78 – a significant increase (78 represents the num-ber of unique elements for a symmetrical 12×12 matrix based on three domains crossed with four time points); see, as an example, the matrix "`Estimated R Matrix for ID 1`" in Figure 6.34).

In this section, we focused on various parameters of the simulated data and the implementation of the model to uncover those parameters. But in a real-life

```
Data mixed_ds2; Set mixed_ds1;
DomainVisit=DomainID*10+Visit;
Run;

Proc Mixed data=mixed_ds2;
Class Visit Treatment ID DomainID DomainVisit;
Model Ymijk = DomainID DomainID*Baseline DomainID*Visit DomainID*Treatment
DomainID*Visit*Treatment / solution NOINT ddfm=kr;
Repeated DomainVisit / Subject=ID Type=UN R rcorr;
LSMeans DomainID*Treatment DomainID*Visit*Treatment / cl diff;
Run;
```

Figure 6.37 Implementation of the completely general model.

situation, interest will likely center on treatment differences. Are the domain scores for one treatment significantly different from another treatment? Are those differences meaningful? In implementations represented by Figures 6.33 and 6.37, the answer to those questions is based on the following LSMeans statement

```
LSMeans DomainID*Treatment DomainID*Visit*Treatment / cl
diff;
```

and will be discussed at length in the next chapter.

6.3 Summary

In this chapter, the ability to detect change (responsiveness) is described in detail, both conceptually and methodologically, and is based on three core principles: (i) change in the target COA (or PRO) scores need to be compared with change in similar measures, (ii) the target COA is sensitive to gains and losses in the concept of measurement, and (iii) such gains and losses in the instrument should be examined for the entire possible range of scores in the population of interest. Grounded in this framework, an analytic model-based implementation on the ability to detect change is presented and quantified for the relationship between changes in the target scale and changes in the anchor scale, which serves as a similar measure. Next, it is shown that correlational analysis by itself may not be enough to provide sufficient evidence of an instrument's ability to detect change and, therefore, should be limited to an ancillary role in this regard. It is also shown that the correlation between score changes between a pair of variables, such as a target COA and an anchor measure, is a complicated function of a set of cross-sectional and longitudinal correlations. Therefore, correlations between score changes on a pair of variables may provide only adjunct evidence on the ability to detect change on a target COA.

The second theme of this chapter, related to the first theme on responsiveness, is an instrument's sensitivity to treatment effects, whose exposition is highlighted and informed through subject matter knowledge, empirical (published) applications, and model-based (simulated) illustrations. Several key facets on the COA's (or PRO's) context of use are needed to ensure that the instrument meets standards for sensitivity to treatment effects. Among them are elements particular to the measure itself, such as its recall period; the study design, such as when and how often COA measurements should be taken; and the structural validity and accompanying scoring of the COA, such as which items go with which domains and how domains are scored. Knowledge of the instrument and its context of use are relevant to understand which domains of a multi-item scale will respond (or not respond) and in which direction (improvement or worsening) to an intervention. Lastly, the chapter provides a framework and an implementation of applying one unified multi-domain longitudinal model, intended for a scale with multiple domains assessed over time, as a way to assess treatment effects and increase the efficiency of the analyses.

References

Bushmakin, A.G., Cappelleri, J.C., Symonds, T., and Stecher, V.J. (2013). Multi-domain longitudinal modeling: an application to the International Index of Erectile Function. *Therapeutic Innovation & Regulatory Science* 47: 57–64.

Cappelleri, J.C., Bushmakin, A.G., Baker, C.L. et al. (2005). Revealing the multidimensional framework of the minnesota nicotine withdrawal scale. *Current Medical Research and Opinion* 21: 749–760.

Cappelleri, J.C., Zou, K.H., Bushmakin, A.G. et al. (2013). *Patient-Reported Outcomes: Measurement, Implementation and Interpretation*. Boca Raton, FL: Chapman & Hall/CRC Press.

Cella, D., Li, J.Z., Cappelleri, J.C. et al. (2008). Quality of life in patients with metastatic renal cell carcinoma treated with sunitinib versus interferon-alfa: results from a phase III randomized trial. *Journal of Clinical Oncology* 26: 3763–3769.

Cohen, J., Cohen, P., West, S.G., and Aiken, L.S. (2003). *Applied Multiple Regression/Correlation Analysis for the Behavioral Sciences*, 3e. Mahwah, NJ: Lawrence Erlbaum Associates.

Cronbach, L.J. and Furby, L. (1970). How should we measure "change" – or should we? *Psychological Bulletin* 74: 414–417.

de Boer, M.R., Terwee, C.B., de Vet, H.C. et al. (2006). Evaluation of cross-sectional and longitudinal construct validity of two vision-related quality of life questionnaires: the LVQOL and VCM1. *Quality of Life Research* 15: 233–248.

Fairclough, D.L. (2010). *Design and Analysis of Quality of Life Studies in Clinical Trials*, 2e. Boca Raton, FL: Chapman & Hall/CRC.

Farivar, S.S., Liu, H., and Hays, R.D. (2004). Another look at the half standard deviation estimate of the minimally important difference in health-related quality of life scores. *Expert Review of Pharmacoeconomics & Outcomes Research* 4: 515–523.

FDA (Food and Drug Administration) (2019). Patient-focused drug development guidance series for enhancing the incorporation of the patient's voice in medical product development and regulatory decision making. Draft Guidance Documents. https://www.fda.gov/drugs/development-approval-process-drugs/fda-patient-focused-drug-development-guidance-series-enhancing-incorporation-patients-voice-medical (accessed 15 April 2020).

Fitzmaurice, G.M., Laird, N.M., and Ware, J.H. (2011). *Applied Longitudinal Analysis*, 2e. Hoboken, NJ: Wiley.

Galecki, A.T. (1994). General class of covariance structures for two or more repeated factors in longitudinal data analysis. *Communications in Statistics – Theory and Methods* 23: 3105–3109.

Gonzales, D., Rennard, S., Nides, M. et al. (2006). Varenicline, an α4β2 nicotine acetylcholine receptor partial agonist, vs sustained-release bupropion and placebo for smoking cessation: a randomized controlled trial. *JAMA* 296: 47–55.

Griffin, D., Murray, S., and Gonzalez, R. (1999). Difference score correlations in relationship: a conceptual primer. *Personal Relationships* 6: 505–518.

Husted, J.A., Cook, R.J., Farewell, V.T., and Gladman, D.D. (2000). Methods for assessing responsiveness: a critical review and recommendations. *Journal of Clinical Epidemiology* 53: 459–468.

Jorenby, D.E., Hays, J.T., Rigotti, N.A. et al. (2006). Efficacy of varenicline, an α4β2 nicotinic acetylcholine receptor partial agonist, vs placebo or sustained-released buproprion for smoking cessation: a randomized controlled trial. *JAMA* 296: 56–63.

Mokkink, L.B., Terwee, C.B., Knol, D.L. et al. (2010). The COSMIN checklist for evaluating the methodological quality of studies on measurement properties: a clarification of content. *BMC Medical Research Methodology* 10: 22.

Norman, G.R., Sloan, J.A., and Wyrwich, K.W. (2004). The truly remarkable universality of a half a standard deviation: confirmation through another look. *Expert Review of Pharmacoeconomics & Outcomes Research* 4: 581–585.

Rosen, R.C., Riley, A., Wagner, G. et al. (1997). The international index of erectile function (IIEF): a multidimensional scale for assessment of erectile dysfunction. *Urology* 49: 822–830.

Rosen, R.C., Cappelleri, J.C., and Gendrano, N. (2002). The International index of erectile function (IIEF): a state-of-the-science review. *International Journal of Impotence Research* 14: 226–244.

Russell, I.J., Crofford, L.J., Leon, T. et al. (2009). The effects of pregabalin on sleep disturbance symptoms among individuals with fibromyalgia syndrome. *Sleep Medicine* 10: 604–610.

Singer, J.D. and Willett, J.B. (2003). *Applied Longitudinal Data Analysis: Modeling Change and Event Occurrence*. New York: Oxford University Press.

Vincent, J.I., Macdermid, J.C., King, G.J.W., and Grewal, R. (2013). Validity and sensitivity to change of patient-reported pain and disability measures for elbow pathologies. *Journal of Orthopaedic & Sports Physical Therapy* 43: 263–274.

Ware, J.E. Jr., Kosinski, M., Bjorner, J.B. et al. (2007). *User's Manual for the SF-36v2® Health Survey*, 2e. Lincoln, RI: QualityMetric.

7

Interpretation of Patient-Reported Outcome Findings

As discussed previously, to be useful to patients and decision-makers (e.g., physicians, regulatory agencies, reimbursement authorities), PRO measures in particular, and COA measures in general, must undergo a validation process to confirm that it is measuring what it is supposed to be measuring and undergo reliability testing to ensure it is reliably measuring what it is intended to measure. But more is needed: PRO (and COA) results must also be interpreted by attaching meaning to them (Cappelleri and Bushmakin 2014; Cappelleri et al. 2013; Cocks et al. 2008; Coon and Cook 2018; de Vet et al. 2011; Marquis et al. 2004; Revicki et al. 2007; Schünemann et al. 2006).

Unlike well-established clinical measurements such as survival and blood pressure, which are generally understood and can be measured directly, the latent (unobserved) concepts captured by PROs (and COAs in general) may be unfamiliar to many healthcare professionals and patients (Cappelleri et al. 2013). Patient-reported outcomes have been used to define and operationalize (through their constitute observed items) latent concepts such as physical functioning or emotional well-being. Unlike survival and blood pressure, there may be insufficient data available or lack of experience or clinical understanding to draw from to properly interpret what, for example, a five-point change means on a 0–100 PRO scale.

Given the prevalence and influence of PROs in medical care, especially in chronic diseases, interpretation of scores and changes in scores from PROs is crucial for understanding the meaning and relevance of these scores for effective decision-making. Useful interpretation of score values (e.g., score values above a certain threshold are considered a successful response) or score changes (e.g., change from baseline to end of study above a certain threshold is considered meaningful improvement) can be valuable in designing studies, evaluating

A Practical Approach to Quantitative Validation of Patient-Reported Outcomes: A Simulation-Based Guide Using SAS, First Edition. Andrew G. Bushmakin and Joseph C. Cappelleri.
© 2023 John Wiley & Sons, Inc. Published 2023 by John Wiley & Sons, Inc.

interventions, educating consumers, and informing health policy makers involved with regulatory, reimbursement, and advisory agencies.

Thus, an inherent and a fundamental issue for PRO measures in particular and COA measures in general centers on the interpretation and meaning of their scores, especially relevant for evaluating the effect of treatment interventions on the concept of interest measured by the PRO and COA measures. Are the scores clinically meaningful? What are the analytic frameworks to determine clinically relevance of PRO and COA scores? In this chapter, the logic and rationale for some of those methods are expressed conceptually, analytically, and computationally through meaningful within-patient change (MWPC) (Section 7.1), clinically important difference (Section 7.2), and responder analysis and cumulative distribution functions (Section 7.3).

7.1 Meaningful Within-Patient Change

7.1.1 Definitions and Concepts

After a study is finalized and treatment effects have been estimated, then the next important step is to understand whether those treatment effects are not only statistically significant but also clinically relevant. "Statistical significance can be achieved for small differences between comparator groups, but this finding does not indicate whether individual patients have experienced meaningful clinical benefit." (FDA 2019).

Unfortunately, historically in the medical literature and other documented sources, there is a discordance on the terminology and methods related on what constitutes meaningful change for an individual patient. Typically, two different types of threshold scores can be established for a target PRO or COA of interest. The first is referenced as minimal clinically important difference (MCID), minimal important difference (MID), clinically important difference (CID), or variations thereof, and linked to the interpretation of the between-group mean difference, commonly used to evaluate treatment difference between two interventions (Coon and Cappelleri 2016; Farivar et al. 2004; King 2011; Mamolo et al. 2015; Maruish 2011; McLeod et al. 2016; McGlothin and Lewis 2014). The second type of threshold is referenced as responder definition (RD) (FDA 2009; Vanier et al. 2021), clinically important responders (CIR) (Coon and Cappelleri 2016; Mamolo et al. 2015), significant change (SC) (Ware et al. 2007), and MWPC (Conaghan et al. 2022; FDA 2019) and is ultimately used to classify subjects based on a change from baseline to a particular post-baseline point in time (with the same threshold change for all subjects) as a responder or not a responder. What compounds the confusion on terminology is that the same term may be used to describe the other type of threshold (e.g., MCID is used to determine individual change), that terms may be applied interchangeably to describe both types of threshold, or the distinction between individual change or group difference is not made explicit (Beaton et al. 2001; Copay et al. 2007; King 2011; Mouelhi et al. 2020; Norman et al. 2004; Revicki et al. 2006, 2008; Wells et al. 2001). In this chapter, however, we will use MWPC to reference a threshold related to within-person change and CID to reference a threshold related to between-group difference.

It should be clear from the previous description, that the purpose and application of the MWPC and the CID are fundamentally different. In the previous chapter (specifically, Section 6.2.2.1) a simulated example for the following clinical study was investigated: (i) data were collected at four post-baseline occasions, (ii) there were two treatments (active treatment and placebo), and (iii) 600 subjects from the population of interest were "recruited" (300 subjects per treatment arm). A longitudinal model was applied to estimate overall mean treatment difference (across time points) and mean treatment differences at every time point by using the LSMeans statement (more on this in Section 7.3). We need first to check whether those mean differences are statistically significant and then, if they are, those mean score treatment differences can be gauged against the CID threshold: If those differences are also equal to or greater than the CID, then it implies that treatment differences are not only statistically significant but also clinically relevant.

In contrast, the use of the MWPC threshold is completely different. In the previous example, we estimated mean differences between active treatment arm and placebo, but "... From a regulatory standpoint, FDA is more interested in what constitutes a meaningful within-patient change in scores from the patient perspective (i.e., individual patient level). The between-group mean difference ... does not address the individual within-patient change that is used to evaluate whether a meaningful score change is observed. A treatment effect is different than a meaningful within-patient change ..." (FDA 2019). This insight implies that, in addition to the estimation of the mean treatment differences, as a way to augment interpretation, additional analyses based on the MWPC threshold should be performed. Typically, those additional analyses are (i) responder analyses using a predetermined MWPC threshold or (ii) examination of all possible thresholds with cumulative distribution functions (more on this in Section 7.3).

As noted, with the CIDs, we interpret whether the mean treatment differences can be described as clinically relevant or not (and "stop" after this), but with MWPCs, we need to perform an additional set of new analyses whose results also require interpretation. For example, say we perform a responder analysis and find that at the last time point in the active treatment arm there are 60% of individuals who responded and in the placebo arm this number is 50%. Is this difference of 10% between treatment arms large enough to be meaningful? Additional clinical insights are needed to evaluate meaningfulness between such responder percentages.

In this chapter, we do not distinguish between change as improvement and change as worsening. There are a few reasons for that. One reason is grounded in symmetry and immutability of a given change of score with respect to physical time: From the standpoint of the follow-up visit, an improvement of, say, five points on a scale from baseline to follow-up equates numerically and symmetrically with, from the standpoint of the baseline visit, a worsening of five points from follow-up to baseline. The second reason is that the assumed linear relationship between change in the target PRO (or COA) scale and change in the anchor measure, which our empirical experience with numerous analyses suggests tends to apply in practice, implies that the magnitude of improvement equals the magnitude of deterioration. The third reason is that, even if such a linear relationship is not justified, our experience suggests that it is usually due to sparseness in at least one of the extreme categories of the anchor measure; if doubt remains, the larger of the two types of changes (be it improvement or worsening) can be taken as the threshold for change (to be conservative).

7.1.2 Anchor-Based Method to Assess Meaningful Within-Patient Change

The anchor-based algorithm to estimate MWPC as a part of the FDA documents first surfaced in 2009 (FDA 2009), where it was referred to as an RD. The following description of the algorithm was given: "... anchor-based approach to defining responders makes use of patient ratings of change administered at different periods of time or upon exit from a clinical trial. These numerical ratings range from *worse* to *the same* and *better*. The difference in the PRO score for persons who rate their condition *the same* and *better* or *worse* can be used to define responders to treatment. Patient ratings of change are less useful as anchors when patients are not blinded to treatment assignment." (FDA 2009).

There are several noteworthy points in this description. First, the anchor is a scale representing change in a subject state with only three categories *worse, the same*, and *better*. Second, the **difference in the scores** for persons who rate their condition *the same* and *better* (or *worse*) represents the RD. That is, it emphasizes the need to adjust the mean score on target measurement for subjects who rated themselves as, say, *better* by the mean score from subjects who rated themselves *the same*. And third is the statement that data for those analyses should be from the study phase when patients are blinded to the treatment assignment, indicating that all available data from all treatment arms during the double-blind phase of a clinical study should be used in analyses.

Let's examine more closely the key elements of the above-described anchor-based methodology. The first element is the external anchor measure itself. An anchor with just three categories to represent change appears to be an attempt to remove categories with qualifiers, such as "A little better" or "Much worse," which are commonly used as a part of the patient global impression of change (PGIC) scales. A positive attribute of having three simple categories of only *worse, the same* and *better* is that no assumptions need to be made about "distance" between categories on the anchor. On the other hand, a negative consequence is that an estimated RD will likely not be study or drug agnostic. Imagine a study with an extremely efficacious drug A, where everybody in active treatment arm improved on this global anchor (i.e., every subject selected *better* category) and in placebo arm stays the same (i.e., every subject selected *the same* category) by the end of the study. Moreover, assume that mean difference of change between the two treatment arms is, say, 10 points on the target PRO scale, and therefore the RD is also 10 points.

Let's picture another study with drug B that is half as efficacious as drug A. As before with drug A, everybody in the active treatment arm B improves on this global anchor (i.e., every subject also selected *better* category) and in placebo arm stays the same (i.e., every subject selected *the same* category). Now assume that the mean difference between changes for these two arms is five points on the same target PRO scale (based on the assumption that the drug B is half as efficacious relative to drug A), and, therefore, the RD is also five points. Thus, using this algorithm can create a lower threshold when data from studies with a less efficacious drug are used and compared with studies with more efficacious drugs. This "side-effect" of this algorithm was corroborated by following statement: "The responder definition is determined empirically and may vary by target population or other clinical trial design characteristics. Therefore, we will evaluate an instrument's responder definition in the context of each specific clinical trial." (FDA 2009).

The second point is that the **difference in the scores** for persons who rate their condition *the same* and *better* (or *worse*) should be used as an RD. Such a calibration (by *the same* category) is analogous to adjusting for placebo in an active intervention study, where it is the relative or placebo-adjusted treatment effect that is important, rather than the unadjusted or absolute effect. Thus, this approach calibrates the relationship between change in target PRO measure and change in anchor external measure. By contrast, a non-calibrated approach will make no such correction and therefore does not adjust for *the same* category on the anchor by subtracting out its corresponding mean change score on the target PRO. This non-calibrated approach, in effect, forces no change on the anchor to correspond to no change on the target PRO and therefore assumes that perfect harmony exists in the relationship between these two measures, which is not generally the case (as the two measures are expected to measure similar but distinct concepts). Note that the same methodological issue was already discussed in Chapter 4 (specifically, see last paragraph in Section 4.1.4.2 and Figure 4.24).

The third point is that all data across the treatment arms should be used. There are two main reasons to use all data. One reason is that we want to create an MWPC that can be used for any subject in any treatment group (be it active or placebo) and, as such, all data from all treatment arms should be used. The other reason is that if we were to use only data from one arm, then there is a high probability that subjects on a very efficacious treatment will largely or completely respond *better* on the anchor (as previously discussed), giving a skewness or imbalance in comparison with the *same* category where data may be sparse or absent.

Shifting our focus to the more recent time of the publication of this book, we note that, while the FDA approach to estimate MWPC has slightly evolved, it has largely stayed methodologically the same. New terminology has been introduced with the RD replaced by the meaningful within-patient change. The other noteworthy fact is that in the 2009 FDA Guidance, there was no mention of MCIDs, MIDs, or CIDs, but in the current draft documents there is a"black box" that references MCIDs and MIDs and emphasizes the contrast on the use of the MCID (MID) vs. MWPC (FDA 2019) (see more on this topic in Section 7.2). Accordingly, the FDA offers the following description on the anchor-based method to estimate MWPC: "Anchor-based methods utilize the associations between the concept of interest assessed by the target COA and the concept measured by separate measure(s), referred to as anchoring measure(s), often other COAs .... The anchor measure(s) are used as external criteria to define patients who have or have not experienced a meaningful change in their condition, with the change in COA score evaluated in these sets of patients." (FDA 2019).

As we can see, there are no substantial methodological changes in the algorithm to define MWPC. We still need to have an independent anchor, and the difference in scores in the target COA (or PRO) between groups of patients who have or have not experienced a meaningful change in their condition (as measured by the anchor) represents what is now referred to as MWPC. It is nearly the same description as that defined in the 2009 FDA Guidance, where the difference in mean scores in the target measurement scale between the groups of persons who rate their condition *the same* and *better* (or *worse*) represented the RD.

The anchor itself is not pre-defined, as it was done in 2009 Guidance, but FDA has some recommendations (with generic examples described in Chapter 2): "Considerations for Anchor Measure(s):

- Selected anchors should be plainly understood in context, easier to interpret than the COA itself, and sufficiently associated with the target COA or COA endpoint
- Multiple anchors should be explored to provide an accumulation of evidence to help interpret a clinically meaningful within-patient score change (can also be a range) in the clinical outcome endpoint score

- Selected anchors should be assessed at comparable time points as the target COA but completed after the target COA
  The following anchors are sometimes recommended to generate appropriate threshold(s) that represent an MWPC in the target patient population:
  - Static, current-state global impression of severity scale (e.g., patient global impression of severity or PGIS)
  - Global impression of change scale (e.g., PGIC)
  - Well-established clinical outcomes (if relevant)
- A static, current state global impression of severity scale is recommended at minimum, when appropriate, since these scales are less likely to be subject to recall error than global impression of change scales; they also can be used to assess change from baseline." (FDA 2019).

To illustrate the assessment of MWPC the following simulated dataset will be used. There are only two treatments: active treatment and placebo. Overall, initially 1000 subjects from the population of interest were "enrolled" for this simulated study (500 subjects per treatment arm). There are two measurements: the PGIS of symptoms anchor scale represented by five categories with "5" representing "very severe" and "1" representing "none" (variable X_{ijk} in the final dataset "mixed_ds_sim") and the target COA (or PRO) represented by the 11-category numerical rating scale (NRS) with values from 0 to 10 (variable Y_{ijk} in the final dataset "mixed_ds_sim"), with higher scores representing less favorable outcomes on the concept of interest. Data were simulated for the four post-baseline observations.

Figure 7.1 represents SAS code to generate the "mixed_ds_sim" dataset, and Figure 7.2 represents data for the first three subjects. The approach we use to generate data was described in detail previously in Chapter 6 and represents a "mixture" of the simulations from Section 6.2.2.1 to Section 6.1.2. Note that the simulation of the anchor data is based on Eq. (6.2) (although in Chapter 6, this equation was used to describe the target COA rather than the PGIS), and simulation of the data for the target COA is based on the following Eq. (7.1) (important to highlight that this equation methodologically is close to the Eq. (6.1) in the previous chapter).

The model for the relationship between values X_{ijk} representing anchor values and Y_{ijk} representing target COA assumes that this relationship can be represented by the following equation:

$$Y_{ijk} = a + bX_{ijk} + e_{ijk} \tag{7.1}$$

where

Y_{ijk} is the value of the target COA for subject i at postbaseline measurement j and treatment k;

```
/* For this example we have initially 1000 subjects (NumberOfSubjectsPerTreatment *
NumberOfTreatments). For every subject we have 4 visits (NumberOfVisits = 4;).There
are 2 treatments arms (NumberOfTreatments = 2;)*/

%Let NumberOfSubjectsPerTreatment = 500; %Let NumberOfVisits      = 4;
%Let NumberOfTreatments = 2;


data mixed_ds;
Retain seed1 1 ; Retain seed2 2 ;
a=1.82;      /* the overall mean */
b=0.19;      /* baseline slope */
/* the time effect at time point j=1,2,3,4*/
Array t{1:4} (0.21 0.17 0.13 0);
/*Array d{1:2} (-0.24 0); */
Array d{1:2} (-0.51 0);
/*the effect of the treatments k=1,2*/
Array r{1:2,1:4} (
 0.05 -0.013 0.1 0 /*interaction effect between active treatment and time point*/
 0     0     0   0 /*interaction effect between placebo and time point */
);
     ID=0;
     Do k=1 to &NumberOfTreatments;
     Do i=1 To &NumberOfSubjectsPerTreatment;
      ID=ID+1;
      Call rannor(seed1,ex); Call rannor(seed2,ey);
      bl_X   = round(3.5 + sqrt(0.4)*ex,1);
      E_Ybl = sqrt(0.3)*ey;
        Do j=1 To &NumberOfVisits;
          X = a  + b*bl_X + t[j]    + d[k]    + r[k,j];
          Visit = j ; Treatment = k;
          Output;
          End;
     End;
     End;
Keep ID Visit Treatment X bl_X E_Ybl;
run;

Proc Print data=mixed_ds NOOBS; Where ID In (1 2 3); Run;
Proc Means data=mixed_ds; Run;
Proc Sort Data=mixed_ds out=_corr_ds; By Visit; Run;

Title "Corr without errors";
Proc Corr data=_corr_ds; By Visit; Run;

data _corr_(type=corr);
input
_TYPE_ $    _NAME_ $  COL1    COL2    COL3    COL4    COL5    COL6    COL7    COL8;
datalines;
CORR       COL1     1       0.76    0.68    0.58    0       0       0       0
CORR       COL2     0.76    1       0.72    0.68    0       0       0       0
CORR       COL3     0.68    0.72    1       0.72    0       0       0       0
CORR       COL4     0.58    0.68    0.72    1       0       0       0       0
CORR       COL5     0       0       0       0       1       0.56    0.41    0.41
CORR       COL6     0       0       0       0       0.56    1       0.56    0.54
CORR       COL7     0       0       0       0       0.41    0.56    1       0.55
CORR       COL8     0       0       0       0       0.41    0.54    0.55    1
MEAN       .        0       0       0       0       0       0       0       0
STD        .        1.2     1.22    1.21    1.29    0.67    0.68    0.70    0.73
N          .        1000    1000    1000    1000    1000    1000    1000    1000
;
Run;

Proc Simnormal data=_corr_ out=err_sim numreal=1000 seed=12345; var Col1-Col8; Run;
Title "Corr of errors";
Proc Corr data=err_sim COV ; Var Col1-Col8; Run;
Proc Transpose data=err_sim out=err_sim_x; Var Col5-Col8; By Rnum; Run;
Proc Transpose data=err_sim out=err_sim_y; Var Col1-Col4; By Rnum; Run;
Data _errors_x; Set  err_sim_x;
ID= Rnum; E_Xijk=Col1;
Keep ID E_Xijk;
Run;
Data _errors_y; Set  err_sim_y;
ID= Rnum; E_Yijk=Col1;
Keep ID E_Yijk;
Run;
Data mixed_ds_sim; Merge mixed_ds  _errors_x _errors_y ;
Xijk   = round(X+E_Xijk,1);
Yijk   = round(0.78 + 1.33*Xijk +E_Yijk,1); bl_Y   = round(1.78 + 1.33*bl_X +E_Ybl,1);
By ID;
Keep Xijk Yijk bl_X bl_Y ID Visit Treatment;
Run;
Data mixed_ds_sim; Set mixed_ds_sim;
Where bl_X In (3 4 5) And Xijk In (1 2 3 4 5) And Yijk In (0 1 2 3 4 5 6 7 8 9 10) And
bl_Y In (0 1 2 3 4 5 6 7 8 9 10);
Run;

Title "Data structure";
Proc Print data=mixed_ds_sim NOOBS; Var ID Visit Treatment bl_X Xijk bl_Y Yijk;
Where ID In (1 2 3);
Run;
```

Figure 7.1 Generating the simulated dataset.

ID	Visit	Treatment	bl_X	Xijk	bl_Y	Yijk
1	1	1	5	3	9	5
1	2	1	5	3	9	5
1	3	1	5	2	9	3
1	4	1	5	3	9	4
2	1	1	3	2	5	4
2	2	1	3	3	5	5
2	3	1	3	2	5	3
2	4	1	3	3	5	5
3	1	1	4	2	7	4
3	2	1	4	3	7	6
3	3	1	4	2	7	5
3	4	1	4	2	7	5

Figure 7.2 Data structure (data for the first three subjects are shown).

X_{ijk} is the value of the anchor for subject i at post-baseline measurement j and treatment k;

e_{ijk} is the error term [assumed to be from a normal distribution with mean 0 and variance σ_j^2, i.e., $e_{ijk} \sim N(0,\sigma_j^2)$];

a is the intercept;

b is the slope associated with variable X_{ijk}.

The same set of assumptions related to the error terms and other parameters made for Eq. (6.1) are also applicable here for Eq. (7.1) (see Section 6.1.2 for details). To model relationships between error terms in this simulation, we use a slightly different approach. The matrix representing correlations (see data step "**data** _corr_(type=corr); ...") has information for error terms for both outcomes (Xijk and Yijk). It is assumed that error terms for variable Xijk covary and error terms for variable Yijk also covary. But error terms for variable Xijk are not related (statistically independent) to error terms for variable Yijk, which is done by assigning zero correlations for relationship between any error term for variable Xijk and error term for variable Yijk. Thus, we have two 4×4 blocks of zeros in the matrix representing correlations between error terms.

As previously noted in Chapter 5, only subjects with certain severity baseline levels – that is, with anchor scores of 3 (Moderate), 4 (Severe), and 5 (Very Severe) – are used in the study (this point is discussed in Chapter 5; see description of the SAS code from Figure 5.90 in Section 5.3.2).

Figure 7.2 shows the general structure of the dataset for the analyses. The first step in the analysis to estimate MWPC is to confirm that the anchor is "sufficiently associated with the target COA." To be statistically correct we should assess their correlations cross-sectionally, at each relevant visit.

Another important point is that "anchors should be assessed at comparable time points as the target COA." In a real study, the anchors and target COA can be collected using different schedules. As a way to avoid methodological complications to deal with different schedules, it is preferable at the design stage of a study to make sure that the anchors and target COA are collected in a way that will later allow, ideally, all of their collected data to be used in the analyses. For example, if a target

COA has a recall period of one week, then the anchor should also, if appropriate, have a recall period of one week. If a target COA assesses a subject state "right now," then the anchor should do the same and ask a subject to evaluate his/her overall status also "right now." If in a study, this target COA assesses a subject state "right now" and is collected every two weeks, but an anchor (overall status "right now") is collected only once a month (every four weeks), then half of the data collected for the target COA will not be used in the analyses to estimate MWPC. In practice, this suggestion may not always be followed because there can be additional (not related to the estimation of the MWPC) reasons why the target COA will be collected more often than the anchor measure(s).

In our simulation, we assume that anchor and target COA are collected at the same visits and have the same recall period. Figure 7.3 shows SAS code

```
Proc Sort Data=mixed_ds_sim out=corr_by_visit; By Visit; Run;
Proc Corr Data=corr_by_visit; Var Xijk Yijk;  By Visit; Run;


Visit=1
                                Simple Statistics
Variable           N        Mean     Std Dev       Minimum       Maximum
Xijk             931     2.51128     0.75820       1.00000       5.00000
Yijk             931     4.11708     1.61786             0       9.00000

Pearson Correlation Coefficients, N = 931
         Prob > |r| under H0: Rho=0
                     Yijk
Xijk              0.61647
                  <0.0001

Visit=2
                                Simple Statistics
Variable           N        Mean     Std Dev       Minimum       Maximum
Xijk             933     2.44266     0.72670       1.00000       5.00000
Yijk             933     3.99786     1.55996             0      10.00000

Pearson Correlation Coefficients, N = 933
         Prob > |r| under H0: Rho=0
                     Yijk
Xijk              0.59145
                  <0.0001

Visit=3
                                Simple Statistics
Variable           N        Mean     Std Dev       Minimum       Maximum
Xijk             932     2.43133     0.75066       1.00000       5.00000
Yijk             932     4.01931     1.58119             0       9.00000

Pearson Correlation Coefficients, N = 932
         Prob > |r| under H0: Rho=0
                     Yijk
Xijk              0.60382
                  <0.0001

Visit=4
                                Simple Statistics
Variable           N        Mean     Std Dev       Minimum       Maximum
Xijk             926     2.29482     0.78397       1.00000       4.00000
Yijk             926     3.82289     1.69098             0       9.00000

Pearson Correlation Coefficients, N = 926
         Prob > |r| under H0: Rho=0
                     Yijk
Xijk              0.62903
                  <0.0001
```

Figure 7.3 Correlations between anchor and target COA by visit.

and results of the correlation calculations. As we can see, correlations between anchor (Variable $Xijk$) and target COA (variable $Yijk$) is about 0.6 at all visits, supporting the statement that anchor and target COA are sufficiently associated.

The simulated dataset at this stage of the analysis is missing the key variables needed to estimate MWPC, which are the changes from baseline in the anchor and target COA. Figure 7.4 adds those additional variables $ChgX$ and $ChgY$ in the dataset and performs the analysis using the repeated measures longitudinal model. The models in Figure 7.4 should look familiar as they were discussed at length earlier in Chapter 6 (specifically in Section 6.1.2). Note that the same assumptions for relationship between anchor and target COA are done here, which were made for Eq. (6.1) in Section 6.1.2.

```
Data mixed_ds_sim; Set  mixed_ds_sim;
ChgX =Xijk-bl_X; ChgY =Yijk-bl_Y;
Run;

Title "Correlations by visit between changes";
Proc Sort Data=mixed_ds_sim out=corr_by_visit; By Visit; Run;
Proc Corr Data=corr_by_visit; Var ChgX ChgY;  By Visit; Run;

Title "MWPC Analsyis (with continuous anchor)";
Proc Mixed data=mixed_ds_sim;
   class Visit ID ;
   model ChgY = ChgX / solution ddfm=kr;
   Repeated  Visit / Subject=ID Type=UN R rcorr;
    Estimate "1 category" ChgX 1 /cl;
    Estimate "2 category" ChgX 2 /cl;
    Estimate " ChgPGIS=-4" Intercept 1 ChgX -4 /cl;
    Estimate " ChgPGIS=-3" Intercept 1 ChgX -3 /cl;
    Estimate " ChgPGIS=-2" Intercept 1 ChgX -2 /cl;
    Estimate " ChgPGIS=-1" Intercept 1 ChgX -1 /cl;
    Estimate " ChgPGIS= 0" Intercept 1 ChgX 0 /cl;
    Estimate " ChgPGIS= 1" Intercept 1 ChgX 1 /cl;
    Estimate " ChgPGIS= 2" Intercept 1 ChgX 2 /cl;
    Estimate " ChgPGIS= 3" Intercept 1 ChgX 3 /cl;
    Estimate " ChgPGIS= 4" Intercept 1 ChgX 4 /cl;
Run;

Title "MWPC Analsyis - Only one (!) observation with ChgX=2";
Proc Freq Data=mixed_ds_sim; Table ChgX; Run;

Title "MWPC Analsyis - Pool observation with ChgX=2 with observations with
ChgX=1)";
Data mixed_mwpc_cat; Set  mixed_ds_sim;
If ChgX=2 Then ChgX=1;
Run;

Title "MWPC Analsyis (with categoric anchor)";
Proc Mixed data=mixed_mwpc_cat;
   class Visit ID ChgX;
   model ChgY = ChgX  / solution ddfm=kr;
   Repeated  Visit / Subject=ID Type=UN R rcorr;
   LSMeans ChgX / cl diff;
Run;
```

Figure 7.4 MWPC estimation implementation.

Before running the models to define MWPC, we noted previously (Chapter 6) that it is customary to also investigate and report correlations between changes from baseline in the anchor and the target COA; this topic was discussed and detailed in Chapter 6 (Section 6.1.2). Here we note only that, if correlations between anchor and target COA (not between changes) are logical and sizable (as in this example – see Figure 7.3), then it is likely that the correlations between changes will also be strong. Numerically correlations of changes could be even larger, as the additional effect of improvements in outcomes in time will also impact correlations (assuming that anchor and target COA are improved during the study). In this simulation, we have exactly this situation – correlations between change scores are numerically slightly larger compared with the correlations between original values of outcomes (compare results from Figure 7.3 and Figure 7.5)

The simulation in Figure 7.4 includes an additional data step ("**Data** mixed_ mwpc_cat;...") between two models to assess MWPC. The first model ("**Proc Mixed** data=mixed_ds_sim;...") uses the anchor (change from baseline

```
Visit=1
Variable          N          Mean      Std Dev         Sum      Minimum      Maximum
ChgX            931       -1.07948      0.89450       -1005     -4.00000      1.00000
ChgY            931       -2.40172      1.84559       -2236     -9.00000      3.00000

Pearson Correlation Coefficients, N = 931
        Prob > |r| under H0: Rho=0
                     ChgY
ChgX            0.64760
                <0.0001


Visit=2
Variable          N          Mean      Std Dev         Sum      Minimum      Maximum
ChgX            933       -1.14791      0.87256       -1071     -4.00000      2.00000
ChgY            933       -2.52304      1.82283       -2354     -9.00000      3.00000

Pearson Correlation Coefficients, N = 933
        Prob > |r| under H0: Rho=0
                     ChgY
ChgX            0.63939
                <0.0001


Visit=3
Variable          N          Mean      Std Dev         Sum      Minimum      Maximum
ChgX            932       -1.16094      0.91758       -1082     -4.00000      1.00000
ChgY            932       -2.50429      1.80850       -2334     -8.00000      3.00000

Pearson Correlation Coefficients, N = 932
        Prob > |r| under H0: Rho=0
                     ChgY
ChgX            0.64621
                <0.0001


Visit=4
Variable          N          Mean      Std Dev         Sum      Minimum      Maximum
ChgX            926       -1.29590      0.92352       -1200     -4.00000      1.00000
ChgY            926       -2.69654      1.91261       -2497    -10.00000      3.00000

Pearson Correlation Coefficients, N = 926
        Prob > |r| under H0: Rho=0
                     ChgY
ChgX            0.65192
                <0.0001
```

Figure 7.5 Correlations between changes from baseline in anchor and outcome by visit.

represented by ChgX) as a continuous variable. And the second model ("**Proc Mixed** data=mixed_mwpc_cat ...") uses the anchor as a categorical variable. But in the simulated dataset "mixed_ds_sim" we have only one (!) observation with ChgX=2, which, if kept in the dataset, will lead to problems with convergence (the methodologically same issue was discussed previously in Chapter 4, specifically in Section 4.1.4.2). To overcome this convergence issue, we simply pool data from this observation with all other data with ChgX=1.

Figures 7.6 and 7.7 represent results of the two models and Figure 7.8 summarizes those results in one graph. It is important to stress the difference between these two models (it was discussed previously in the context of the ability to detect change). The model with the continuous anchor imposes the linear relationship between change in the target COA and change in the anchor. In Figure 7.6, the solution is represented by intercept ("Intercept -0.9972...") and one slope ("ChgX 1.3095..."). In contrast, the model with the anchor as a categorical variable does not make any assumption about the relationship or functional form between changes in the target COA and the anchor. In Figure 7.7, the solution is represented by the intercept ("Intercept -0.9972...") and the six (regression) coefficients corresponding to the six observed categories for the change in the anchor, with last category being the reference. For example, for a change of −4 in the anchor measure, the corresponding coefficient is represented by the following line

```
ChgX    -4    -6.5299    0.2757    2598    -23.68    <.0001
```

in the output section under "Solution for Fixed Effects."

Figure 7.8 demonstrates that, in this simulation, results of both models are practically identical, supporting the use of the model with change in the anchor as a continuous variable as the primary model, which simplifies interpretation of MWPC. To estimate MWPC based on this model we need to define what constitutes the meaningful change in the anchor. "Sponsors should provide evidence for

```
              Solution for Fixed Effects
                      Standard
Effect        Estimate   Error     DF    t Value   Pr > |t|
Intercept     -0.9972   0.04905   1571   -20.33    <0.0001
ChgX           1.3095   0.02318   3590    56.49    <0.0001

                                          Estimates
                      Standard
Label         Estimate   Error     DF   Pr > |t|   Alpha   Lower      Upper
1 category     1.3095   0.02318   3590  <0.0001    0.05    1.2641     1.3550
2 category     2.6190   0.04636   3590  <0.0001    0.05    2.5281     2.7099
ChgPGIS=-4    -6.2353   0.07729   3146  <0.0001    0.05   -6.3868    -6.0837
ChgPGIS=-3    -4.9258   0.05891   2307  <0.0001    0.05   -5.0413    -4.8103
ChgPGIS=-2    -3.6163   0.04517   1266  <0.0001    0.05   -3.7049    -3.5276
ChgPGIS=-1    -2.3067   0.04106    951  <0.0001    0.05   -2.3873    -2.2262
ChgPGIS= 0    -0.9972   0.04905   1571  <0.0001    0.05   -1.0934    -0.9010
ChgPGIS= 1     0.3123   0.06481   2650  <0.0001    0.05    0.1852     0.4394
ChgPGIS= 2     1.6218   0.08408   3303  <0.0001    0.05    1.4570     1.7867
ChgPGIS= 3     2.9313   0.1049    3541  <0.0001    0.05    2.7256     3.1371
ChgPGIS= 4     4.2409   0.1266    3614  <0.0001    0.05    3.9926     4.4891
```

Figure 7.6 Results of the estimation of the MWPC with anchor as a continuous predictor.

Solution for Fixed Effects

Effect	Chg X	Estimate	Standard Error	DF	t Value	Pr > |t|
Intercept		0.3464	0.1154	3459	3.00	0.0027
ChgX	-4	-6.5299	0.2757	2598	-23.68	<0.0001
ChgX	-3	-5.3252	0.1366	3326	-38.97	<0.0001
ChgX	-2	-3.9646	0.1169	3200	-33.91	<0.0001
ChgX	-1	-2.6308	0.1126	3113	-23.37	<0.0001
ChgX	0	-1.3771	0.1086	2980	-12.68	<0.0001
ChgX	1	0	.	.	.	.

Least Squares Means

Effect	Chg X	Estimate	Standard Error	DF	Pr > |t|	Alpha	Lower	Upper
ChgX	-4	-6.1834	0.2535	2465	<0.0001	0.05	-6.6806	-5.6863
ChgX	-3	-4.9788	0.08392	3375	<0.0001	0.05	-5.1433	-4.8142
ChgX	-2	-3.6181	0.04883	1647	<0.0001	0.05	-3.7139	-3.5223
ChgX	-1	-2.2844	0.04473	1288	<0.0001	0.05	-2.3721	-2.1966
ChgX	0	-1.0306	0.05410	2085	<0.0001	0.05	-1.1367	-0.9245
ChgX	1	0.3464	0.1154	3459	0.0027	0.05	0.1202	0.5727

Differences of Least Squares Means

Effect	Chg X	_ChgX	Estimate	Standard Error	DF	Pr > |t|	Alpha
ChgX	-4	-3	-1.2046	0.2508	2372	<0.0001	0.05
ChgX	-4	-2	-2.5653	0.2513	2386	<0.0001	0.05
ChgX	-4	-1	-3.8991	0.2530	2412	<0.0001	0.05
ChgX	-4	0	-5.1528	0.2557	2447	<0.0001	0.05
ChgX	-4	1	-6.5299	0.2757	2598	<0.0001	0.05
ChgX	-3	-2	-1.3607	0.07652	3109	<0.0001	0.05
ChgX	-3	-1	-2.6944	0.08142	3310	<0.0001	0.05
ChgX	-3	0	-3.9482	0.08965	3417	<0.0001	0.05
ChgX	-3	1	-5.3252	0.1366	3326	<0.0001	0.05
ChgX	-2	-1	-1.3337	0.03889	3172	<0.0001	0.05
ChgX	-2	0	-2.5875	0.05452	3460	<0.0001	0.05
ChgX	-2	1	-3.9646	0.1169	3200	<0.0001	0.05
ChgX	-1	0	-1.2538	0.04411	3182	<0.0001	0.05
ChgX	-1	1	-2.6308	0.1126	3113	<0.0001	0.05
ChgX	0	1	-1.3771	0.1086	2980	<0.0001	0.05

Figure 7.7 Results of the estimation of the MWPC with anchor as a categorical predictor.

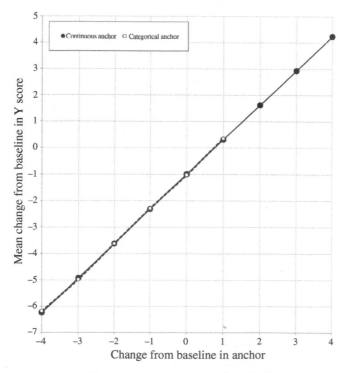

Figure 7.8 MWPC analyses: results of the modeling with anchor as a continuous predictor vs. results with anchor as a categorical predictor.

what constitutes a meaningful change on the anchor scale by specifying and justifying the anchor response category that represents a clinically meaningful change to patients on the anchor scale, e.g., a two-category decrease on a five-category patient global impression of severity scale." (FDA 2019). Depending on what constitutes the meaningful change in the anchor, the value of 1.3 ("1 category 1.3095...") or 2.6 ("2 category 2.6190...") can be proposed as MWPC based on the results from Figure 7.6. Note that no modeling is done to establish "a clinically meaningful change to patients on the anchor scale." Patient input and clinical insights are needed to establish what value is meaningful for the anchor.

Our experience is that these two models (with continuous vs categorical anchor) have been in general agreement for most, if not all, categories with a substantial number of observations. Only for the extreme categories may some departure from linearity be observed (e.g., see Figure 6.10 in Chapter 6), especially when the number of observations is sparse). But what if we have some notable departure from linearity even for categories with a considerable number of observations? In this case, obviously, the model with continuous anchor should not be used as the primary model, and the model with the anchor as a categorical variable should take precedence.

The first step is to evaluate the number of observations available for the modeling for every category. In Figure 7.4, the FREQ procedure ("Proc Freq Data=mixed_ds_sim;...") produces total frequencies over the entire study (see Figure 7.9 for output). As shown, the vast majority (~91.5%) of observations are linked to change in the anchor values of 0 (734 observations), −1 (1593), and −2 (1077). It is, therefore, logical to assume that differences between those categories should be investigated to assess MWPCs. In Figure 7.7 (with a categorical anchor) in the section titled as "Differences of Least Squares Means," the difference between category 0 and category −1 is -1.2538 and difference between category 0 and category −2 is -2.5875. In this simulation, those values are quite similar to the corresponding results in Figure 7.6 (with a continuous anchor; respectively, 1.3095 and 2.6190; note that absolute values should be compared). As noted, in a practical situation when linearity is not supported, values from the model with a categorical anchor would have to serve as estimations of MWPCs.

ChgX	Frequency	Percent	Cumulative Frequency	Cumulative Percent
-4	14	0.38	14	0.38
-3	215	5.78	229	6.15
-2	1077	28.94	1306	35.09
-1	1593	42.80	2899	77.89
0	734	19.72	3633	97.61
1	88	2.36	3721	99.97
2	1	0.03	3722	100.00

Figure 7.9 Overall frequencies for the change from baseline in anchor.

7.1.3 Cumulative Distribution Functions to Supplement Anchor-Based Methods

In the previous section the anchor-based approach to define MWPC was described. The FDA document also suggests "Using Empirical Cumulative Distribution Function and Probability Density Function Curves to Supplement Anchor-Based Methods. The empirical cumulative distribution function (eCDF) curves and the probability density function (PDF) curves can be used to supplement anchor-based methods. The eCDF curves display a continuous view of the score change (both positive and negative) in the COA-based endpoint score from baseline to the proposed time point on the horizontal axis, with the vertical axis representing the cumulative proportion of patients experiencing up to that level of score change. An eCDF curve should be plotted *for each distinct anchor category* as defined and identified by the anchor measure(s)" (FDA 2019). Figure 7.10 gives an illustrative example of a set of eCDF curves.

Let's generate and investigate eCDFs based on our simulated example from the previous section. The SAS code from Figure 7.11 produces eCDF curves for the changes from baseline in the target COA for every category change from baseline in the anchor score from baseline to visit 4. Note that we use dataset "mixed_ mwpc_cat," which was used in the modeling with a categorical anchor. Figure 7.12 displays eCDF curves for our simulated example. We first highlight the noticeable difference from the usual appearance of eCDF curves represented by generally smooth continuous monotonic function (as shown, for example, by

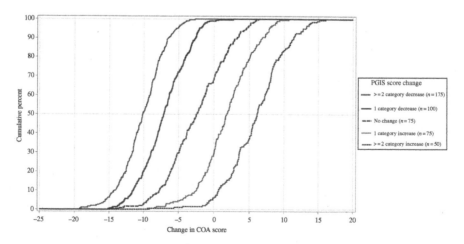

Figure 7.10 Example of empirical cumulative distribution function curves of change in COA score from baseline to primary time point by change in Patient Global Impression Severity Score. *Source:* Adapted from FDA (2019).

```
Data _cdf_; Set mixed_mwpc_cat;
Where Visit=4;
Keep ChgX chgY;
Run;
Proc Freq data=_cdf_; Tables ChgX; Run;
Proc Sort Data=_cdf_; By ChgX;        Run;

proc template;
   define style tmp_cdf; parent=styles.listing;
      style GraphReference    / LINETHICKNESS=1 ContrastColor=lightgray;
      style GraphGridLines     / LINETHICKNESS=1;
      style GraphDataDefault / LINETHICKNESS=5 ContrastColor=black linestyle =1;
      style GraphData1 /        ContrastColor=black      Linestyle=1;
      style GraphData2 /        ContrastColor=black      Linestyle=2;
      style GraphData3 /        ContrastColor=black      Linestyle=3;
      style GraphData4 /        ContrastColor=black      Linestyle=4;
      style GraphData5 /        ContrastColor=black      Linestyle=5;
      style GraphData6 /        ContrastColor=black      Linestyle=6;
   end;
run;

ods listing style=tmp_cdf;
Title "CDF; change in original units";
ods graphics on /HEIGHT=600PX WIDTH=1000PX IMAGEFMT=BMP;
Proc Univariate data=_cdf_ ;
Class chgX; var chgY;
cdfplot chgY/overlay NOFRAME
vref=0 to 100 by 50        HAXIS=-10 to 5 by 1        href=-10 to 5 by 1;
Output OUT=median MEDIAN=MedianChange;
Run;
ods graphics off;

Proc Print Data=median NOOBS; Var ChgX MedianChange; Run;
```

Figure 7.11 Example of the generation of the eCDF curves.

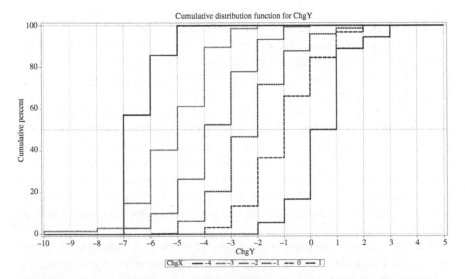

Figure 7.12 Example of empirical cumulative distribution function curves of change in the target COA score from baseline (variable ChgY) to visit 4 by change in the anchor score (ChgX).

Figure 7.10). In this example, we rather see a well-defined step function. This is simply a result of the scoring of the target COA used in the simulation. Recall that we defined responses to be represented by the 11-category NRS with possible discrete scores of 0, 1, 2, ..., 9, 10. Therefore, changes from baseline also will be represented by integers.

The updated and expanded (draft) FDA documents state the following: "The meaningful within-patient threshold of the target COA should be explored by the eCDF of the anchor category where the patients are defined and judged (by the anchor measure) as having experienced meaningful change in their condition .... Note that the median change is indicated by the red line in this example (*note from authors: a gray horizonal line, instead of a red line, corresponds to the 50th percentile in* Figure 7.10). The number of PGIS category increases and decreases defines the example's curves. In some instances, not all two (or 1 or 0) category changes are the same. This should be considered when choosing an anchor summary and interpreting these figures and data." (FDA 2019).

Our interpretation is that implied differences between eCDF curves at 50th percentile may be considered as plausible candidate thresholds to represent MWPCs. In the example represented by Figure 7.10, the distances between eCDFs at the 50th percentile are relatively close to each other (assessing this graph visually gives distances between 3–5 points). In real studies, though, those median differences between eCDFs are likely to be even more different, as acknowledged previously in the FDA statement. Our experience indicates that those descriptive differences, rather than not being the same "in some instances," are generally not the same for real data (and even in our current simulation).

Previously we discussed that it is very likely that zero or no change on the anchor will not correspond to zero change on the target COA. Note that in Figure 7.10, among subjects who did not change on anchor, a majority of them (about 70–80%) actually improved on the target COA. In our simulated example (see Figure 7.12), we also have about 70% of subjects who did not change on anchor (ChgX = 0) but improved on target COA (variable ChgY). Moreover, it should not be anticipated that the eCDF curve representing subjects with no change on anchor will intersect at the 50th percentile for cumulative percent at exactly 0 value for X-axis. Or that it will always correspond to an improvement on the target COA (as do Figures 7.10 and 7.12). There could be occasions when zero change on the anchor will correspond to worsening on the target COA (e.g., Bennett et al. 2009).

Although it is recommended to create an eCDF "for each distinct anchor category," it does not necessarily mean that a difference on mean change scores on the COA measure between any two anchor categories should be given the same weight during the interpretation of the results. As in modeling with the anchor as a categorical variable, it is important to evaluate the numbers of observations

ChgX	Frequency	Percent	Cumulative Frequency	Cumulative Percent
-4	7	0.76	7	0.76
-3	67	7.24	74	7.99
-2	311	33.59	385	41.58
-1	367	39.63	752	81.21
0	156	16.85	908	98.06
1	18	1.94	926	100.00

Figure 7.13 Number of subjects by the anchor change category (variable ChgX).

(subjects) represented by every eCDF curve (note that the number of the subjects was also reported in Figure 7.10). Figure 7.13 indicates that most subjects in our simulated example at visit 4 reported no change in the anchor (156 subjects or 16.85%), improvement by one category from baseline to visit 4 (367 subjects or 39.63%), and improvement by two categories (311 subjects or 33.59%), which as a group represents 90% of all data.

Based on the number of available observations (subjects) for every eCDF, the differences between *median* changes corresponding to categories 0, −1, and −2 should play a supplementary role in the assessment of MWPCs. Figure 7.14 (results of the "**Proc Print** Data=median NOOBS;...") shows that median change on the target COA corresponding to zero change on the anchor is −1, median change corresponding to the one-point improvement on the anchor is −2, and median change corresponding to the two-point improvement on the anchor is −4. If we assume that a one-category change on the anchor represents meaningful change, then the value of 1 (an absolute value of difference between median changes of −2 and −1 corresponding to changes of −1 and 0 on anchor) or the value of 2 (an absolute value of difference between median changes of −4 and −2 corresponding to changes of −2 and −1 on anchor) can be used to as supplementary assessments representative of MWPC for the target COA. For example, those two values can be viewed as a range for MWPCs. Recall that in anchor-based model (see Figure 7.6), the estimated MWPC was 1.3 (1.3095), which falls inside this range. If we assume that a two-category change on the anchor represents meaningful change, then the value of 3 (an absolute value of difference between median changes of −4 and −1 corresponding to changes of −2 and 0 on anchor)

ChgX	Median Change
-4	-7.0
-3	-5.0
-2	-4.0
-1	-2.0
0	-1.0
1	0.5

Figure 7.14 Median change corresponding to the anchor changes.

can be used as MWPC, which is close to the value of 2.6 from the anchor-based model (see Figure 7.6).

When producing and analyzing eCDFs it is important to point out that using eCDFs median changes associated with categories of change on the anchor is also a *model* of some kind, one which assumes that the differences at 50% percentile represent meaningful changes on target COA. Another fundamental difference between the eCDF and the anchor-based model described in the previous Section 7.1.2 is that "the eCDF does not take into account estimation uncertainty and is not a test" (FDA 2019). In other words, eCDFs simply visualize descriptive changes in outcome in a subgroup of subjects at a single time point in a study versus our anchor-based model, which uses all available data from all subjects at all time points. Moreover, eCDFs are based on "completers" only, that is, subjects who had values for both outcomes (anchor and COA) collected at the selected visit.

As noted at the beginning of this section, it is also recommended to plot PDFs. Figure 7.15 provides the implementation of the analyses, while Figure 7.16 depicts PDFs for the same data used to produce Figure 7.12. Generally, given a well-chosen anchor and well-designed COA, the eCDF curves (as depicted by Figures 7.10 and 7.12) are expected to be clearly and largely separated, with overlapping only at the edges of the distributions. If some eCDF curves overlap unexpectedly, say at around 50% percentile, then FDA recommends inspecting PDF plots for further insights. Still, it should be noted that, even for our simulated dataset with a practically "perfect" relationship between change in anchor and change in COA (as shown by Figures 7.8 and 7.12), the interpretation of the PDF curves could pose some challenges (Figure 7.16).

```
ods graphics on /HEIGHT=600PX WIDTH=1000PX IMAGEFMT=BMP;
Title "PDF kernel; change in original units";
Proc Template;
  define statgraph densityplot;
    begingraph;
      entrytitle "PDF (kernel)";
      layout overlay / xaxisopts=(griddisplay=on
        gridattrs=(color=lightgray pattern=dot))
        yaxisopts=(griddisplay=on
        gridattrs=(color=lightgray pattern=dot));
      densityplot chgY / kernel() name="densityplot" group=ChgX;
      discretelegend "densityplot" / title="ChgX";
      endlayout;
    endgraph;
  end;
Run;
Proc Sgrender template=densityplot data=_cdf_; Run;
```

Figure 7.15 Example of the generation of the PDF curves.

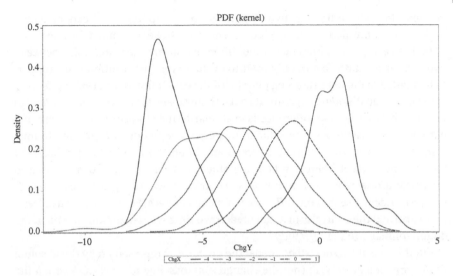

Figure 7.16 Example of probability density function curves of change in the target COA score from baseline (variable ChgY) to visit 4 by change in the anchor score (ChgX).

7.2 Clinical Important Difference

7.2.1 Meaningful Within-Patient Change Versus Between-Group Difference

In Section 7.1.1, we partially quoted the "black box" describing difference between MWPC and between-group difference. But it is important enough for it to be quoted in full. "It is important to recognize that individual within-patient change is different from between-group difference. From a regulatory standpoint, FDA is more interested in what constitutes a meaningful within-patient change in scores from the patient perspective (i.e., individual patient level). The between-group difference is the difference in the score endpoint between two trial arms that is commonly used to evaluate treatment difference. Between-group differences do not address the individual within-patient change that is used to evaluate whether a meaningful score change is observed. A treatment effect is different from a meaningful within-patient change. The terms minimally clinically important difference (MCID) and minimum important difference (MID) do not define meaningful within-patient change if derived from group-level data and therefore should be avoided. Additionally, the minimum change may not be sufficient to serve as a basis for regulatory decisions." (FDA 2019).

The above citation is packed with important methodological statements that clarify the difference between MWPCs and CIDs and are crucial for practical applications. The following two sentences "It is important to recognize that individual within-patient change is different from between-group difference" and "The between-group difference is the difference in the score endpoint between two trial arms that is commonly used to evaluate treatment difference" are partially related to the long-standing practice of the estimation of treatment effects or between-group difference in clinical trials. Historically, the outcome in a model to estimate between-group difference is customarily the change from baseline in a particular COA with baseline value of this COA, treatment, and (in longitudinal studies) time (or visit), and time-by-treatment interaction serving as predictors of the treatment effect (there can be some other covariates such as center). But, to understand how well treatment works, we are not evaluating the mean change from baseline per se, but the difference of mean changes between the active treatment arm and the control arm at the predefined time point (generally at end of the double-blind period of the study).

Yet, if in the above-described model the outcome is represented by the absolute COA score at a given visit (not the change from baseline for this COA), then the between-treatment difference will be the same (even p-values will be the same). It seems that this can be the source of some confusion about which threshold should be used to assess between-treatment difference: CID or MWPC. The FDA document clearly states (which the authors agree with) that whatever model is used (change in scores from baseline or scores themselves as the outcome), the MWPC should not be used to evaluate clinical relevance of the between-treatment difference. Moreover, the document also warns that "Between-group differences do not address the individual within-patient change that is used to evaluate whether a meaningful score change is observed."

The sentences "A treatment effect is different from a meaningful within-patient change" and "The terms minimally clinically important difference (MCID) and minimum important difference (MID) do not define meaningful within-patient change if derived from group-level data and therefore should be avoided" emphasize that the value of a CID threshold is not interchangeable with the value of the MWPC threshold (and vice versa). Hence, if a CID value is known for a scale, then this value cannot be used to define a responder on the individual patient level; it can be used only to assess clinical relevance of between- group differences.

7.2.2 Anchor-Based Method to Assess Clinically Important Difference

Although the set of draft FDA documents (as of this writing) does not specify any procedure for the estimation of the CID, it is logical to assume that the methodology suggested for MWPC (i.e., anchor-based approach) can be adapted also for the CID. The main difference will be that the relationship between the target COA and the anchor scores (not the changes from baseline) will be investigated in those analyses.

The key assumption for modeling relationship between the anchor (variable Xijk) and the target COA (variable Yijk) is that it can be represented by a "simple" regression discussed in Section 7.1.2 (specifically Eq. (7.1)). In fact, in Chapter 5 (Section 5.4, which describes known-groups validity assessment) the same model was implicitly assumed and described in detail for the relationship between a patient global impression of symptoms severity (variable $M2$ in Chapter 5 with four categories from "None" to "Severe") and a target COA (variable $M1$ in Chapter 5; represented by the NRS with values from 0 to 10). Moreover, the results of this model can provide evidence of not only known-groups validity but also estimations of the CID.

Another difference from the anchor-based model for MWPC assessment is that all available data starting with the baseline can be used in CID estimation. In MWPC analyses, only post-baseline observations (changes from baseline) are used. Note that in Section 5.4, the dataset used for analyses included all data starting with baseline observations. However, the data in this chapter thus far (see Figure 7.2) were simulated for post-baseline visits only. Now, Figure 7.17 updates the dataset "mixed_ds_sim" to have additional observations representing baseline scores (the dataset "mixed_cid"). Figure 7.18 shows the updated data structure for the first subject (compare this structure with Figure 7.2).

Figure 7.19 represents the implementation of the model to estimate CID with the anchor measure as a continuous variable according to Eq. (7.1) and, separately, with anchor as a categorical variable, which relaxes the assumption of linearity. As noted previously, these two models were discussed in Chapter 5, Section 5.4.1. The only difference here is that we adapt the implementation of the model for the current dataset with different variable names and an anchor with five categories. Figures 7.20 and 7.21 show the results of the analyses; Figure 7.22 summarizes their results. We see that both models give very close results,

```
/*Create dataset with baseline observations only*/
Proc SQL;
Create table bl as
Select ID, avg(bl_X) as Xijk, avg(bl_Y) as Yijk, avg(bl_X) as bl_X, avg(bl_Y) as bl_Y,
0 as Visit, Treatment
From mixed_ds_sim
Group by ID, Treatment;
Quit;

Title "Means at baseline";
Proc Means data=bl;Var Yijk; Run;

/*Merge baseline data with original data*/
Data mixed_cid; Set bl mixed_ds_sim;    Run;
Proc Sort data=mixed_cid; By ID Visit; Run;

Title "Data structure (with baseline observation)";
Proc Print data=mixed_cid NOOBS; Var ID Visit Treatment bl_X Xijk bl_Y Yijk;
Where ID In (1);
Run;
```

Figure 7.17 Creating a dataset for the CID analysis.

ID	Visit	Treatment	bl_X	Xijk	bl_Y	Yijk
1	0	1	5	5	9	9
1	1	1	5	3	9	5
1	2	1	5	3	9	5
1	3	1	5	2	9	3
1	4	1	5	3	9	4

Figure 7.18 Analysis dataset data structure for the CID analysis (only data for the first subject are shown).

```
Title "CID Analsyis (continuous anchor)";
Proc Mixed data=mixed_cid;
   Class Visit ID ;
   Model Yijk = Xijk  / solution ddfm=kr;
   Repeated  Visit / Subject=ID Type=UN R rcorr;
    Estimate "1 category" Xijk 1 /cl;
    Estimate " X= 1" Intercept 1 Xijk 1 /cl;
    Estimate " X= 2" Intercept 1 Xijk 2 /cl;
    Estimate " X= 3" Intercept 1 Xijk 3 /cl;
    Estimate " X= 4" Intercept 1 Xijk 4 /cl;
    Estimate " X= 5" Intercept 1 Xijk 5 /cl;
Run;

Title "Frequencies";
Proc Freq  data=mixed_cid; Tables Xijk; Run;

Title "CID Analsyis (categorical anchor)";
Proc Mixed data=mixed_cid;
   Class Visit ID Xijk;
   Model Yijk = Xijk  / solution ddfm=kr;
   Repeated Visit / Subject=ID Type=UN R rcorr;
   LSMeans Xijk / cl diff;
Run;
```

Figure 7.19 CID analysis: implementation of models.

				Estimates				
Label	Estimate	Standard Error	DF	t Value	Pr > |t|	Lower	Upper
1 category	1.5094	0.01760	3957	85.77	<0.0001	1.4749	1.5439
X= 1	2.4400	0.04433	3305	55.04	<0.0001	2.3531	2.5269
X= 2	3.9493	0.02886	2239	136.84	<0.0001	3.8927	4.0059
X= 3	5.4587	0.01790	1037	304.97	<0.0001	5.4236	5.4938
X= 4	6.9681	0.02067	1266	337.13	<0.0001	6.9276	7.0087
X= 5	8.4775	0.03396	2094	249.62	<0.0001	8.4109	8.5441

Figure 7.20 Results of the CID analysis with anchor as a continuous variable.

supporting the linearity assumption (compare this figure with Figure 5.97 in Chapter 5). From those results, we can conclude that for the target COA in this simulation the value of 1.5 ("1 category 1.5094...") corresponding to a one-category difference in the anchor can be assumed to represent CID.

In the last paragraph of Section 7.1.2, we discussed a possible situation of departure from linearity during the estimation of MWPC. Again, though, it is the experience of the authors that these two models for CID estimation (with continuous vs.

```
                          Least Squares Means
                       Standard
Effect   Xijk   Estimate   Error      DF    t Value   Pr > |t|    Lower    Upper
Xijk      1      2.6090    0.05939    3417   43.93    <0.0001     2.4926   2.7254
Xijk      2      3.9412    0.03445    3058   114.40   <0.0001     3.8737   4.0088
Xijk      3      5.4511    0.02247    1430   242.65   <0.0001     5.4070   5.4952
Xijk      4      6.9210    0.02627    1143   263.46   <0.0001     6.8695   6.9725
Xijk      5      8.8932    0.07589     917   117.18   <0.0001     8.7443   9.0421

                      Differences of Least Squares Means
Effect   Xijk   _Xijk    Estimate    Pr > |t|      Lower       Upper
Xijk      1       2       -1.3322    <0.0001      -1.4400     -1.2245
Xijk      2       3       -1.5099    <0.0001      -1.5743     -1.4455
Xijk      3       4       -1.4699    <0.0001      -1.5356     -1.4042
Xijk      4       5       -1.9722    <0.0001      -2.1295     -1.8149
```

Figure 7.21 Results of the CID analysis with anchor as a categorical variable.

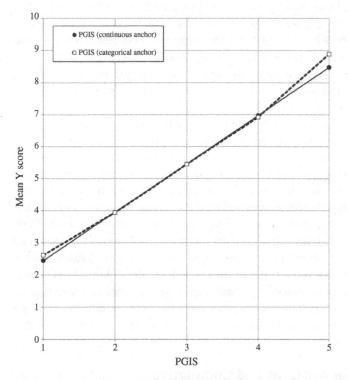

Figure 7.22 Results of the CID analysis: model with anchor as a continuous variable vs. model with anchor as a categorical variable.

categorical anchor) are generally in agreement for most categories with a substantial number of observations. However, in the case when a model with a continuous anchor cannot be used as the primary model, the second model with the anchor measure as a categorical predictor should be again given priority.

X_{ijk}	Frequency	Percent	Cumulative Frequency	Cumulative Percent
1	372	7.98	372	7.98
2	1654	35.49	2026	43.48
3	1906	40.90	3932	84.38
4	663	14.23	4595	98.61
5	65	1.39	4660	100.00

Figure 7.23 Overall anchor frequencies.

In Figure 7.19, the FREQ procedure ("**Proc Freq** data=mixed_cid;…") produces total frequencies (see Figure 7.23 for output). As we can see, the vast majority (more than 90%) of observations correspond to anchor categories of 2 (1654 observations), 3 (1906), and 4 (663) – and differences between those categories should be investigated to assess CIDs. In Figure 7.21 in its section titled as "Differences of Least Squares Means," the difference between category 2 and category 3 is -1.5099 and the difference between category 3 and category 4 is -1.4699. In this example, those values are almost exactly the same as the value produced by the model with the anchor as a continuous variable. But, again, in the hypothetical situation when linearity is not supported, those values can be used as estimations of CIDs.

There are also other approaches cited in the literature to define meaningful thresholds (MWPCs or CIDs). Among the most popular of them are distribution-based approaches. For example, one such variant is to simply use half a standard deviation on the COA (PRO) scores (Norman et al. 2003) or to use one standard error of measurement as the estimation of the clinically relevant cutoff (Wyrwich et al. 1999). It is generally accepted, however, that these methods have no direct relation to what a subject perceives as a meaningful change or difference, which is clearly stated by FDA: "Distribution-based methods (e.g., effect sizes, certain proportions of the standard deviation and/or standard error of measurement) do not directly take into account the patient voice and as such cannot be the primary evidence for within-patient clinical meaningfulness. Distribution-based methods can provide information about measurement variability." (FDA 2019). As such, we recommend to use distribution-based approaches only as secondary evidence, as an adjunct to anchor-based methodology.

7.3 Responder Analyses and Cumulative Distribution Functions

7.3.1 Treatment Effect Model

It is important to point out that mean treatment differences are generally the preferred method to analyze outcomes collected during a clinical study: "COA data often are ordinal or continuous in nature. Sponsors should consider analyzing

COA-based endpoints as continuous or ordinal variables rather than as a responder (i.e., dichotomized from either ordinal or continuous COA data) to avoid misclassification errors and potential loss of statistical power. There tends to be more precision in the evaluation of medical product effects on continuous variables (i.e., *based on a comparison of means*)" (FDA 2019). This recommendation is generally accepted (Cappelleri 2021; Collister et al. 2021a, 2021b; Weinfurt 2021).

An interesting duality arises from the previous quote when considered in tandem with a dichotomized responder outcome (yes, no) eventually emanating from an MWPC analysis. On the one hand, the estimation of a treatment effect is encouraged to be assessed based on the original scores (i.e., "the between-group difference is the difference in the score endpoint between two trial arms that is commonly used to evaluate treatment difference." (FDA 2019)) and dichotomized responder analyses are discouraged. On the other hand, for interpretation of those differences, a set of additional analyses rooted in responder analysis is proposed – that is, responder analysis stemming from an MWPC evaluation or, even more generally, Cumulative Distribution Functions (CDFs), which will be discussed in the next sections.

Figure 7.24 shows the implementation of the modeling framework for the current simulated dataset. Note that we start with the dataset "`mixed_ds_sim`" generated by Figure 7.4 and keep only relevant portions for the longitudinal analysis of variables. The two models and their implementation – the first model with the scale score at each visit as the outcome (absolute score) and the second model with the change scale score from baseline to follow-up visit as the outcome (change score) – were discussed in much detail in the previous Chapter 6 in Section 6.2.2.1 and therefore will not be repeated here.

Figure 7.25 shows the estimated means for the overall treatment difference across visits and for the treatment difference at every visit based on the first

```
Data trt_eff; Set  mixed_ds_sim; Keep ID Visit Treatment Yijk bl_Y ChgY; Run;

Title "Longitudinal Analysis for Y";
Proc Mixed data=trt_eff;
   class Visit Treatment ID ;
   model Yijk = bl_Y Visit Treatment Visit*Treatment   / solution ddfm=kr;
   Repeated  Visit / Subject=ID Type=UN R rcorr;
   LSMeans Treatment Visit*Treatment / cl diff;
Run;

Title "Longitudinal Analysis for change from baseline in Y";
Proc Mixed data=trt_eff;;
   class Visit Treatment ID ;
   model ChgY = bl_Y Visit Treatment Visit*Treatment   / solution ddfm=kr;
   Repeated  Visit / Subject=ID Type=UN R rcorr;
   LSMeans Treatment Visit*Treatment / cl diff;
Run;
```

Figure 7.24 Longitudinal model for treatment effects.

Least Squares Means

Effect	Visit	Treatment	Estimate	Standard Error	DF	t Value	Pr > |t|	Alpha	Lower	Upper
Treatment		1	3.6905	0.05983	936	61.68	<0.0001	0.05	3.5731	3.8079
Treatment		2	4.2772	0.06060	930	70.58	<0.0001	0.05	4.1583	4.3961
Visit*Treatment	1	1	3.8190	0.07301	937	52.31	<0.0001	0.05	3.6757	3.9622
Visit*Treatment	1	2	4.4083	0.07378	930	59.75	<0.0001	0.05	4.2635	4.5531
Visit*Treatment	2	1	3.6764	0.07024	934	52.34	<0.0001	0.05	3.5386	3.8143
Visit*Treatment	2	2	4.3131	0.07109	929	60.67	<0.0001	0.05	4.1736	4.4526
Visit*Treatment	3	1	3.7495	0.07143	936	52.49	<0.0001	0.05	3.6093	3.8897
Visit*Treatment	3	2	4.2828	0.07224	930	59.28	<0.0001	0.05	4.1410	4.4246
Visit*Treatment	4	1	3.5171	0.07690	931	45.74	<0.0001	0.05	3.3662	3.6680
Visit*Treatment	4	2	4.1046	0.07754	922	52.93	<0.0001	0.05	3.9524	4.2568

Differences of Least Squares Means

Effect	Visit	Treatment	_Treatment	Estimate	Standard Error	DF	t Value	Pr > |t|	Alpha	Lower	Upper
Treatment		1	2	-0.5867	0.08522	933	-6.88	<0.0001	0.05	-0.7539	-0.4195
Visit*Treatment	1	1	2	-0.5894	0.1038	934	-5.68	<0.0001	0.05	-0.7932	-0.3856
Visit*Treatment	2	1	2	-0.6366	0.09999	932	-6.37	<0.0001	0.05	-0.8329	-0.4404
Visit*Treatment	3	1	2	-0.5333	0.1016	933	-5.25	<0.0001	0.05	-0.7328	-0.3338
Visit*Treatment	4	1	2	-0.5875	0.1093	927	-5.38	<0.0001	0.05	-0.8019	-0.3731

Figure 7.25 Estimated means for variable Y_{ijk} (model with target COA score as the outcome).

Effect	Visit	Treatment	Estimate	Least Squares Means Standard Error	DF	t Value	Pr > |t|	Alpha	Lower	Upper
Treatment		1	-2.8302	0.05983	936	-47.30	<0.0001	0.05	-2.9476	-2.7128
Treatment		2	-2.2435	0.06060	930	-37.02	<0.0001	0.05	-2.3624	-2.1246
Visit*Treatment	1	1	-2.7017	0.07301	937	-37.00	<0.0001	0.05	-2.8450	-2.5584
Visit*Treatment	1	2	-2.1124	0.07378	930	-28.63	<0.0001	0.05	-2.2572	-1.9676
Visit*Treatment	2	1	-2.8442	0.07024	934	-40.49	<0.0001	0.05	-2.9821	-2.7064
Visit*Treatment	2	2	-2.2076	0.07109	929	-31.05	<0.0001	0.05	-2.3471	-2.0681
Visit*Treatment	3	1	-2.7712	0.07143	936	-38.79	<0.0001	0.05	-2.9114	-2.6310
Visit*Treatment	3	2	-2.2379	0.07224	930	-30.98	<0.0001	0.05	-2.3797	-2.0961
Visit*Treatment	4	1	-3.0036	0.07690	931	-39.06	<0.0001	0.05	-3.1545	-2.8527
Visit*Treatment	4	2	-2.4161	0.07754	922	-31.16	<0.0001	0.05	-2.5683	-2.2639

Figure 7.26 Estimated means for variable ChgY (model with change from baseline in the target COA score as the outcome).

(absolute score) model in Figure 7.24. Figure 7.26 shows estimated means for the change from baseline based on the second (change score) model. As noted earlier, treatment differences produced by both models will be exactly the same (including all outputted values, such as standard errors, degree of freedom, p-values, etc.), and thus they are shown only once (Figure 7.25).

If the primary time point is at visit 4, then the difference between active treatment (treatment 1) and comparator (treatment 2) is -0.5875 (p-value <0001). In this simulation, the lower scores on the target COA, the better the outcome on the concept of interest; therefore, a negative difference means that subjects in the active treatment arm have, on average, lower (i.e., more favorable) least square means relative to the comparator arm. Now, is this difference of about a half of a point on the 11-category COA (or PRO) scale meaningful? We will try to answer this question in the upcoming sections.

7.3.2 MWPC Application: A Responder Analysis

In the Section 7.1, the MWPC was estimated for the target COA (or PRO). The most straightforward use of this threshold is to perform a responder analysis. Figure 7.27 shows the estimation of the number of responders using two different estimations (1.3 and 2.6) for the MWPC at visit 4. Note that the same dataset "trt_eff" used for estimation of the treatment effects in the previous section (Section 7.3.1) is also used here as the input for our responder analysis. The results presented in Figure 7.28 represent standard 2×2 tables, which provide absolute and relative numbers of responders (Responder=1) and not responders (Responder=0) by treatment arm (Treatment=1 represents the active treatment arm and Treatment=2 represents the comparator arm).

The relevant numbers for interpretation of the COA are the percentages of the responders by treatment arm. In the first analysis with MWPC = 1.3, the percentage of responders is 78.92 for treatment 1 and 68.98 for treatment 2, a difference of 9.94%. For the second analysis with MWPC = 2.6, the corresponding percentages are 58.71 and 50.76, a difference of 7.95%. As we can see, both analyses give similar results in terms of differences, with the percent of responders

```
Title "Responder analysis based on MWPC=1.3";
Data _trt_cdf_;
Set trt_eff;
If chgY ne . Then Do;
   Responder=0;
   If chgY<=-1.3 Then Responder=1;
End;
Where Visit=4;
Keep Treatment chgY Responder;
Run;

Proc Freq Data=_trt_cdf_; Tables Responder*Treatment; Run;

Title "Responder analysis based on MWPC=2.6";
Data _trt_cdf_; Set trt_eff;
If chgY ne . Then Do;
   Responder=0;
   If chgY<=-2.6 Then Responder=1;
End;
Where Visit=4;
Keep Treatment chgY Responder;
Run;

Proc Freq Data=_trt_cdf_; Tables Responder*Treatment; Run;
```

Figure 7.27   Using FREQ procedure to estimate number of responders by treatment arm.

```
Responder analysis based on MWPC=1.3
Table of Responder by Treatment
Responder      Treatment
Frequency|
Percent  |
Row Pct  |
Col Pct  |        1|       2|   Total

       0 |      98 |     143 |     241
         |   10.58 |   15.44 |   26.03
         |   40.66 |   59.34 |
         |   21.08 |   31.02 |

       1 |     367 |     318 |     685
         |   39.63 |   34.34 |   73.97
         |   53.58 |   46.42 |
         |   78.92 |   68.98 |

Total          465       461       926
             50.22     49.78    100.00

Responder analysis based on MWPC=2.6
Table of Responder by Treatment
Responder      Treatment
Frequency|
Percent  |
Row Pct  |
Col Pct  |        1|       2|   Total

       0 |     192 |     227 |     419
         |   20.73 |   24.51 |   45.25
         |   45.82 |   54.18 |
         |   41.29 |   49.24 |

       1 |     273 |     234 |     507
         |   29.48 |   25.27 |   54.75
         |   53.85 |   46.15 |
         |   58.71 |   50.76 |

Total          465       461       926
             50.22     49.78    100.00
```

Figure 7.28   Responder analysis results.

differing by approximately 10% between arms. To interpret this difference in a real-life situation, we need to know more about this study. If a comparator arm is represented by placebo, do we anticipate to have a large placebo effect? Such is the case in psychiatric studies, for example (Jones et al. 2021) or, for ethical reasons, is the comparator an approved drug for the same illness (as routinely occurs in oncology studies)?

In our simulation, a mean improvement from baseline to visit 4 is 3 (-3.0036; see Figure 7.26) points for treatment 1 and 2.4 (-2.4161) points for treatment 2. In a clinical research setting, these results are indicative of a large comparator effect when, although a large improvement from baseline is observed in the active treatment arm, considerable improvement is observed in the comparator arm as well. Suppose those results come from a study with a new treatment under investigation where the comparator is the standard-of-care active drug for an illness. Then a most plausible conclusion here would be that the treatment effect of a new drug is not only statistically significant (recall that treatment difference of -0.5875 was significant; see Figure 7.25) but also clinically relevant, even if the difference between the percentage of responders between treatment arms is only about 10%.

But what about a CID for this scale? Can it be applied here to assess clinical relevance? Recall that the FDA does not encourage that CIDs be used primarily for interpretation of treatment effect. Reinforcing that, this simulated example can provide insights on why CIDs should not play such a primary role. The treatment effect for this simulated study was approximately 0.6 (-0.5875) points, which is noticeably smaller than an estimated CID of 1.5 (see Section 7.2.2) points for this scale. If we were to use this CID value to judge clinical relevance of this treatment effect, then the answer will be in the negative – a lack of clinical relevance.

7.3.3 Using CDFs for Interpretation of Results

"When analyzing a COA-based endpoint as either a continuous or an ordinal variable, it is important to evaluate and justify the clinical relevance of any observed treatment effect. Sponsors should plan to evaluate the meaningfulness of within-patient changes to aid in the interpretation of the COA-based endpoint results by submitting a supportive graph (i.e., eCDF) of within-patient changes in scores from baseline with separate curves for each treatment arm. The graph will be used to assess whether the treatment effect occurs in the range that patients consider to be clinically meaningful." (FDA 2019).

As indicated in the above text, for interpretation of the treatment effects it is suggested to extend beyond responder analysis and to evaluate eCDFs curves by treatment arm, which have become visually appealing aids (Cappelleri and Bushmakin 2014; McLeod et al. 2011). Figure 7.29 provides the implementation of

```
Data _cdf_; Set trt_eff; Where Visit=4; Keep Treatment chgY; Run;

Proc Template;
  define style tmp_cdf; parent=styles.listing;
      style GraphFonts from GraphFonts /
      'GraphDataFont'=("<sans-serif>,<MTsans-serif>",10pt)
      'GraphUnicodeFont'=("<MTsans-serif-unicode>",10pt)
      'GraphValueFont'=("<sans-serif>,<MTsans-serif>",15pt)
      'GraphLabelFont'=("<sans-serif>,<MTsans-serif>",20pt)
      'GraphFootnoteFont'=("<sans-serif>,<MTsans-serif>",8pt)
      'GraphTitleFont'=("<sans-serif>,<MTsans-serif>",20pt,bold);
        style GraphReference   / LINETHICKNESS=1 ContrastColor=lightgray;
        style GraphGridLines   / LINETHICKNESS=1;
        style GraphDataDefault / LINETHICKNESS=5
        ContrastColor=black   linestyle =1;

        style GraphData1 /      ContrastColor=black      Linestyle=1;
        style GraphData2 /      ContrastColor=black      Linestyle=2;
  end;
Run;

ods listing style=tmp_cdf;
Title "CDF; treatment differences";
ods graphics on /HEIGHT=1200PX WIDTH=2000PX IMAGEFMT=BMP;
Proc Univariate data=_cdf_ ;
Class Treatment;
var chgY;
cdfplot chgY / overlay NOFRAME VAXIS= 0 to 100 by 10
vref = 50.76  58.71  68.98  78.92
HAXIS= -10 to 5 by 1 href = -2.6 -1.3;
Run;
ods graphics off;
```

Figure 7.29 eCDF curves implementation.

the analyses to generate eCDF curves (the same dataset "trt_eff" used in Section 7.3.1 is used to produce eCDFs), and Figure 7.30 shows the generated eCDF graph.

As a way to support the clinical relevance of the estimated treatment effect, the eCDF curves should demonstrate (i) "consistent separation between the treatment arms" and that (ii) "the treatment effect occurs in the range patients consider to be clinically meaningful" (FDA 2019). Let's examine these two conditions as applied to Figure 7.30. The first criterion is that there should be consistent separation between eCDF curves. But in which dimension? For example, the two lines are clearly separated along the *Y*-axis (vertical axis, Cumulative Percent). Nevertheless, it seems the curves touch each other at integer numbers such as, for example, −5, −4, etc., along the *X*-axis (ChgY).

When examining eCDF figure, it is important to understand that those eCDF lines are simply the graphical depiction of the responder analyses using a variety of values to define a responder. In the 2009 FDA PRO guidance, it was clearly described as follows: "Alternatively, it is possible to present the entire distribution of responses for treatment and control group, avoiding the need to pick a responder criterion .... Such cumulative distribution displays show a continuous plot of the percent change from baseline on the *X*-axis and the percent of patients

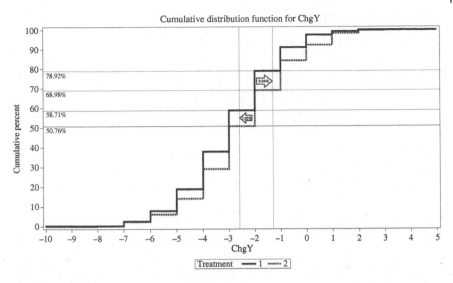

Figure 7.30 eCDF curves by treatment arm.

experiencing that change on the Y-axis .... A variety of responder definitions can be identified along the cumulative distribution of response curve" (FDA 2009).

To show this link in Figure 7.30, we include two vertical reference lines corresponding to the MWPC threshold of 1.3 and 2.6 (see coded line "href = -2.6 -1.3" in Figure 7.29). It clearly shows that the percentages of responders and differences between those percentages correspond to the responder analysis using MWPC thresholds of −1.3 and −2.6 discussed in the previous Section 7.3.2 (see Figure 7.28). As such, it is the opinion of the authors that the statement about "consistent separation between the treatment arms" should be interpreted as a consistent difference between percentages of responders corresponding to the treatment arms.

The difference between percentages of responders among treatment arms can also be viewed as the difference between eCDF curves. To calculate differences between eCDF curves, we can simply calculate differences between percentages of responders using "a variety of responder definitions." Figure 7.31 shows the implementation of the analyses to calculate differences between percentages of responders. In essence, to do this, the code from the Figure 7.27 is modified to produce and summarize results for the variety of RDs from −10 to 5 (i.e., the limits for the variable ChgY in Figure 7.30).

Figure 7.32 shows the percentages of responders. This figure is practically the same as Figure 7.30 with one small but important methodologically difference. For example, if the responder is defined as anybody improving by at least two points (i.e., −2 points or more extreme), then the percentages of responders are 58.71% in treatment arm 1 and 50.76% in treatment arm 2. If the responder is

```
PROC DELETE DATA=WORK.Percentages; RUN;

proc lua restart; submit;
for RespDef=-10, 5, 0.1
do
sas.submit[[
Data _trt_cdf_; Set trt_eff;
If chgY ne . Then Do;
    Responder=0;
    If chgY<=@RespDef@ Then Responder=1;
    End;
Where Visit=4;
Keep Treatment chgY Responder;
Run;

Proc Freq Data=_trt_cdf_; Tables Responder*Treatment/out=FreqPct outpct; Run;

Data trt1; Set FreqPct;
Responder_Pct_Trt_1=PCT_COL;
Where Responder=1 And Treatment=1;
Keep Responder_Pct_Trt_1;
Run;

Data trt2; Set FreqPct;
Responder_Pct_Trt_2=PCT_COL;
Where Responder=1 And Treatment=2;
Keep Responder_Pct_Trt_2;
Run;

Data ResponderDiff; Merge trt1 trt2;
Responder_Pct_Diff=Responder_Pct_Trt_1 - Responder_Pct_Trt_2;
Responder_Definition=@RespDef@;
Keep Responder_Definition Responder_Pct_Trt_1 Responder_Pct_Trt_2 Responder_Pct_Diff;
Run;

proc append base=Percentages data=ResponderDiff; run;
]]
end

endsubmit;
run;

Proc Template;
  define style tmp_cdf;  parent=styles.listing;
      style GraphFonts from GraphFonts /
      'GraphDataFont'=("<sans-serif>,<MTsans-serif>",10pt)
      'GraphUnicodeFont'=("<MTsans-serif-unicode>",10pt)
      'GraphValueFont'=("<sans-serif>,<MTsans-serif>",15pt)
      'GraphLabelFont'=("<sans-serif>,<MTsans-serif>",20pt)
      'GraphFootnoteFont'=("<sans-serif>,<MTsans-serif>",8pt)
      'GraphTitleFont'=("<sans-serif>,<MTsans-serif>",20pt,bold);
      style GraphReference   / LINETHICKNESS=1 ContrastColor=lightgray;
      style GraphGridLines   / LINETHICKNESS=1;
      style GraphDataDefault / LINETHICKNESS=5
      ContrastColor=black    linestyle =1;
      style GraphData1 /       ContrastColor=black       Linestyle=1;
      style GraphData2 /       ContrastColor=black       Linestyle=2;
  end;
run;
ods listing style=tmp_cdf;
Title "Responder anaysis: Percentages by treatment arm";
ods graphics on /HEIGHT=1200PX WIDTH=2000PX IMAGEFMT=BMP;
Proc Sgplot data=Percentages;
  series x=Responder_Definition y=Responder_Pct_Trt_1;
  series x=Responder_Definition y=Responder_Pct_Trt_2;
  xaxis values=(-10 to 5 by 1); yaxis values=(0 to 100 by 10);
  refline -2.6 -1.3 / axis=x;   refline 50.76  58.71 68.98 78.92  / axis=y;
Run;

Title "Responder anaysis: Differences";
ods graphics on /HEIGHT=600PX WIDTH=2000PX IMAGEFMT=BMP;
Proc Sgplot data=Percentages;
  series x=Responder_Definition y=Responder_Pct_Diff;
  xaxis values=(-10 to 5 by 1);  yaxis values=(-1 to 10 by 1);
  refline -2.6  -1.3 / axis=x;  refline 0 7.95 9.94 / axis=y;
Run;
ods graphics off;
```

Figure 7.31 Generating the entire distribution of responses.

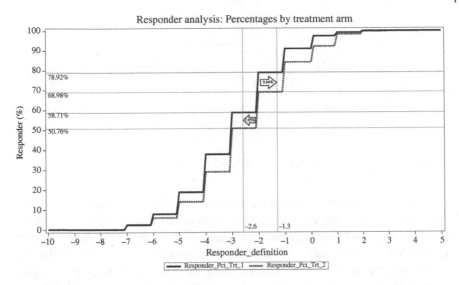

Figure 7.32 Responder analyses results.

defined as anybody improving by at least 1.9 points, then the number of responders in treatment arm 1 is 78.92% and 68.98% in treatment arm 2. This result occurs because in Figure 7.31 we calculated percentage of responders in steps of 0.1 points. The graph from Figure 7.32 will be exactly the same as the eCDF from Figure 7.30 if we were to run analyses with infinitely small steps. In this simulation, the following code line (Figure 7.31) "`for RespDef=-10, 5, 0.1`" defines step size (and as a result the number of responder analyses). The authors encourage readers to run this analysis with even smaller steps, replacing `0.1` by, say, `0.01` to see a difference in produced plots.

Figure 7.33 shows the differences in percentages of responders between treatment arms. Recall that we need to show "consistent separation between the treatment arms" and that "the treatment effect occurs in the range patients consider to be clinically meaningful." Figure 7.33, which defines responder difference as the difference in the percent of responders in active treatment arm minus control treatment arm, demonstrates that differences are consistently non-negative for all definitions of the responder threshold. If eCDF curves intersect or there is no consistent separation, then differences between percentage of responders will be not only positive but also negative. Thus, having all differences to be non-negative supports "consistent separation between the treatment arms." In real life, though, there may be some negative differences at either extreme of the responder thresholds and to support the "consistent separation between the treatment arms" the responder differences do not have to be non-negative necessarily for all responder thresholds (or definitions) but should be non-negative for most responder thresholds.

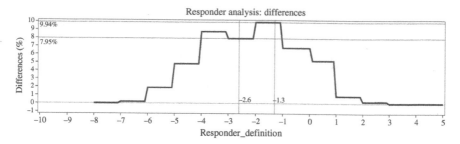

Figure 7.33 Differences in percentages of responders between treatment arms.

The next requirement is to demonstrate that "the treatment effect occurs in the range patients consider to be clinically meaningful." Again, Figure 7.33 shows that the largest differences between treatment arm occurs in the region around the two MWPC candidates (−1.3 and −2.6). In fact, in this simulation, the largest responder difference of 9.94% corresponds to the MWPC definition of 1.3 points (threshold of −1.3) on the target COA. In this graph, additional MWPC definitions based on CDFs can also be added (see Section 7.1.3). Recall that values of 1, 2, and 3 points are implied to be representative of MWPC based on supplementary CDF analyses. Note that in Figure 7.33 those values are represented by the additional vertical lines corresponding to values of −3, −2, and −1 for the Responder_ Definition variable. To add those additional values to Figure 7.33 simply replace "refline -2.6 -1.3 / axis=x;" in Figure 7.31 with "refline -3.0 -2.6 -2.0 -1.3 -1.0/ axis=x;." The conclusion remains the same even with those additional MWPC values: "the treatment effect occurs in the range patients consider to be clinically meaningful."

We started this section with the FDA statement that "Sponsors should plan to evaluate the meaningfulness of within-patient changes to aid in the interpretation of the COA-based endpoint results by submitting a supportive graph (i.e., eCDF) of within-patient changes in scores from baseline with separate curves for each treatment arm." (FDA 2019). We recommend to produce and submit not only supportive eCDF graphs but also supportive graphs representing differences of the eCDF curves as shown in this section. To conclude this section, it is important to stress again that "the eCDF does not take into account estimation uncertainty and is not a test" (FDA 2019) and, as such, no statistical inferences should be attached to those supportive graphs.

7.4 Summary

Useful interpretation of score values or score changes on COAs, including PROs, can be valuable in designing studies, evaluating interventions, educating consumers, and informing health policy makers involved with regulatory, reimbursement, and advisory agencies. Unlike certain "objectives" outcomes like blood pressure, subjective outcomes often lack the historical, empirical, and clinical thread to draw from for meaningful interpretation. This chapter provides a conceptual, an analytical, and a computational framework to assess MWPC and clinical important differences on PRO and other COA scores in order to enrich their interpretation and relevance in the context of an intervention study.

Using all available data, the anchor-based methodology espoused in this chapter is elucidated and applied to distinguish MWPC and CID for interpretation of treatment effects. In addition, responder analyses and cumulative distribution functions are described as an extension and adjunct to supplement meaningful within-patient change.

Responder analysis is a determined attempt to understand whether the effect of an intervention, shown to be statistically significant on a PRO or other COA measurement scale, has clinical significance. While it has defenders (Lewis 2004), its limitations have been reported (Cappelleri and Chambers 2021; Collister et al. 2021a; Senn 2003; Uryniak et al. 2011). Limitations include the expected reduction in statistical power when moving from a continuous to binary outcome, misclassification error, and, when not assessed empirically and justifiably, the potential for an arbitrary cutoff score to distinguish responders from non-responders. For a quantitative or continuous outcome, responder analysis is best positioned as a descriptive display in the assessment and reporting of clinical meaningfulness of the treatment effect and as an adjunct to – as a complement and supplement to – the main statistical analysis and inference based on the full original scale of measurement using established statistical methods (e.g., repeated measures or random coefficient models when the data are longitudinal) (Cappelleri and Chambers 2021; Collister et al. 2021a; Senn 2003; Uryniak et al. 2011).

Cumulative distribution plots are most compelling and best suited for interpretation when there is minimal overlap in the curves between treatments. When there is some or considerable overlap, the cumulative treatment curves interact and interpretation gets clouded. In such a case, judgment is needed on what cutoff scores are considered clinically most plausible.

References

Beaton, D.E., Bombardier, C., Katz, J.N. et al. (2001). Looking for important change/difference in studies of responsiveness. *Journal of Rheumatology* 28: 400–405.

Bennett, R.M., Bushmakin, A.G., Cappelleri, J.C. et al. (2009). Minimally clinically important difference in the fibromyalgia impact questionnaire (FIQ). *Journal of Rheumatology* 36: 1304–1311.

Cappelleri, J.C. (2021). Further reduction in statistical power for responder analysis of patient-reported outcomes with measurement error. *Journal of Clinical Epidemiology* 140: 200–201.

Cappelleri, J.C. and Bushmakin, A.G. (2014). Interpretation of patient-reported outcomes. *Statistical Methods in Medical Research* 23: 460–483.

Cappelleri, J.C. and Chambers, R. (2021). Addressing bias in responder analysis of patient-reported outcomes. *Therapeutic Innovation & Regulatory Science* 55: 989–1000.

Cappelleri, J.C., Zou, K.H., Bushmakin, A.G. et al. (2013). *Patient-Reported Outcomes: Measurement, Implementation and Interpretation*. Boca Raton, FL: Chapman & Hall/CRC Press.

Cocks, K., King, M.T., Velikova, G. et al. (2008). Quality, interpretation and presentation of European Organisation for Research and Treatment of Cancer quality of life questionnaire core 30 data in randomized controlled trials. *European Journal of Cancer* 44: 1793–1798.

Collister, D., Bangiwala, S., Walsh, M. et al. (2021a). Patient reported outcome measures in clinical trials should be initially analyzed as continuous outcomes for statistical significance and responder analyses should be reserved as secondary analyses. *Journal of Clinical Epidemiology* 134: 95–102.

Collister, D., Bangiwala, S., Guyatt, G. et al. (2021b). Response to Weinfurt and Cappelleri on "Patient reported outcome measures in clinical trials should be initially analyzed as continuous outcomes for statistical significance and responder analyses should be reserved as secondary analyses". *Journal of Clinical Epidemiology* 140: 1–2.

Conaghan, P.G., Dworkin, R.H., Schnitzer, T.J. et al. (2022). WOMAC meaningful within-patient change: Results from three studies of tanezumab in patients with moderate-to-severe osteoarthritis of the hip or knee. *Journal of Rheumatology* 49: 615–621.

Coon, C.D. and Cappelleri, J.C. (2016). Interpreting change in scores on patient-reported outcome instruments. *Therapeutic Innovation & Regulatory Science* 50: 22–29.

Coon, C.D. and Cook, K.F. (2018). Moving from clinical significance to real-world meaning: methods for interpreting change in clinical outcome assessment scores. *Quality of Life Research* 27: 33–40.

Copay, A.G., Subach, B.R., Glassman, S.D. et al. (2007). Understanding the minimum clinically important difference: a review of concepts and methods. *The Spine Journal* 7: 541–546.

Farivar, S.S., Liu, H., and Hays, R.D. (2004). Half standard deviation estimate of the minimally important difference in HRQOL scores? *Expert Review of Pharmacoeconomics and Outcomes Research* 4: 515–523.

FDA (Food and Drug Administration) (2009). Guidance for industry on patient-reported outcome measures: use in medical product development to support labeling claims. *Federal Register* 74 (235): 65132–65133.

FDA (Food and Drug Administration) (2019). Patient-focused drug development guidance series for enhancing the incorporation of the patient's voice in medical product development and regulatory decision making. Draft Guidance Documents. https://www.fda.gov/drugs/development-approval-process-drugs/fda-patient-focused-drug-development-guidance-series-enhancing-incorporation-patients-voice-medical (accessed 15 April 2020).

Jones, B.D.M., Razza, L.B., Weissman, C.R. et al. (2021). Magnitude of the placebo response across treatment modalities used for treatment-resistant depression in adults: a systematic review and meta-analysis. *JAMA Network Open* https://doi.org/10.1001/jamanetworkopen.2021.25531.

King, M.T. (2011). A point of minimal important difference (MID): a critique of terminology and methods. *Expert Review of Pharmacoeconomics & Outcomes Research* 11: 171–184.

Lewis, J.A. (2004). In defence of the dichotomy. *Pharmaceutical Statistics* 3: 77–79.

Mamolo, C.M., Bushmakin, A.G., and Cappelleri, J.C. (2015). Application of the itch severity score in patients with moderate-to-severe plaque psoriasis: clinically important difference and responder analysis. *Journal of Dermatological Treatment* 26: 121–123.

Marquis, P., Chassany, O., and Abetz, L. (2004). A comprehensive strategy for the interpretation of quality-of-life data based on existing methods. *Value in Health* 7: 93–104.

Maruish, M.E. (ed.) (2011). *User's Manual for the SF-36v2 Health Survey*, 3e. Lincoln, RI: QualityMetric Incorporated.

McGlothlin, A.E. and Lewis, R.J. (2014). Minimal clinically important difference: defining what really matters to patients. *JAMA* 312: 1342–1343.

McGlothlin, A.E. and Lewis, R.J. (2014). Minimal clinically important difference: defining what really matters to patients. *JAMA* 312: 1342–1343.

McLeod, L.D., Coon, C.D., Martin, S.A. et al. (2011). Interpreting patient-reported outcome results: US FDA guidance and emerging methods. *Expert Reviews of Pharmacoeconomics & Outcomes Research* 11: 163–169.

McLeod, L.D., Cappelleri, J.C., and Hays, R.D. (2016). Best (but of forgotten) practices: expressing and interpreting meaning and effect sizes in clinical outcome assessments. *American Journal of Clinical Nutrition* 103: 685–693. Correction: 2017; 105:241.

Mouelhi, Y., Jouve, E., Castelli, C., and Gentile, S. (2020). How is the minimal clinically important difference established in health-related quality of life instruments? Review of anchors and methods. *Health and Quality of Life Outcomes* 18: 136.

Norman, G.R., Sloan, J.A., and Wyrwich, K.W. (2003). Interpretation of changes in health-related quality of life: the remarkable universality of half a standard deviation. *Medical Care* 41: 582–592.

Norman, G.R., Sloan, J.A., and Wyrwich, K.W. (2004). The truly remarkable universality of a half a standard deviation: confirmation through another look. *Expert Review of Pharmacoeconomics & Outcomes Research* 4: 581–585.

Revicki, D.A., Cella, D., Hays, R.D. et al. (2006). Responsiveness and minimal important differences for patient reported outcomes. *Health and Quality of Life Outcomes* 4: 70.

Revicki, D., Erickson, P.A., Sloan, J.A. et al. (2007). Interpreting and reporting results based on patient-reported outcomes. *Value in Health* 10: S116–S124.

Revicki, D., Hays, R.D., Cella, D., and Sloan, J. (2008). Recommended methods for determining responsiveness and minimally differences for patient-reported outcomes. *Journal of Clinical Epidemiology* 61: 102–109.

Schünemann, H.J., Akl, E.A., and Guyatt, G.H. (2006). Interpreting the results of patient reported outcomes in clinical trials: the clinician's perspective. *Health and Quality of Life Outcomes* 4: 62.

Senn, S. (2003). Disappointing dichotomies. *Pharmaceutical Statistics* 2: 239–240.

Uryniak, T., Chan, I.S.F., Fedorov, V.V. et al. (2011). Responder analyses: a PhRMA position paper. *Statistics in Biopharmaceutical Research* 3: 476–487.

Vanier, A., Sébille, V., Blanchin, M., and Hardouin, J.-B. (2021). The minimal perceived change: a formal model of the responder definition according to the patient's meaning of change for patient-reported outcome data analysis and interpretation. *BMC Medical Research Methodology* 21: 128.

de Vet, H.C.W., Terwee, C.B., Mokkink, L.B., and Knol, D.L. (2011). *Measurement in Medicine: A Practical Guide*. New York: Cambridge University Press.

Ware, J.E. Jr., Kosinski, M., Bjorner, J.B. et al. (2007). *User's Manual for the SF-36v2® Health Survey*, 2e. Lincoln, RI: QualityMetric Incorporated.

Weinfurt, K.P., (2021). Analyzing and interpreting patient-reported outcome measures in clinical trials: comment on Collister et al. *Journal of Clinical Epidemiology* 140: 202.

Wyrwich, K.W., Tierney, W.M., and Wolinsky, F.D. (1999). Further evidence supporting an SEM-based criterion for identifying meaningful intra-individual changes in health-related quality of life. *Journal of Clinical Epidemiology* 52: 861–873.

Index

Note: Page numbers followed by "*f*" denotes figure and "*t*" denotes table respectively.

a

ability to detect change 16, 24–25, 251
  analysis implementation 255–263
  anchoring scale scores 252
  assessment 252, 268
  for COA 251
  correlation analysis to support 263–267
  dataset structure for 258*f*
  definitions and concepts 252–254
  FDA defines 252
  property 253
  review 252
active treatment arm 274, 280, 297, 299, 301
advanced comprehensive theory 69
analysis of correlations 83
anchor-based methods 101, 298–309, 306*f*
  as categorical predictor 308*f*
  to clinically important difference 316–320
  continuous predictor 307*f*, 308*f*
  cumulative distribution functions to 310–315

  for MWPC assessment 317
  and target COA 304–306, 305*f*
anchoring scale scores 252
  longitudinal values for 255*f*
anchor measure 25
"artificial" construct 268
average score 54

b

Bentler's Comparative Fit Index (CFI) 188, 222
Best Linear Unbiased Prediction (BLUP) 93
between-group difference, meaningful within-patient change *vs.* 315–316
between-observer reliability 112–113
between-subjects variance estimation 94, 94*f*
bifactor model 219–227, 220*f*
  fit summary 222*f*
  implementation 221, 221*f*
  standardized loading 223*f*, 224
  unstandardized loading 223*f*
  variances of error terms 223*f*
binary logistic regression 60

A Practical Approach to Quantitative Validation of Patient-Reported Outcomes: A Simulation-Based Guide Using SAS, First Edition. Andrew G. Bushmakin and Joseph C. Cappelleri.
© 2023 John Wiley & Sons, Inc. Published 2023 by John Wiley & Sons, Inc.

bivariate model   221
Bounds statement   192, 194, 195,
   203, 206

C
CALIS procedure   86, 92
   confirmatory factor analysis
      using   184
   during convergence process   192
   to estimate covariances between latent
      factors   185
   estimated means using   120
   estimated variances using   97*f*
   input file for   227
   vs. MIXED procedure   92
   model implementation using   127
   partial output of   120*f,* 122*f*
   "Variance" statement   118
casual/formative indicators   15
categorical variables   258, 267, 276, 307,
   312, 317, 319*f*
   continuous variable *vs.*   319*f*
causal framework, random-effects model
   using   90
causal models   85, 88
   confirmatory factor analysis
      model *vs.*   182
ceiling effect   19, 56, 254
centrally *vs.* locally appraised outcomes
   113–114, 116*f*
   observed scores   118, 122
   true scores   116, 116*f,* 117*f,* 122–123
change from baseline   98, 99
classical measurement theory   180
classical test theory (CTT)   51, 79
   educational or psychological
      phenomena   55
   formula   52
   overview   52–55
   and Rasch model   76
Class statement   239

clinically important difference (CID)
   analysis   316, 317*f*
   anchor-based methods to   316–320
   as categorical variable   319*f*
   as continuous variable   318*f*
   dataset data structure for   318*f*
   implementation of models   318*f*
clinical outcome assessment (COA)   2,
   51, 61, 231
   ability to detect change for   251, 263
   categories   3
   content/construct validity   231, 253
   definitions   3*f*
   educational testing and   73
   instruments   24
   types   2
clinical trial data, for validation   35–39
   advantage   37
   challenges   36
   newly developed scale for use in   47
   planning   36
clinician-reported outcome   2, 111, 251
close-ended questions   9
cognitive interviews   11–12
common variance   47, 48, 153, 171
comprehensive psychometric
   evaluation   16
concept elicitation   8, 11, 12
concept identification, PRO measure
   4–9
   and cognitive interviewing   12
   concepts of interest   4
   context of use   5
   endpoint model   5, 6*f*
   literature and instrument review
      5–6
   patient-centered input   6–9
concept of interest   4, 7, 22, 55, 252,
   254, 301
   PRO measure   97
concept saturation   8

conceptual framework 5, 9, 20, 35
  development process with 13–15
  multi-item domain 45
  postulated measurement
    model on 46
  for PRO instrument 14–15, 14*f*
  qualitative research and 21
concurrent validity 24
confirmatory factor analysis (CFA) 21,
    38, 39, 44, 46–48, 152, 195, 272
  Cronbach's coefficient alpha for 213
  exploratory factor analysis and 184
  with standardized variables 190*f*, 191
  using polychoric correlations
    227–230
confirmatory factor analysis (CFA)
    model 179–183, 181*f*, 210*f*, 229*f*
  bifactor model. *See* bifactor model
  vs. causal models 182
  with domains represented by single
    item 192–204
  first-order 185
  fit statistics 187*f*
  formative *vs.* reflective model
    213–218
  implementation 183–192, 184*f*, 194,
    200, 210*f*
  latent factor and error 180*f*
  measurement part of 181*f*, 182
  with one domain 228*f*
  partial output of 196*f*, 199*f*,
    202*f*–203*f*
  second-order. *See* second-order
    CFA model
  with single item domains 195*f*, 197*f*
  with single variables 193*f*
  specifications 186*f*
  structural part of 182, 182*f*
  using CALIS procedure 184
confirmatory validation workflow 35,
    43–45, 44*f*

construct of interest. *See* concept of
    interest
construct validity 17, 23–24, 151
  aspect 151, 152
  assessments 151
  clinical outcome assessment 231
content validity 17, 23, 35
context of use 5
continuous variables 258, 317, 318*f*
  vs. categorical variable 319*f*
convergence status 209
convergent/divergent validity 23, 41,
    152, 231–236, 247
  assessment 36, 231–232
  continuous simulated 235*f*
  and discriminant validity 232
  evaluation in clinical study
    232–236
correlation coefficient 20
correlation matrix 160, 161, 161*t*, 167
  eigenvalues using 168*f*
  parallel analysis and 169,
    171–175, 172*f*
  scree plot based on 178*f*
correlations 266*f*
  to ability to detect change 263–267
  between changes, deconstructing
    268–270
  covariance and 288*f*
  estimation of 263*f*
  item-to-total 147*f*, 148
  for latent factors 157*f*
  between latent factors and
    variables 159*f*
  Pearson 267
  polychoric 143, 145*f*, 146, 146*f*
  between score change 268, 269*f*,
    270, 270*f*
  Spearman 267
  between variables 236*f*
  variances and 191

CORR procedure   99, 99*f*
  output   135*f*
  "POLYCHORIC" option in   143, 145*f*
  using Cronbach's coefficient alpha
    130, 131*f*
covariance parameter estimates
    92*f*, 289*f*
  using mean scores   109*f*
covariances:
  and correlation matrices   288*f*
  of error terms   274
  matrix using error terms   259*f*
  variances and   134
"Cov" statement   119, 125, 185, 194, 225
criterion validity   24, 152, 242–247
  assessment   242, 243*f*, 245*f*, 246*f*
Cronbach's coefficient alpha   22, 39, 46,
    84, 129–148, 142*f*, 188
  for confirmatory factor analysis   213
  CORR procedure using   130, 131*f*
  dataset and estimating   130*f*, 137*f*
  dichotomous items   139–148
  domain with perfectly correlated
    items   135*f*
  exploratory factor analysis   188
  formula   129
  independent items and
    estimating   131*f*
  for internal consistency
    reliability   213
  item-to-total correlations   138–139,
    143, 145*f*, 147*f*
  Kuder–Richardson 20 (KR-20)
    143, 144*f*
  Likert-type scales   129–139
  negative   132*f*, 133*f*
  reporting   139
  standardized   136
  value   139
cross-cultural validity   24, 152
cross-sectional data   37, 48

CTT-based scoring *vs.* IRT-based scoring
    69–78
  estimated abilities   70*f*, 78*f*
  raw scores and *T*-scores   71, 72*t*
cumulative distribution functions (CDF)
    310–315
  empirical. *See* empirical cumulative
    distribution function
  for interpretation   325
  responder analyses and   320–330
  treatment effect model   320–323

d

dataset structure   89*f*
deconstructing correlation between
    changes   268–270
dichotomous items   139–148
difference in the scores   298, 299
discriminant validity   41, 152,
    231–236, 247
  assessment   231–232
  convergent validity and   232
  evaluation in clinical study   232–236
distributional characteristics   18*t*, 19–20
distribution-based methods   320
disturbances   116, 123, 206
domain-level concept   47
domain score   138, 254
  ICC for   110
  variances   129
double-blind phase   298

e

educational testing   73
effect/reflective indicators   14
eigenvalues   161–163 162*f*, 165
  for initial factor solution   170*f*
  observed and simulated   167*f*
  for rotated factor pattern   170*f*
  by UNIVARIATE procedure   173
electronic administration (ePRO)   13

empirical cumulative distribution
function (eCDF) curves   310, 310*f*
of change   311*f*
generation   311*f*
implementation   326*f*
median changes   313*f*, 314
by treatment arm   327*f*
endogenous variables   185, 195
endpoint model   5, 6*f*
equivalent-forms reliability   84
error terms   180, 182, 185, 201, 205,
239, 274
covariance matrix using   259*f*
covariance of   274
model relationships between   303
variance   256
variance–covariance matrix for
259, 277
error variables   185, 186
estimated abilities:
CTT-based *vs.* IRT-based scoring
70*f*, 78*f*
Rasch model   74
raw scores and   77, 77*f*
using NLP procedure   62*f*, 63, 66, 74,
75*f*, 76*f*
using SCOREMETHOD   70*f*
Estimate statements   259
estimations:
of correlation   263*f*
difficulties   60*f*
least-square means for change   266*f*
meaningful within-patient
change   305*f*
means using CALIS procedure   120
MIXED procedure   275
model parameters   289*f*
polychoric correlations   143, 145*f*,
146, 146*f*
variance–covariance matrix   277*f*, 290*f*
variances using CALIS procedure   97*f*

European Medicines Agency (EMA)   1, 4
exogenous variables   185, 186, 195,
197*f*, 216
exploratory factor analysis   21, 38,
47–48, 153–179
and confirmatory factor analysis   184
Cronbach's alpha and   188
factors loadings   175–179
implementation   159–165, 160*f*
initial factor solution   160*f*, 162*f*
with manifest variables   177*f*
model   153–159, 154*f*, 155*f*
scree plot   165–168, 166*f*
using FACTOR procedure   159
using parallel analysis. *See* parallel
analysis
external measure   25, 298

f

factor analysis   153
confirmatory. *See* confirmatory factor
analysis
exploratory. *See* exploratory factor
analysis
factor loading   180
FACTOR procedure, with parallel
analysis   165, 166*f*, 173
field testing   35
first-order confirmatory factor
analysis   185
first-order latent domains   204–213
focus groups   7–8
Food and Drug Administration (FDA)
1, 12, 37, 39, 47, 95, 231–233,
237, 242, 252–254, 297–298,
300, 310, 312, 314–316, 320,
325–326, 330
formative indicators   19
formative model   15
vs. reflective model   213–218, 213*f*
full causal model   153

g

gold standard   24
group/nuisance factors   224, 225

h

healthcare professional training   2
health-related quality of life (HRQoL)
    4, 15, 214
  definition   2
  "hybrid" CFA model   215
hypothesis testing   152

i

independent variables   161
indicators   14
individual within-patient change   25
intensive qualitative analysis   35
intercept *vs.* slope   119, 120, 121*f*, 126
inter-interviewer reliability   112–113
internal consistency reliability   22, 44,
    49, 84, 129, 136, 138, 232
  Cronbach's coefficient alpha for   213
internal reliability   83, 84
interpretation:
  anchor-based methods. *See* anchor-
    based methods
  CID analysis. *See* clinically important
    difference analysis
  cumulative distribution functions
    310–315, 320–330
  meaningful within-patient change
    295, 325. *See also* meaningful
    within-patient change
inter-rater reliability   84
interviewer-based scales   111–113
intraclass correlation coefficient
    (ICC) estimation   22–23, 39, 85,
    87*f*, 90*f*
  purpose   102
  random-effects model for   90–95
  single measurement for   41

test–retest reliability   104
  using MIXED procedure   91–93, 107
item development   9–11
item response theory (IRT)   51, 79, 152
  estimated abilities   60*f*, 61*f*
  estimated difficulties,
    frequencies of   60*f*
  implementation   59
  Rasch model. *See* Rasch model
item test–retest, test–retest reliability *vs.*
    109–111
item-to-item correlations   84
item-to-total correlations   138–139, 143,
    145*f*, 147*f*
item tracking matrix   12

k

known-groups validity   23–24, 152,
    237–242, 238*f*, 239*f*, 247, 317
Kronecker product   283, 287
Kuder–Richardson 20 (KR-20)
    143, 144*f*

l

latent factors   156–158, 157*f*
  correlations for   157*f*, 168–171
  estimation of   61, 63
  first-order   204–207
  item score and   66
  and variables   159*f*
  variances   182, 184
latent variables   51, 54, 55, 153, 185
least-square means   240*f*, 260, 261*f*, 266*f*
Likert-type scales   129–139
linear function   264
"Lineqs" statement models   118, 125,
    184, 185, 194, 198
locally *vs.* centrally appraised outcomes
    113–114, 116*f*, 117*f*
  observed scores   118, 122
  true scores   116, 116*f*, 117*f*, 122–123

logistic regression 152
LSMeans statement 239, 292
LUA language 280

m
manifest variables 185
maximum log-likelihood method 62
mean 98, 99
    covariance parameter estimates
        using 110
    estimation 119
    and range for simulated scores 259*f*
    and variance 106
"mean and covariance structures"
    model 118
meaningful within-patient change
    (MWPC) 25, 38, 48, 296
    anchor-based method to
        298–309, 317
    application 323–325
    vs. between-group
        difference 315–316
    definitions and concepts 296–298
    estimation implementation 305*f*,
        307*f*, 308*f*
    MCIDs and MIDs 300
measurement error model 85–87, 85*f*,
    106, 127*f*
    accounting for 113–122, 116*f*
    estimated variance for 89
    implementation 86*f*, 89*f*
    for individual items 110
    initial 180
    and ordinary regression 120, 121*f*
    partitioning 116*f*
    with two observations 122–129, 122*f*
    for two time points 88*f*
    variance 87, 89, 94, 119, 124
measurement model 14, 18*t*, 47, 48
    aspects 21
    structure 20–22, 24

measurement scale 251
    ability to detect the change 251
    confirmatory factor analyses 272
    validity 251
measurement theory 51, 84
    classical test theory 51
    estimations 93
    item response theory 51
measurement, true relationship between
    113–129. *See also* measurement
    error model
meta-regression 95
minimally clinically important
    difference (MCID) 300, 316
minimum important difference (MID)
    300, 316
mixed methods research 9
MIXED procedure:
    CALIS procedure *vs.* 92
    estimated variances using 97*f*
    estimating parameters by using 278*f*
    estimation 275
    ICC estimation using 91–93, 107
    time effects 276
    vertical structure for 91*f*, 237*f*, 238
multi-item domains 84, 110, 129,
    192–193
    score 258
    sensitivity to treatment 279–292
    simultaneous assessments 283*f*
    test–retest reliability 84
    "true" outcomes for 281*f*–282*f*
multi-item multi-domain scales:
    conceptual framework 45
    confirmatory validation 35, 43–45
multivariate normal distribution 268

n
natural environment (field test) 48
NLP procedure, estimated ability using
    62*f*, 63, 66, 74, 75*f*, 76*f*

NOINT option 284, 287
non-calibrated approach 299
non-interventional study 97
numeric rating scale (NRS) 252

o

observable constructs 51
observed scale score 52–54, 83
   "true" score and 118, 123
observed variables 120, 153, 154,
   160, 180
  latent factors and 182
observer-based scales 111–113
observer-reported outcomes 2, 251
one-on-one interviews 7–8
one-parameter non-linear model 58
open-ended questions 9
ordered polytomous item
    responses 58
ordinary regression 120, 121*f*

p

paper-based PRO measure 13
parallel analysis 165
  exploratory factor analysis
    using 169*f*
  FACTOR procedure with 165,
    166*f*, 173
  with reduced correlation matrix
    171–175, 172*f*
  scree plot and critical values 170*f*
parallel tests, theory of 54–55
PARMS statement 94
patient global impression of change
    (PGIC) 37, 38*f*, 98–99,
    99*f*–100*f*, 299
  "no change" category 101
  target PRO measure 102*f*
patient global impression of severity
    (PGIS) scale 37, 38*f*, 97, 98
  appropriateness 38

patient-reported outcome (PRO) 1–2.
    See also PRO measure (PROM)
  conceptual framework 14*f*
  interpretation. *See* interpretation
  multi-item scales 22, 23, 78
  and non-PRO 5
  and PGIC scales 99*f*, 100*f*
  and PGIS scales 98
patient-reported outcome
    assessments 2
Patient-Reported Outcomes
    Measurement Information System
    (PROMIS®) 6–9, 57
Pearson correlation coefficients 140,
    141, 267, 268
  and polychoric correlations
    estimations 143
performance-based outcome tools 251
performance outcome assessments 2, 3
person-item (or Wright) maps 79
  construction 64*f*
  CTT-based scoring *vs.* IRT-based
    scoring 69–78
  implementation 58–69
  item response theory 56–58
Phase II clinical trial 272
pilot testing 35
placebo 274, 280, 297, 299, 300
placebo-adjusted treatment effect
    237, 299
polychoric correlations 143, 145*f*, 146*f*
  confirmatory factor analysis using
    227–230
  estimations 143, 145*f*, 146, 146*f*
post-baseline data 97–101
posteriori method 61
predictive validity 24
preliminary psychometric evaluations 16
probability density function (PDF)
    curves 310, 314*f*, 315*f*
promax rotation method 164*f*

PRO measure   1, 84, 242
  categories   2
  cognitive interviews   11–12
  concept identification   4–9
  concept of interest   4, 97
  conceptual framework   14–15, 14*f*
  context of use for   5
  development   4–15
  developmental phase of validating.
    See validation workflow
  for electronic administration   13
  gold standard   24
  item development   9–11
  measurement properties on   251
  paper-based   13
  psychometric validation. *See*
    psychometric validation
  responsiveness. *See* responsiveness
  sensitivity. *See* sensitivity
proxy-based scales. *See* observer-based
    scales
psychometric theory   78
psychometric validation   15–26, 36, 270
  ability to detect change   24–25
  construct validity   23–24
  distributional characteristics   19–20
  evaluations   16–17
  interpretation   25–26
  measurement model structure   20–22
  properties   17–26, 18*t*–19*t*
  purposes   37
  reliability   22–23
  statistical analysis plan   17

q
qualification   5
qualitative research method   5, 7, 9
  and conceptual framework   21
quantitative research methods   7
quantitative validation workflow   35,
    43, 45–47

r
random-effects model   90–95
  between-patient and within-patient
    variances   92*f*
  between-subjects variance estimation
    94, 94*f*
  using causal framework   90
random intercept model   91
Rasch model   21, 51, 57, 74, 79
  classical test theory and   76
  estimating abilities   74
  implementation   59*f*
  person-item maps   58
raw scores   71
  estimated abilities   75*f*, 77*f*
  and estimated abilities   77, 77*f*
  and *T*-scores   72*f*, 73*f*
reflective model   14, 52
  formative *vs.*   213–218
REG procedure:
  intercept and slope   129*f*
  simple regression using   127
regression models   284
reliability   22–23
  between-observer   112
  Cronbach's coefficient alpha
    129–148
  definition   16
  domain scores   109
  inter-reviewer   112
  measurement error model. *See*
    measurement error model
  measurements   83
  repeatability   83
  single-item measure   84
  test–retest. *See* test–retest reliability
  types   83
reproducibility reliability. *See* test–retest
    reliability
responder analysis   325–327, 329, 329*f*
responsiveness   16, 24, 251

root mean square error of approximation (RMSEA) 188

r-squared values 160, 161, 161*t*

s

SAS software 26–27
  log, warning message in 201–202
scales:
  hybrid type 112
  observer-based and interviewer-based 111–113
scale validation 83
scatter plot 63
score change:
  correlation between 268, 270, 270*f*
  and correlations 269*f*
  estimated relationship between 264, 267, 267*f*
scree plot 165–168, 166*f*, 170*f*
  on reduced correlation matrix 178*f*
second-order CFA model 204–213, 205*f*
  first-order latent factors 204–207
  implementation 206*f*, 208*f*, 216, 218*f*
  parameters 218*f*
  standardized loadings for 207*f*, 212*f*
  with two first-order latent factors 208*f*
  unstandardized loadings 206*f*, 207, 211*f*, 212*f*
sensitivity 17, 42, 251. *See also* sensitivity to treatment
sensitivity to treatment 270–292
  decision making 272
  effect of 271, 276
  multi-domain scale 279–292
  single domain, effect for 273–279
simple linear regression 128
single-item domains 194*f*
  CFA implementation with 195*f*, 197*f*

single-item scales 39–43, 104
skewness 300
slope, intercept *vs.* 119, 120, 121*f*, 126
Spearman-Brown prophecy formula 104–109, 148
Spearman correlation coefficients 267
standardized Cronbach's coefficient alpha 136
standardized loadings 190–191, 190*f*
  bifactor model 223*f*, 224
  second-order CFA model 207*f*, 212*f*
structural validity 24, 151
subjective realm 73
supportive evidence 20
symmetry property 130

t

target COA 301, 303–304
  anchor and 304–306, 305*f*
  improvement on 312*f*
test–retest reliability 22–23, 39, 48, 84, 148
  assessment 95–104, 148
  intraclass correlation coefficient 104
  vs. item test–retest 109–111
  measurement error model 85–87, 85*f*
  multi-item scales 84
  observer/interviewers for 113
  post-baseline data 97–101
  pre-treatment/pre-baseline period 95–97
  single-item scale 104, 148
  Spearman-Brown prophecy formula 104–109
  time period between observations 101–104

two time points   87–90
validation workflow for assessment
      39–40, 40*f*
Translatability assessments   13
treatment-by-time interaction effects   276
treatment effect model   320–323,
      325, 326
"true" score   52, 83, 86, 92
   central and local measurements   116,
      116*f*, 117*f*, 122–123
   distributed uniformly   96*f*
   error terms and   54
   estimation   93*f*, 107
   latent   57–58
   and measurement errors   89, 106,
      118*f*, 122
   and observed scores   118, 124
   relationship between measurements
      113–129
   with two observations   125*f*,
      126*f*, 128*f*
   unbiased estimate of   54
   unobserved   118
   variances   85, 87, 93
T-scores   71
   raw summed scores and   72*f*, 73*f*

u

UN@AR   287, 290
UN@CS   287
unidimensional construct of interest
      22, 54, 61, 79
unique variance   153
unobservable constructs   51, 52
unobserved variables   116, 122
unstandardized loadings   189*f*, 191
   bifactor model   223*f*
   second-order CFA model   206*f*, 207,
      211*f*, 212*f*
UN@UN   283, 287, 290

v

validation process   4
   of measurement scale   270, 272
validation workflow:
   clinical trial data   35–39
   confirmatory, multi-item multi-domain
      43–45, 44*f*
   cross-sectional studies   48
   field tests   48
   new multi-item multi-domain scale
      45–48, 46*f*
   of optional analyses   43*f*
   quantitative   35, 43, 45–47
   for required analyses   42*f*
   single-item scales   39–43
   for test-retest reliability assessment
      39–40, 40*f*
validity   16, 18*t*, 83
   measurement scale   251
   types   151
variability   86
variables, latent factors and   159*f*
variance–covariance matrix   89, 129,
      188, 239
   calculations of   277*f*
   for error terms   277
   estimation   277*f*, 290*f*
   Kronecker product of   283
   off-diagonal elements in   131, 132
   with set of variables   130*f*
   special type   283
   unstructured   287
variances   83, 163
   and covariances   134
   disturbance   118
   domain score   129
   of error terms   206, 239
   estimations   87, 97*f*, 108, 191
   latent factors   182, 184, 185
   latent true score   118

variances (*cont'd*)
  measurement error   87, 89, 94, 119, 124
  predefined *vs.* estimated   191*f*
  true score   85, 87
  types   153
  using observed and averaged
    scores   108*f*

"VARIANCE" statement   118, 185,
    194, 198
VARIMAX rotation   163

W

weekly averaging approach   41
within-group changes   272